Edited by
Martin J. Leahy

Microcirculation Imaging

D1556527

Related Titles

Wolfbeis, O. S. (ed.)

Fluorescence Methods and Applications

Spectroscopy, Imaging, and Probes

2008
ISBN: 978-1-57331-716-0

Ntziachristos, V., Leroy-Willig, A., Tavitian, B. (eds.)

Textbook of in vivo Imaging in Vertebrates

2007
ISBN: 978-0-470-01528-5

de Leon, M. J., Snider, D. A., Federoff, H. (eds.)

Imaging and the Aging Brain

2007
ISBN: 978-1-57331-659-0

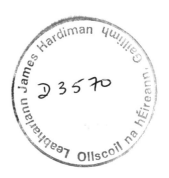

Edited by Martin J. Leahy

Microcirculation Imaging

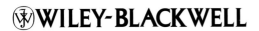

The Editor

Prof. Dr. Martin J. Leahy
Tissue Optics and Microcirculation
Imaging Facility
National Biophotonics and Imaging
Platform Ireland (NBIPI)
School of Physics
NUI Galway
Ireland

Cover
1. Live imaging of the developing
vasculature in Tg(Flk1-myr::mCherry) X
Tg(Flk1-H2B::EYFP) mice using confocal
microscopy (for more details, see Fig. 2c
in Chapter 12 by Irina V. Larina and Mary
E. Dickinson). 2. The working principles of
sidestream dark-field (SDF) imaging (for
more details, see Fig. 2 in Chapter 2 by
M.J. Milstein *et al.*). 3. Three-dimensional
image of an experimental tumor (KHT)
growing in a mouse (for more details, see
Fig. 6 in Chapter 13 by Stuart Foster).
4. Blood flow changes during stroke: relative
cerebral blood flow 10 min after occlusion of
the middle cerebral artery in a rat (for more
details, see Fig. 12 in Chapter 8 by Bryers
et al., with kind permission by SPIE and
A.K. Dunn, University of Texas). 5. Micro-
CT image data (20 μm isotropic voxels) of
the vascular bed of a rat heart, which was
filled with a contrast agent (Microfil) and
was imaged *in situ*. For more details, see
Fig. 15 in Chapter 14 by Timothy L. Kline
and Erik L. Ritman).

Library of Congress Card No.: applied for

**British Library Cataloguing-in-Publication
Data**
A catalogue record for this book is available
from the British Library.

**Bibliographic information published by the
Deutsche Nationalbibliothek**
The Deutsche Nationalbibliothek
lists this publication in the Deutsche
Nationalbibliografie; detailed bibliographic
data are available on the Internet at
<http://dnb.d-nb.de>.

© 2012 Wiley-VCH Verlag & Co. KGaA,
Boschstr. 12, 69469 Weinheim, Germany

Wiley-Blackwell is an imprint of John Wiley
& Sons, formed by the merger of Wiley's
global Scientific, Technical, and Medical
business with Blackwell Publishing.

Print ISBN: 978-3-527-32894-9
ePDF ISBN: 978-3-527-65122-1
ePub ISBN: 978-3-527-65121-4
mobi ISBN: 978-3-527-65120-7
oBook ISBN: 978-3-527-65123-8

Cover Design   Adam-Design, Weinheim
Typesetting Laserwords Private Limited,
Chennai, India
Printing and Binding Markono Print Media
Pte Ltd, Singapore

Contents

Preface

This book brings together the main techniques used for imaging the small blood vessels, which supply nutritional oxygen and remove waste products from the cells of the body. The rapid development of new techniques to image the microcirculation (vessels <100 μm in diameter) in two and three dimensions was the main driver for publishing this book. The macrocirculation of the cardiovascular system enjoys a special place in medicine and is well catered for with imaging modalities that are ever present in our hospitals. X-ray CT, ultrasound, MRI, and PET all play an important role in diagnosis and treatment of the disorders of the large vessels. However, there is growing realization that some of the diseases that most threaten the quality and quantity of life in the developed world, such as diabetes and cancer, have their origins in the microcirculation. Therefore, new techniques with appropriate resolution were required to image these smaller vessels, and these largely depend on the rapid developments in photonics.

It is impossible to present all techniques that have been applied to microcirculation in this book. The editor is grateful to the (unknown) reviewers of the original proposal for their suggestion to supplement the biophotonics techniques well known to him with MRI and high-frequency ultrasound. The result is a more thorough covering of the field, although I am open to further suggestions for additions in future editions. Researchers, practitioners, and professionals in the fields of diabetes, cancer, wound healing, biomedical optics, and biophotonics, as well as professionals in other disciplines, such as laser physics and technology, fibre optics, spectroscopy, and biology, will find the book a useful resource. Graduate and undergraduate students studying biomedical physics and engineering, biomedical optics and biophotonics, and medical science would benefit greatly from consulting this reference.

Several Irish and international grants supported this project, particularly the National Biophotonics & Imaging Platform Ireland, funded by the Irish Government under the national development plan (NDP) 2007–2013 HEA PRTLI IV. I greatly appreciate the cooperation, contributions, patience, and support of all the contributors, my colleagues from the School of Physics at NUI Galway, the Department of Physics at the University of Limerick, the Royal College of Surgeons, and the

National Biophotonics and Imaging Platform. Last, but not least, I would like to thank my family for their support and understanding during my work on this book.

NUI, Galway   *Martin J. Leahy*
March 2012

List of Contributors

Rick Bezemer
University of Amsterdam
Department of Translational
Physiology
Academic Medical Center
Meibergdreef 9
1105 AZ Amsterdam
The Netherlands

J. David Briers
Kingston University
Cwm Gorllwyn
SA35 0DN
UK

Daniel De Backer
Université Libre de Bruxelles
Department of Intensive Care
Erasme Hospital
Route de Lennik
1070 Brussels
Belgium

Mary E. Dickinson
Baylor College of Medicine
Department of Molecular
Physiology and Biophysics
One Baylor Plaza
Houston TX 77030
USA

Ingemar Fredriksson
Linköping University
Department of Biomedical
Engineering
581 85 Linköping
Sweden

Song Hu
Washington University
in St. Louis
Optical Imaging Laboratory
Department of Biomedical
Engineering
One Brookings Drive
St. Louis
MO 63130-4899
USA

Can Ince
University of Amsterdam
Department of Translational
Physiology
Academic Medical Center
Meibergdreef 9
1105 AZ Amsterdam
The Netherlands

Christian M. Kerskens
Trinity College Institute of
Neuroscience
Trinity College Dublin
Lloyd Institute
Dublin 2
Ireland

Timothy L. Kline
Mayo Clinic
Department of Physiology and
Biomedical Engineering
Physiological Imaging Research
Laboratory
200 First Street SW
Rochester
MN 55905
USA

Kirill V. Larin
University of Houston
Department of Biomedical
Engineering
4800 Calhoun Rd.
Houston
Texas 77204
USA

Irina V. Larina
Baylor College of Medicine
Department of Molecular
Physiology and Biophysics
One Baylor Plaza
Houston TX 77030
USA

Marcus Larsson
Linköping University
Department of Biomedical
Engineering
581 85 Linköping
Sweden

Martin J. Leahy
Tissue Optics and
Microcirculation Imaging Facility
National Biophotonics and
Imaging Platform Ireland
(NBIPI)
National University of Ireland
Galway
School of Physics
University Road
Galway
Ireland

Adam Liebert
Nalecz Institute of Biocybernetics
and Biomedical Engineering
Polish Academy of Sciences
Department of Biophysical
Measurements and Imaging
Trojdena 4
02-109 Warsaw
Poland

Roman Maniewski
Nalecz Institute of Biocybernetics
and Biomedical Engineering
Polish Academy of Sciences
Department of Biophysical
Measurements and Imaging
Trojdena 4
02-109 Warsaw
Poland

Paul M. McNamara
Tissue Optics and
Microcirculation Imaging Facility
National Biophotonics and
Imaging Platform Ireland
(NBIPI)
National University of Ireland
School of Physics
Galway
Ireland

James F.M. Meaney
Centre for Advanced Medical
Imaging (CAMI)
St. James's Hospital
James's Street
Dublin 8
Ireland

Dan M.J. Milstein
University of Amsterdam
Department of Translational
Physiology
Academic Medical Center
Meibergdreef 9
1105 AZ Amsterdam
The Netherlands

Gert E. Nilsson
WheelsBridge AB
Lövsbergsvägen 13
58937 Linköping
Sweden

Marie-Louise O'Connell
Tissue Optics and
Microcirculation Imaging Facility
National Biophotonics and
Imaging Platform Ireland
(NBIPI)
National University of Ireland
School of Physics
Galway
Ireland

Jim O' Doherty
Royal Surrey County Hospital
Department of Medical Physics
Egerton Road
Guildford GU2 7XX
UK

Richard M. Piech
Trinity College Institute of
Neuroscience
Trinity College Dublin
Lloyd Institute
Dublin 2
Ireland

Erik L. Ritman
Mayo Clinic
Department of Physiology and
Biomedical Engineering
Physiological Imaging Research
Laboratory
200 First Street SW
Rochester
MN 55905
USA

Terence J. Ryan
University of Oxford
Green College
Oxford
UK

Wiendelt Steenbergen
University of Twente
Biomedical Photonic Imaging
Group
MIRA Institute for Biomedical
Technology and Technical
Medicine
PO Box 217
7500 AE Enschede
The Netherlands

Tomas Strömberg
Linköping University
Department of Biomedical
Engineering
581 85 Linköping
Sweden

F. Stuart Foster
Sunnybrook and Health Sciences
Centre and the University of
Toronto
Department of Medical
Biophysics
2075 Bayview Avenue
Toronto
M4N3M5 Ontario
Canada

Hrebesh M. Subhash
Oregon Health and Science
University
Department of Biomedical
Engineering
School of Medicine
3303 SW Bond Avenue
Portland OR 97239
USA

Jean-Louis Vincent
Université Libre de Bruxelles
Department of Intensive Care
Erasme Hospital
Route de Lennik
1070 Brussels
Belgium

Lihong V. Wang
Washington University
in St. Louis
Optical Imaging Laboratory
Department of Biomedical
Engineering
One Brookings Drive
St. Louis
MO 63130-4899
USA

Ruikang K. Wang
University of Washington
Biophotonics and Imaging
Laboratory
Department of Bioengineering
3720 15th Avenue Northeast
Seattle
Washington 98195
USA

Stanislaw Wojtkiewicz
Nalecz Institute of Biocybernetics
and Biomedical Engineering
Polish Academy of Sciences
Department of Biophysical
Measurements and Imaging
Trojdena 4
02-109 Warsaw
Poland

1

A Historical Perspective of Imaging of the Skin and Its Gradual Uptake for Clinical Studies, Inclusive of Personal Reminiscences of Early Days of Microcirculation Societies

Terence J. Ryan and Martin J. Leahy

Modern microscopy of microcirculation was conceived by the observers of especially the seventeenth century, but gestation was in the hands of the national and continental Microcirculatory Societies that began in the decade 1954–1964. They were a meeting point between the laboratory investigator of microcirculation and the clinician. Zweifach [1] reviewing historical aspects of microcirculation research wrote "The usage of the term 'microcirculation' in an organic context is of comparatively recent vintage, first appearing consistently in the literature during the 1950s." Global collaboration with a strong clinical input began with World Congresses of Microcirculation first held in Toronto in 1975, then in San Diego in 1979, next in Oxford in 1984, and every four to five years since then. As an Oxford clinician specializing in care of the skin, T. J. R. was roped in at the deep end of nonclinical pursuit of microcirculation on several occasions. However, this began by a chance observation that if one pushes tissue fluid away by indenting the skin with a steel probe, one gets much better visualization of the skin capillary bed [2, 3]. It has long been known that one sees at the surface of the skin only what its optical properties allow. Excised epidermis from white skin placed over a printed page is transparent enough to read through it. Melanin of pigmented skin prevents such visualization. The redness of blood provides *in vivo* pinkness, but blue blood in veins is a consequence of blue light being scattered more than red. This does not stop the practised clinician from easily recognizing the condition when black skin is flushed. Newton [4] discussed the decomposition of white light, and Doppler [5] made known that the effect of movement toward or away from the observer influenced the color observed. For several centuries, any observation of complex surfaces reflecting light was clarified by applying transparent oils to that surface.

1.1
Early History

George P. Fulton [6], Professor of Biology at the Boston University, writing on the historical perspective of the founding of the American Microcirculatory Society, lists Harvey and Lord Lister amongt the early influences on microcirculation, but it

Microcirculation Imaging, First Edition. Edited by Martin J. Leahy.
© 2012 Wiley-VCH Verlag GmbH & Co. KGaA. Published 2012 by Wiley-VCH Verlag GmbH & Co. KGaA.

was interest in microscopy and improved microscopes in the seventeenth century that led to the first observations of blood flow by better imaging. The discoverers and forerunners of imaging were fascinated when they applied their new magnifying devices, and detecting transparency in some living tissues saw for the first time the movement of the content of the small capillaries. These early observations especially on red cells were well reviewed for the journal *Blood Cells* by Bessis and Delpechi [7]. As stated in that review, three men, Malpighi, Leeuwenhoek, and Swammerdam, made the most of the improvements in magnifying lenses in the early seventeenth century and noted red particles in blood capillaries in transparent tissues. Of these, van Leeuwenhoek of Delft (1632–1723) gained the most publicity by getting his observations published by the Royal Society of London [8]. Indeed, it was the tax collector, van Leeuwenhoek, who contributed one of the greatest innovations through his hobby by producing a very short focal length lens. This avoided chromatic aberrations, which plagued compound microscopes of the day, and yet produced sufficient magnification to reveal the structure of the blood cell (Figure 1.1) and its movement within organs and organisms if they were sufficiently transparent. It was this innovation that allowed Malpighi to confirm Harvey's theory that blood circulates from the arterial to the venous side via these small capillaries, and indeed, it can be considered the discovery of the microcirculation.

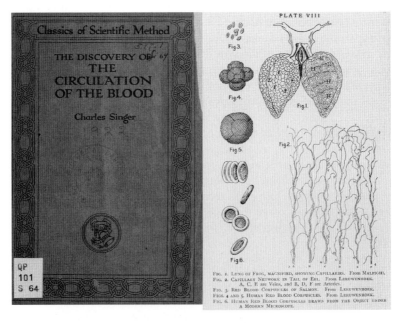

Figure 1.1 The discovery of the circulation of the blood, the shape of the red blood cell, and, most importantly, the microcirculation (*after The Discovery of the Circulation of the Blood*, Charles Singer, G. Bell and Sons Ltd., London, Ref. [9]).

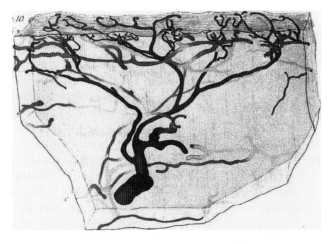

Figure 1.2 The late nineteenth century drawings of Spalteholz, illustrating the distinctive candelabra pattern of the blood supply of the skin.

van Leeuwenhoek, like several other observers, noted blood circulating in the capillaries of the louse intestine. He also noted the flexibility of the red cell, with shape change to facilitate, he supposed, their passing through small capillaries. Probably, however, he was observing clumped red cells, known as *rouleaux*, rather than single red cells. Furthermore, he was not an anatomist and could not even distinguish muscle tendon from nerve, until a critical anatomist, Swammerdam, on several visits, somewhat to his annoyance, took over his project.

Malpighi of Bologna (1628–1694) was a more casual observer, probably with less passion for red cells than for microscopes. He had observed these particles a few years earlier in fish gills, in dog and frog lungs, and in the hedgehog. Compared to van Leeuwenhoek, he was not an enthusiastic publisher of his findings, the importance of which was only recognized long after his death [10]. The only other significant technology of the time was the use by Leeuwenhoek of a fine glass capillary pipette to draw blood from the vessels of the louse, which could then be more easily manipulated under the microscope.

In the nineteenth century, anatomists studying cadavers provided clear images of the smallest blood vessels, and Spalteholz [11] provided some of the best imaging by injecting colored gelatin solutions into the arteries (Figure 1.2), showing clearly the candelabra pattern of the skin's blood supply.

The challenge was finding transparent tissues that could be placed under a microscope and a short-distance high-power lens that limited all but totally im-mobile tissues and thus except for the nail fold, excluded humans from observation. It was the window of glass, or the lighter and less breakable Perspex placed in the skin of the rabbit's ear or the cheek pouch of the hamster or in the dorsal skin of the mouse, that allowed long-term and frequent observations of life events and allowed greater understanding of the role of the skin's circulation. Sandison

[12, 13] and Clark and Clark [14, 15] in their series of publications from 1918 to 1942 first in the tadpole tail and then in the rabbit ear window provided some of the best ever descriptions of observations on visualizing the blood supply of the wounded skin. However, the hamster cheek pouch favored by Herman Berman in the United States and by Sanders and Shubik [16] in the United Kingdom had a vascular bed that could not be criticized for being a wound. It was the preparation that convinced one that the epidermis was the governing body of its capillary bed [17].

It was Starling [18] at the University College London (1896) who made the physiologist aware of pressure, both hydrostatic and oncotic, inside and outside of the capillary, thereby determining one of its most important functions, viz, control of permeability, and opening up the topic of *"exchange."* August Krogh, Professor of Zoophysiology, in Copenhagen, by receiving the Nobel prize and authoring *Anatomy and Physiology of the Capillaries* (1922) [19] not only convinced the scientist and the clinician of the importance of microcirculation but also attracted a new generation of investigators, many of whom were clinicians. He was the teacher of those who refined for human studies modern microscopy and cinephotomicroscopy including Melvin Knisely, at the University of Chicago and the Medical University of South Carolina, who, by improved lighting using quartz conduction [20] and increasing the working distance of the high-power lenses demonstrated how blood flow could be best observed in the human by examining the conjunctival blood vessels. His special interest was the changes that occurred in malaria. The conjunctiva remains the most transparent organ, requiring no anesthesia and being immobilized by looking at a single point. It was the development of long-working-distance lenses that facilitated easy examination with which to astonish a new recruit and introduce the wonders of the microcirculation in the human. Knisely showed that in malaria, the blood became "sludged" [21].

1.2
The Microcirculatory Societies

The American Microcirculatory Society was founded at a 1954 meeting of anatomists in Galveston. Most presentations were on *in vivo* microscopy (Conference report 1954) [6, 22].

In the 1960s, many discussions were held with the founders of the American Microcirculatory Society and with like-minded Europeans about collaboration and the setting up of Microcirculation Societies. The Europeans held preliminary conferences in Lund (1959), Hamburg (1960), Pavia (1962), and Jerusalem (1964). The range and the breadth of the field can be read in the Karger of Basel series *Biblio Anatomica* and became further apparent at the 4th European Conference in 1966 organized by the Cambridge anatomist Alexander Monro [23] at Cambridge with the Oxford experimental pathologist, a colleague of Lord Florey, Gordon Sanders as President. These early meetings suffered from the technologies of the time, as described by Alexander Monro [24] when writing about the meeting in Pavia.

"I am sure my Italian friends will forgive me when I say that the organisation of over 150 participants to give the 115 papers on the programme, met with some difficulties-not really anyone's fault- but just one of those things; and one which eventually resulted in all the Italians being asked to read their papers by title only: this must have been very disappointing for them but thanks to their self sacrifice the visitors were able to get home on time! Simultaneous translation into four languages had been arranged, but the opening session for the principle speakers started with a problem, for the slide projectionist was late and when he switched on the lamp, the wrong voltage had been connected and he had no spare: half an hour later the first American-sized slide was inserted but it did not fit, and we watched-fascinated-while progressive cracks in the glass were followed across the screen. The projector was taken out of service in order that it could be dismantled. No other slides were shown that morning. Those who had hoped to show their slides insisted that they should have equivalent time in the afternoon, but as I was the chairman at that session I insisted that we should endeavour to keep more closely to the published timetable. At last a compromise was found, but inevitably everything was late, and when the speakers read their papers faster than they had intended originally, the translators could not keep up in all languages, because some were not so concise as others. Fortunately tolerance and good humour prevailed and all the social events were superb. We started with a blessing from a Cardinal and finished with a banquet at which an enormous fish was displayed before we devoured it. I believe the dancing continued until the dawn, to a piano expertly played by Dr Krahl, from Maryland USA who had paid his way through medical school by use of this talent."

As a medical student in Oxford in the 1950s, one would attend Florey's formidable lectures and find that his first love was not penicillin but lymphatics. Something seen in his lectures but not seen in his well-known text [25] was a cine film made by Sanders, Florey, and Ebert, in 1940, which introduced slow motion to illustrate shape change of red cells in capillaries using the rabbit's ear chamber and in which they also clearly demonstrated capillary endothelial contraction. It was this film that inspired Alexander Monro to take up the field of blood vessel study. In the same laboratory, John Casley-Smith did his D. Phil on lymphatics with Florey as supervisor after World War II and John became the leader of the field of lymphatic study in Australia and later globally [26]. Sanders led the studies on microcirculation, and many learned the technologies from him.

On the other side of the road from William Dunn School of pathology was the post graduate centre where any visitor would be taken. The glasses of sherry were not small and the conversation was intense with persons such as the haematologist (and biographer of Florey and Fleming) Gwyn Macfarlane to listen to. Gwyn would choose an obscure topic like the origin of the term non-undeodorized cowcake given to his cattle and half an hour of discussion would follow. Gordon would have demonstrated

> *technologies before lunch and would snooze in the afternoon while his visitor practiced the technology. The day would end on the high table at Lincoln College. 40 years later one Japanese visitor would still recount the day in his lectures as one of the most challenging he had experienced: not yet proficient in English and wedged between a professor of Aviation and a professor of Saxon English for at least two hours.*
>
> *Terence Ryan was invited by Gordon Sanders in 1965 into the world of microcirculation experts. Gordon was a heavy sherry and wine imbiber at lunch and dinner so observations were only done in the morning. Oddly some of his best dinners at his home were given for the American microcirculation experts, Edward Bloch and John Irwin both of whom were teetotal so Gordon and Terence Ryan often had whole bottles to consume.*

The British Microcirculation Society (BMS) was founded in 1965 at a meeting of The Royal Microscopical Society, demonstrating again the importance of the subject of imaging but still tied to microscopes. Its history was recorded by Alexander Monro [24].

> *The committee meeting that created the British Microcirculation Society was, for someone as junior as Terence Ryan, rather hair raising. Lord Florey had consented to be a member but did not turn up. The mild Gordon Sanders could not control the pedantic Alexander Munro who argued every point of the newly developing rules of the society and Sir Henry Barcroft walked out in a huff. We all had to pay for our lunch which was expensive (Figure 1.3).*
>
> *It was not a happy occasion; the proceeding committee meeting being one of discord! The costs to individuals was carefully allocated and is seen in the handwriting of its first President Gordon Sanders, a close colleague of Howard Florey in Oxford and well known for his meticulous studies of blood supply in the Rabbits Ear Chamber and Hamster cheek Pouch.*

The various continental and national societies were always international in outlook. Thus the committee that organized the European Society for Microcirculation in 1988 had Su Chien, United States, and M. Tsuchiya, Japan, as advisory members.

Hemorheology had as its main concern the fact that the diameter of the red cell was more than the width of the capillary lumen, and shape changes had to be understood if rapid flow were to occur, especially when red cells and the even larger white cells were grouped together.

Sadly, the tall and gangly Knisely allowed his enthusiasm to make him long winded so that his late-in-life guest lectures and after-dinner speeches to the new microcirculatory societies went on far too long. The topic of "sludging" and the appearance of rouleaux formation of red cells helped to introduce the subject of blood rheology to the Microcirculation Societies, which were inaugurated when rheology was much debated, and the experts on this were the burly figure of Copley contrasting with the asthenic Oxford figure, Scott Blair, editor of *Biorheology*,

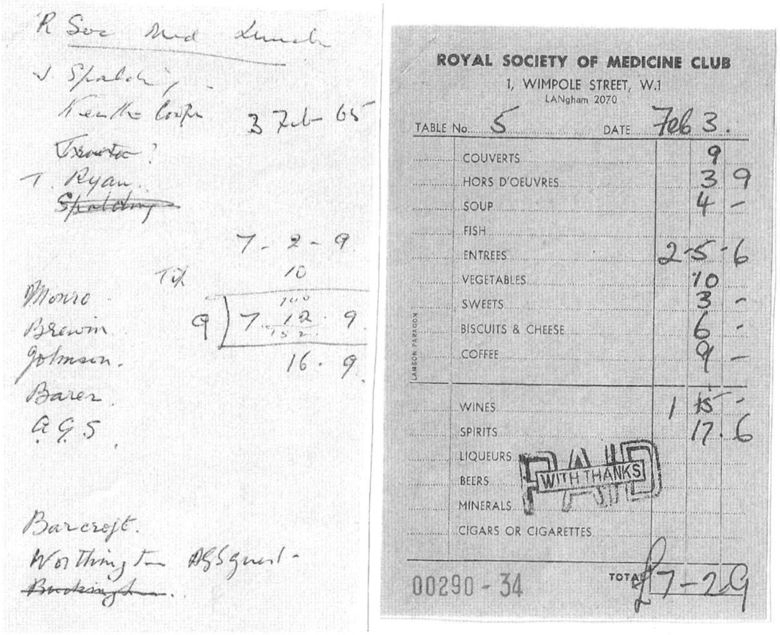

Figure 1.3 The lunch bill for the first meeting of the new committee of the British Microcirculation.

in which were published the early proceedings of the BMS edited by Terence Ryan. There was also a certain amount of modeling of red cells to show how the geometrical and elastic properties of one red cell during flow would affect the same properties of the immediately following cell. Such modeling by engineers (viz Lighthill of Imperial College London) [27] so that red cells looked like a series of square boxes lost some listener's respect for modeling because they seemed to have no visual resemblance to the real thing. The study of the vascular tree in different organs, and the circulation through it, raised increasing concern about the clinical relevance of statements made by those who had never observed the microcirculation *in vivo*. Each new observation raised new questions, many of which could only be answered by better imaging. Alexander Monro gave several talks to the BMS during its first 25 years about early measurements of red cell velocity, first in the eel by Leeuwenhoek in 1689 and then in the frog by Stephen Hales in 1733. He himself had rheology and microscopy as interests. In developing cine techniques for measuring individual red cell flow and shape change, Alexander Monro in 1969 [28] put much effort into using a narrow collimated beam with energy ranging from 0.23 to 200 J from the Strobex model 135 manufactured by Chadwick-Helmuth Co Inc. The further development of blood flow measurement depended on velocity techniques such as dual slit devices, allowing measurement of the time taken to move between two points. Advances in the sensitivity of computerized measurement improved accuracy and the recording of measurement. Later reviews [29] reveal a much

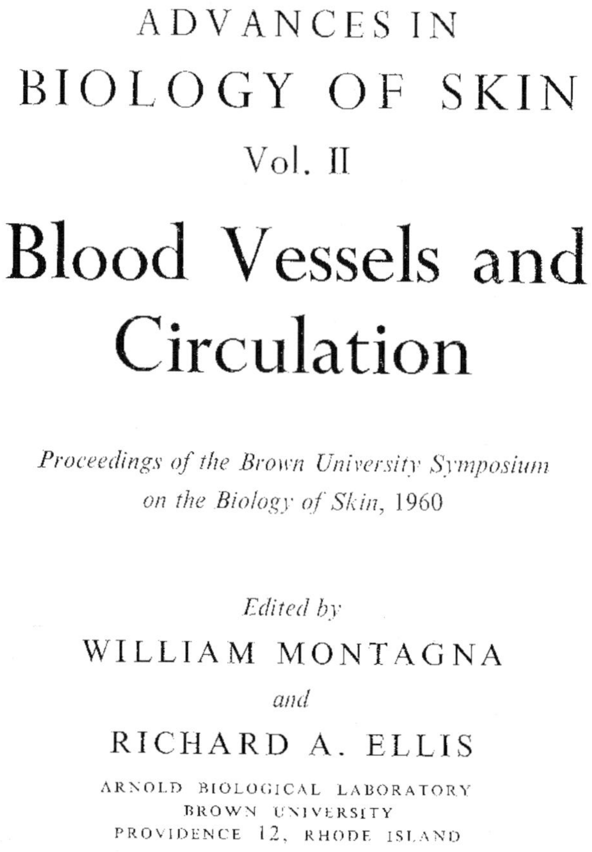

ADVANCES IN

BIOLOGY OF SKIN

Vol. II

Blood Vessels and Circulation

Proceedings of the Brown University Symposium
on the Biology of Skin, 1960

Edited by

WILLIAM MONTAGNA

and

RICHARD A. ELLIS

ARNOLD BIOLOGICAL LABORATORY
BROWN UNIVERSITY
PROVIDENCE 12, RHODE ISLAND

Figure 1.4 The Brown University Symposium on the Biology of the Skin in 1960 was a landmark for identifying the importance of the blood vessels and circulation of the skin.

altered and complex field, and few of the early observations that filled the early meetings of the 1960s have much relevance.

For those interested in the skin, the most influential event was the 1960 Brown University Symposium on the Biology of the Skin, the publication of which was *Advances in the Biology of the Skin, Blood Vessels and Circulation* (Figure 1.4) [30].

Therein was discussed injection of skin with India ink and alkaline phosphatase reaction studies by Winkelmann and his team of the Mayo Clinic as well as by Richard Ellis of Brown University. R. L. de C. H. Saunders reviewed the recent development of X-ray projection microscopy of the skin. George Odland from Seattle reviewed the recent advances in ultrastructure that had been led by Palade [31] and of the skin by Hibbs *et al.* [32]. This publication included an excellent review of capillary microscopy in normal and diseased skin by Michal J. Davis and James Lawler. The skin's capillaries had first been examined as a special interest using reflected light by Lombard in 1912 [33], and Gilje in 1953 [34] was the first to effectively examine diseases such as psoriasis. Davis and Lorincz [35] showed that removal by stripping with Sellotape of the keratin layer overlying the vascular bed greatly increased the visibility of the capillaries and subpapillary vessels. Alrick B. Hertzman described the convective transfer of heat to the surface whence it is lost by radiative, convective, conductive, and evaporative pathways, with which developed our understanding of the correlation between blood flow and temperature. Grahame Weddell introduced the topic of the innervations of cutaneous blood vessels.

Grahame Weddell was later to become Professor of anatomy in Oxford. Because of his interest in cutaneous nerves he became the centre of attention of the Leprosy World of investigators. He lived in one of Europe's oldest leprosy hospitals. Immigrants from Africa and Asia were housed in the department of dermatology in Oxford so that fresh material could be available. Grahame was a jovial and generous to his junior collaborators but would be in bed by 9 p.m.! He spoke about himself as being worthy of "no more than B+", but he became the centre of a World Class centre for Leprosy research after his retirement from Anatomy and this was based in the Department of Dermatology which at that time had graduated from a septic ward in the old infirmary to the isolation hospital outside the city boundaries. Graduation to nearer the centre of Oxford would occur in 1992 well after Leprosy was shown no longer to be a public health problem. The role of the microcirculation in this disease was shown to account for the localisation of the causative organism in the nose and its dissemination from the nasal cavity. Several studies showed that cooling, hypoxia and impaired fibrinolysis were characteristics of nasal septal blood supply all encouraging the M Leprae to thrive at that site in endothelium [36].

The increasing awareness of the importance of the blood supply of clinicians in Europe was slow to gel. Clinical investigation of the circulation of the skin by Sir Thomas Lewis [37] in the 1920s, a pupil of Starling, led to some detailed reports in *Clinical Science*, which remain a wonderful read. He described very thoroughly the axon flare, the white blanch reaction, reactive hyperemia, and other changes in blood flow. Besides being a good scientist and a clinician, he wrote beautiful English. He recognized that there were different responses to injury of the vascular tree within the skin at different levels within the vascular tree. It was his young colleague Sir George Pickering with whom Terence Ryan worked in 1958 when, as Regius Professor of Medicine, he was completing his book on "high blood pressure." He insisted that whatever one wrote should be in good basic English and he shortened the title of Ryan's thesis to "The blood supply of the skin" from something with seventeenth century length. A brief chapter on the history of imaging using capillary microscopy [38] was part of the first major publication for dermatologists, being a supplement of the *British Journal of Dermatology* in 1969, edited by Terence Ryan, followed by Volume 2 of the series *Physiology and Pathophysiology* of the skin [39], and a review of the lymphatic system [40] and

Microvascular Injury [41]. The emphasis of this book was on the clinical need for observations of skin blood supply, and the title was chosen to encourage the field of microvascular research to read an essentially clinical book.

The clinical relevance of microcirculation studies were frequently debated, and it was often stated (by, for example, Ben Zweifach (personal communication after reading *Microvascular Injury*)) that the best basic science was being generated in the United States but its applied clinical relevance was a feature of European work. Ben Zweifach was the doyen of microcirculation for longer than any other significant scientist. First working with chambers, they demonstrated preferential channels through the capillary bed in the early 1930s [42], and he continued publishing for 50 years. A scientist rather than a clinician, he hosted the second World Congress in San Diego.

> *TJR remembers there was a stall in the exhibition hall of a Chinese memory enhancing drug which Ben Zweifach and his wife with Mrs Anne Ryan set aside evidence and decided after only a little discussion to give it a go; seemingly 20 years later still effective especially in Ben's case who was much the elder of the three! The site of this 2nd World congress was shared with three other conferences. The normality of dress of the microcirculationists was distinctive in La Jolla in comparison with that of the bulging at the waist of a Fat Boys congress, the grouping and glamorous arm waving of the Chair Leaders Congress and the bearded gentlemen in shorts attending an Anthropology Congress.*

After the successful first meeting of the BMS with the Royal Microscopical Society, it was decided to have a meeting of the BMS in Oxford. Terence Ryan, as local organizer, along with the orthopedic surgeon Joseph Trueta, who came to Oxford fleeing Spain after the Civil War and had been the first to study angiography [43], to image the kidney to delineate renal vasospastic responses after crush injury of the legs, relevant to the bombing injuries in London and Coventry during World War II. He was keen to demonstrate imaging of blood supply in bone while Terence Ryan along with the plastic surgeon Tom Patterson imaged the skin. Tom used vital dyes to produce bright green or blue pigs in the study of skin grafts. These colorful pigs were one of the most popular exhibits of early meetings. They became the animals whose skin seemed most like that of humans for several studies by several investigators in Oxford.

In 1967, at a meeting at the Royal Postgraduate Medical School [44], the cardiovascular group demonstrated one of the first instruments to measure forward and reverse flow using a 3 mm diameter nylon tube on which was mounted an electromagnetic velocity-sensing element, and Eva Kohner showed how useful fluorescence photography was for the study of diabetes, allowing the capillary bed of the retina to be studied and the natural history of retinopathy and response to treatment to be assessed. The full potential of high-quality fluorescein angiography and high-speed cine fluorescence photography was demonstrated at several of the

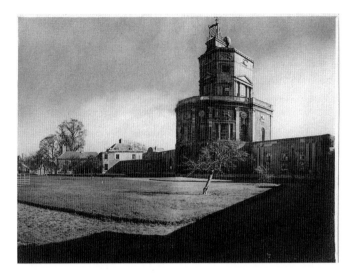

Figure 1.5 The eighteenth century Radcliffe Observatory *The Tower of the Winds*. This was brought by Mr Morris, the Oxford car manufacturer, as a laboratory to support the nearby County Hospital *The Radcliffe Infirmary*. Few places were more unsuitable for such work, but as the Nuffield Institute of Medicine, it produced world class information on the vascular system in newborn sheep and pioneered angiography. It was later host to the 3rd World Congress on Microcirculation and the First European Laser Doppler Users meeting.

Society's meetings and at a meeting organized at The Institute of Opthalmology by Norman Ashton in 1973 [45].

It was at about this time that blood flow in the newborn was being measured in sheep in the highly inconvenient laboratory of the adapted Radcliffe Observatory (Figure 1.5) bought by Mr Morris, later to become Lord Nuffield and the funder of Oxford's new clinical School of Medicine, to provide the County Hospital with some laboratory space [46]. Here, Dawes headed the Nuffield Institute for Medical Research and depended on the superb technology of a number of inventions for measuring blood flow in larger blood vessels. Ardran developed cine radiography in the same building. George Cherry, recruited from New Orleans to develop measurement in Oxford's Department of Dermatology enlisted Ardran's help to become one of the first to use the technologies of microangiography to illustrate altered blood supply in wounds in the pig skin [47]. It was a collaboration also with the Radcliffe Observatory scientists at The Nuffield Institute for Medical Research.

This all took place in an 18th century three story building designed to observe the sun and the stars and converted into a vascular laboratory for the study of the major changes occurring in mother and foetus at birth. The pregnant sheep was the model. Herein Gustav Born of platelet fame and John Vane of Prostaglandin Nobel Prize fame began their careers. The sheep had to be enticed up a spiral staircase. The

> *Laboratory was shared by Ardrans radiography with cine film hanging from the top of the spiral staircase and smoke drums hanging out to dry. There was room for friction and sharing included keeping a crocodile in a bath to study the swallowing reflex, so it was said, but actually to mark a room in the centre of the sheep laboratory complex as belonging to radiology.*

Terence Ryan's group was interested in the development of human skin and its blood supply after birth, perhaps under the influence of cooling. They performed these studies on newborn at the Royal Free Hospital in London and found the newborn skin to be more transparent but less mature in the flexures [48]. This is technically easier with the improvements in long-distance viewing. In 1912, Lombard [33], one of the first to note that it was possible to view capillaries in human skin [49], examined the nail fold capillaries of the third fingers of infants immobilized by strapping to allow observations through a short working distance lens.

Besides the newborn, it was important to understand the changes occurring in aging skin in which considerable loss of the capillary bed is a feature. External sources of light penetrate to deep dermis more readily in skin that has a much thinned upper dermis and mid dermis and as a result measure much deeper blood vessels of much larger lumen (reviewed by Ryan [50, 51]).

1.3
A Tour of Microcirculatory Centers in 1968

The status of the imaging field in 1968 can be illustrated by the tour of microcirculation laboratories prepared for Terence Ryan that year. Newly based in his vascular laboratory at the Institute of Dermatology at London University, it became clear that he needed to learn more; it was advised that he should do a world tour to visit the best centers on the way to and back from marriage in Australia. This started in Boston with Herman Berman and Hamster cheek pouch skills and then visiting the frost bitten rabbits of Kulka [52], also in Boston, demonstrating the effect of cold on blood supply using angiography before going to see the variety of viscometers used by the physician Roe Wells. A brief visit to the ophthalmologists, at the Massachusetts General Hospital, showed their current interest in the value of the pericyte as a support to retinal capillaries and their loss in diabetes [53].

The American Microcirculation Society meeting that year was in Atlantic City with 23 000 other biology-related organizations, and from there it was a flight with Edward Bloch to Cleveland where he proudly presented his most pristine laboratory. Not a speck of dust was allowed to spoil his film making, using high-speed cinephotomicrography and a television system for spectrophotometric scanning. Figure 1.6 illustrates the program he would set up for a visitor.

After preparing a paper [54] on microvascular stasis from cooling of the skin, during a short tour at the Mayo Clinic, Terence Ryan then went on to Seattle. The visit to Curt Wiederhielm's bats wings in Seattle was a demonstration that there

"Methods will be considered whereby the visible events that occur in microvascular systems and their adjacent tissues in living animals can be recorded rapidly and how quantitative data can be extracted from the recorded images.   Two types of instrumentation will be considered for recording these events namely instruments that permit the securing of sequential optical images in short periods of time and instruments that permit the transformation of optical into electronic images.

The devices for recording optical images in short segments of time,   milli- or microseconds,   will be considered under the following categories: (1) The types of cameras that are available and applicable for recording microscopic images of living tissues.   (2) Illumination. (3) Optics.   (4) Instrumentation for maintaining the homeostasis of illuminated living tissue.   (5) Cinephotographic films.   (6) Instruments for timing the recorded image.   (7) New Information that has been secured from the microvascular system by using "high-speed" cinephotography. (8) Limitations of "high-speed" cinephotography.   And, (9) suggestions for future studies.

The transformation of optical into electronic images will be considered in respect to: (1) The principles that are involved in electronic image processing.   (2) Types of electronic image sensors. (3) Electronic image sensors that have been used to study microvascular systems: vidicon television systems; image orthicon television systems; image converters.   (4) Devices that have potentialities for studying living tissue at the microscopic level: "image transformers" and "flying spot" microscopes.   (5) The response of electronic sensors in respect to the electromagnetic spectrum.   (6) Optical image resolution versus electronic image resolution.   (7) Electronic image amplification and electronic image contrast.   (8) Electronic image formation rates and image repetition rates.   (9) The recording of electronic images.   (10) Quantitation of electronic images. (11) Electronic images resulting from optical images or spectra.   (12) Information from living organs that has been secured from electronic image processing devices.   And,(13) limitations of electronic image processing as related to the dynamics of microvascular systems.

Image analysis will be considered in respect to analysis by the human sensor and from motion picture film.

Figure 1.6 Edward Bloch's equipment in a laboratory in Cleveland, USA. Inn1968, this was the most advanced technology of the time. Anyone wishing to be up to date in microcirculatory studies would try to visit it. Edward Bloch provided a program of instruction.

are some teaching sessions lasting only a couple of hours that can change one's understanding of a field forever.

In 1831, Hall [55] described the transparency of the hibernating bat's wing. Paget, six years later [56], used it to study inflammation, and Jones in 1852 [57] noted the contractility of the veins in the bat's wing. After its reintroduction by Nicoll and Webb in 1946 [58], it was a popular preparation in the United States during the 1950s–1960s [59] until rabies became a recognized risk.

The bat's wing was second only to Ryan's first look at the conjunctiva as an impressive introduction to the visualization of blood vessels and lymphatics. Here was a hibernating animal that did not need anesthetics, whose transparent wing when spread out under the microscope revealed adnexa such as sebaceous glands, complete with blood supply and lymphatic drainage, which kept the wing well greased when flying. Following any, even slight, manipulation, one learned just how many cells, red and white, were flowing into and along lymph vessels.

It was the topic of bat wings that provided the most worrying lecture Ryan ever attended. This was a plenary lecture by Paul Nicholl at the World Congress in

> *San Diego, (1979). He had at one time found a bat in his attic and while throwing it out of the window noticed the sun shining through the wing showing up blood vessels. Sitting with him at breakfast and at the 9 am lecture, he was clearly very ill from cardiac pain but insisted on giving the prestigious lecture remaining seated and died shortly afterwards.*

Following some pure clinical dermatology visits in the United States on that tour, Terence Ryan went on to Sydney where Dintenfass and Palmer had some wonderful low technologies for visualizing red cell flow, such as along scratch marks on glass slides, and Dintenfass [60] also had a huge knowledge and passion for the clinical effects of high blood viscosity. The tour continued through Asia, lecturing on skin blood supply in Singapore, Calcutta, and Delhi, and ended at a European Microcirculation Congress (1968) in Gothenburg organized by the surgeon Charlie Gelin. He had worked in Boston, on the topic of rheology. He was the organizer of the first European meeting in 1959. Here, in 1968, the main interest was rheology and the effect of dextran in humans on lowering blood viscosity and making microcirculatory flow faster. Hildegard Maricq, attending this meeting, had become the leading exponent of nail fold capillary measurement and had greatly improved the imaging of the human nail fold by selecting transparent nail folds for study, and later, with widefield photography and cinephotography, used this increasingly for the study of both scleroderma and schizophrenia [61]. Maricq with her collaborators tried to introduce controls and population surveys as comparisons for problems such as Raynauds syndrome in which there is vasospasm on even slight cooling or from vibration from industrial tools.

Meeting almost annually at microvascular conferences, Hildegard was noted for focus on the human nail fold, her mixed American and Estonian accent, as well as for getting lost; for example, going the wrong direction on the Great Wall of China when returning to the conference bus. For those wishing to image the skin, the nail fold capillary had been the topic of study throughout the twentieth century. Nail fold enthusiasts such as Bosley tried to make sense of variability in the normal population at the First European Congress in Hamburg in 1960. He published [62] with the Nobel Prize winner Sherrington's protégé, William Gibson, who was still publishing in 2010, the year he died at the age of 94. Eli Davis of Jerusalem was another nail fold enthusiast and the author of a splendid atlas of the human nail fold [63]. He was host to the European Microcirculation Conference in 1964. Terence Ryan arranged an opportunity for viewing skin disease through the capillary microscope first in Oxford in 1966, and then in London (1969) at conferences for dermatologists. Over the years, a number of dermatologists had shown that although, apart from the nail fold healthy human skin was not transparent, skin pathology such as that of the legs with venous disease often had surprising transparency but morphologically, very abnormal shapes and sizes [34, 64].

1.4
TV Video Projection

Better microscopy was developed when Intaglietta assisted with TV video projection observers of the skin such as Fagrell and Bollinger [65], especially in case of venous disorders of the leg that they reviewed, and he had also provided assistance to Xiu Rui Juan for the clinical application that included remarkable studies conducted in China on the effects of Chinese Medicine [66].

She had a laboratory in Beijing, which trained many young Chinese investigators. Her interests began during the revolution when working at the center of a meningitis epidemic and observing in neonates the effects of shock on the blood supply of the skin.

> *Madame Xui (Figure 1.7) appeared on the World forum in 1984 at the World Congress of Microcirculation. Educated at a Christian Missionary School, after qualification as a medical practitioner she found herself expelled to the countryside at the very difficult time of the Cultural Revolution. There was a meningitis epidemic and the death toll of infants was very high. She noted that on one hill side the babies were surviving. She noted that their fingers were pink, whereas those of that died were blanched. Persuading the authorities that it was necessary for a relaxation of rules and the import of American microscopes, she demonstrated that treatment of shock by ephedrine shut down the capillary bed in the infant nail fold, while Chinese Medicine practiced on the hillside did not. Adapting these technologies using television microscopy to both finger and toenail fold has continued to be found valuable for the promotion of Chinese medicine.*

Technological developments in the study of the microcirculation during the decade 1960–1970 were reviewed by Intaglietta and Messmer [67] as a period of "rapid advances in electronic instrumentation, led by investigators such as Wiederheilm, Baez, Wayland, and Johnson and to the development of quantitative methods for the measurement of pressure, diameter, and flow velocity. Progress in television and the introduction of video equipment for consumer use in the 1970s allowed Intaglietta and coworkers to introduce the electronic techniques for obtaining dynamic information directly from the microvascular video image. From the beginning of the 1980s, the advances in fluorescence microscopy used in conjunction with low-light-level video cameras have expanded the range of phenomena accessible to *in vivo* microscopy to include tissue injury, tissue metabolism, and biochemistry." The Japanese, led by Tsuchiya [68] at Keio University in Tokyo, focused on the gastrointestinal tract in animals and humans, with beautiful imaging of lymph flow through Peyer's patches. They hosted the 4th World Congress of Microcirculation (Figure 1.8).

Scattered around the world were studies of the brain. William Feindel and his Canadian colleagues had previously introduced brain studies at the 4th European meeting in Cambridge in 1966, and Russian investigators demonstrated studies on

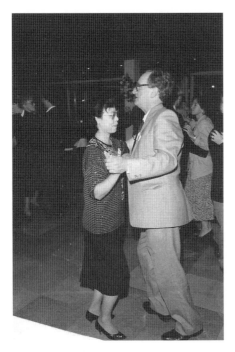

Figure 1.7 Madam Xui Rui-Juan, while singing a Methodist Hymn learned in her childhood in China, dancing with Terence Ryan to a Jazz band at a European Microcirculation Meeting in Maastricht. She had a laboratory in Beijing, which trained many young Chinese investigators. Her interests began during the revolution when working at the center of a meningitis epidemic and observing the effects of shock in neonates on the blood supply of the skin.

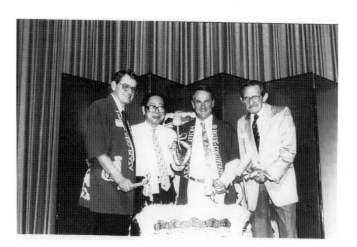

Figure 1.8 At 4th World Congress of Microcirculation in Tokyo. From left to right Phil Harris (incoming President) Masharu Tsuchiya (President, 4th World Congress of microcirculation), Terence J Ryan (President 3rd World Congress), and Ben Zweifach (President 2nd World congress) opening a ceremonial container of Saki.

Table 1.1   Methods used on the study of the microcirculation.

Introductory comments	Harold Wayland
Flow, pressure, and dimension measurements in the microcirculation image time and image transformation	Edward H. Bloch
Edge clamped mesenteric preparation	Wallace G. Frasher, Jr.
Methods of investigating plasma skimming	A. A. Palmer
Dynamic pressure grams of the pulmonary microcirculation	John W. Irwin
Subcutaneous tissue pressure	J. F. Merlen
Estimation of relative blood flow by impedance plethysmography	J. F. Merlen and J. Coget
Optical methods of measuring erythrocyte velocity in living animals	P.A.G. Monro
Methods for *in vivo* measurements of tubular urine flow, flow resistance, compliance, and fluid reabsorption in mammalian kidney	Michael Steinhausen
Measurement of capillary filtration and permeability; optical measurements of transcapillary and interstitial transport	Curt Wiederhielm
Autoradiographic investigations of capillary permeability	G. Freytag
In vivo studies of fluid movement across single capillaries	B. W. Zweifach
The use of fluorescence microscopy in the study of capillary permeability	S. Witte
Studies of vascular geometry	
The microvascular architecture	S. S. Sobin
Selective pulmonary angiography in microcirculatory studies in man	Wilhelm Bolt
Data processing techniques for the microcirculation digital video data handling	Robert Nathan
Online analog computers in microcirculatory studies	Paul C. Johnson

Source: Courtesy of Harold Wayland Cambridge 1987.

the brain at all meetings up to 1968. Feindel made sure that we were well informed at the First World Microcirculation Congress in Toronto [69]. All these depended on the microscope. Wayland, an engineer adviser to all the microcirculation studies and a great traveler (always accompanied by his wife as a passionate collector of and lecturer on playing cards), repeatedly expressed the view that new technologies were needed. At earlier meetings, he focused, as did Alexander Munro, on measuring red cell velocity *in vivo*. At the 4th European Conference on Microcirculation, Harold Wayland [70] organized a symposium on *Methods Used in the Study of Microcirculation*. Table 1.1 lists the content.

All studies of the skin require sampling at rest compared to that under some stimulus such as posture change, pin prick, heating, the application of vasodilators [71], such as methylnicotinate, and vasoconstrictors such as steroid creams, or cooling.

At the 1968 Microcirculation Congress in Gothenberg, fibrinolysis autography was also demonstrated and was adapted for a number of studies of blood vessel behavior in the skin for a few years. It was an indicator of functional changes in the endothelium in response to a number of stimuli. The fact that endothelium in the skin was under the influence of the epidermis was demonstrated by the discovery in the epidermis of a plasminogen activator inhibitor as a controller of endothelial fibrinolysis. It was demonstrated by incubating frozen sections of skin on a bed of fibrin [72, 73].

> *Once diabetes mellitus became a hot topic for the study of its microvascular pathology and skin fibrinolysis it was studies of the eye that provided most insight into microvascular change. Animals made diabetic by streptotocin included the pig. These pigs became giants and examining their eyes while keeping them anaesthetised provided Oxford's Professor of Opthalmology with a temporary overdose of halothane!*

The technologies before 1969 were described and published by the BMS [74] and Ryan *et al.* [75]. This second manual on microcirculatory techniques included descriptions of photoplethsysmograhy and thermoclearance techniques favored, respectively, by Ramsay and Challenor as well as the technique of fibrinolysis autography. A passion for studying vascular systems can be inhibited by the size and immobility of the humans when trying to position them under an imaging device.

Animal preparations require correct supervision to satisfy animal rights. Barnhill and Ryan [76] found the chorioallantoic membrane to be an exciting model not only because of easy viewing but also because it did not require consent of animal rights activists. Indeed, the only disadvantage of having this preparation in a dermatological ward was the rare appearance of a chick tweeting under a patient's bed after a nocturnal hatching.

1.5
The Third World Congress of Microcirculation

> *At a European conference in Denmark 1970 Terence Ryan became a treasurer, for the first time, of the European Society (a hand over of £370) Finances were linked to Karger, the Swiss publisher by whom microcirculation Proceedings Biblio Anatomica were long published by Karger, and readers will find most of the history of 1970s' imaging therein. The Swiss franc did very well and Ryan received undeserved thanks for an accumulation of wealth when he gave the post up. When Harold Wayland chaired an International Liaison Committee to decide the location of the third World Congress, the BMS put Terence Ryan's name forward. Being a clinician, the American Scientists would have preferred the distinguished scientist Charles Michel to be President, but he was × European Society for Microcirculation. Terence Ryan was thrown thus in the deep end hosting the conference in the city of Oxford with no large conference facilities but a new Hospital with an Academic block that*

had previously been unused and unprepared lecture theatres, for audiences of 600, 450, and 200. Getting in quick, space was made use of that was never again used for conferences. The Americans were not impressed when the conference organiser employed went bankrupt. Eventually, the dermatology team organised the conference very successfully, 900 people attended a barbecue at Terence and Anne's home, Anne sewed all the curtains for the conference center, participants dined simultaneously in three College halls and took over Blenheim Palace for a reception and ate afterwards at Green College in a tent with crystal chandeliers.

It was Howard Florey's second wife Margaret who opened the the World Congress of Microcirculation in 1984 to speak of his interest in the lymphatic system. His pupil John Casely-Smith chaired the lymphatic session. Phillip Shubik who had pioneered imaging of cancers in the hamster cheek pouch gave a memorial lecture on Gordon Sanders, which included Sanders' film using the versions of Malpighi's compound microscope that became popular in early Hanoverian London. Possibly, this was the event that indicated that microcirculation and microscopy had come of age.

It became necessary to make more formal liaison between many groups. This had been well done by the American Clinical Physiologist and resident surgeon in Linköping, Sweden, David Lewis, whose wit aggregated the societies and ensured smooth flow (Figure 1.9). Terence Ryan took over such liaison after the 1984 congress.

At the 1984 World Congress, Alfred Bollinger revealed much improved cine fluorescence in human peripheral circulatory disorders.

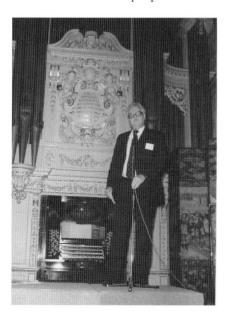

Figure 1.9 David Lewis speaking in the Great Library and Organ Room of Blenheim Palace before handing over his successful role as Chairman of the Liaison Committee for Microcirculation Societies. "If I had known I was going to be here I would have brought my library Ticket!" As an American surgeon living in Linköping, the home of Perimed, and a distinguished researcher into shock and many other circulation phenomena, he was also a favorite after-dinner speaker over several decades of microcirculatory events.

1.6
Perfusion Monitoring and the Advent of the Laser Doppler

It was at this meeting in 1984 that continuous, noninvasive, real-time, blood perfusion monitoring, laser Doppler flowmetry was first demonstrated to a global microcirculation audience by Allen Holloway and Ăke Oberg (Figure 1.10). The paper by Holloway and Watkins [77] was by that time well known, and Oberg *et al.* had published their seminal paper the year of the congress [78]. The technique had previously used Leeuwenhoek's glass, tubes but in 1975, it was Stern who developed it as a tool for tissue microcirculation [79]. Stern proposed that when coherent light impinges on the skin, some of it will be scattered by moving red blood cells and some by static tissue. If this light (which is spectrally broadened due to the Doppler effect) is brought to the surface of a sensitive photodetector, optical beating will produce an audio frequency photocurrent output. Spectral analysis of the photocurrent produced by backscattered He–Ne red laser light from the fingertip showed a clear difference between normal flow and occlusion of the brachial artery. The feasibility of real-time monitoring was demonstrated using the root-mean-square (RMS) of the photocurrent signal as a flow indicator. This method was shown to be sensitive to the microcirculatory response to temperature, posture, respiratory pattern, and emotional stimulation. Furthermore, it was proposed that "Because it provides information about the flow velocity distribution, it has the potential ability to analyse the distribution of flow in the different microvascular compartments" [79].

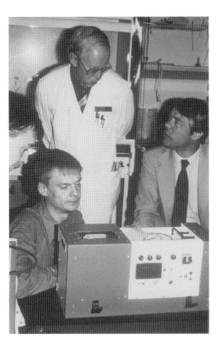

Figure 1.10 Admiring the first commercial laser Doppler flowmeter from Med-Pacific (around 1978). Left to right: Gert Nilsson Hans Pettersson (research engineer at IMT, Linkoping), Åke Öberg (Professor in biomedical engineering IMT), and Allan Holloway (inventor of the LDF equipment, University of Washington, Seattle, USA).

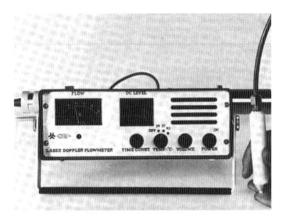

Figure 1.11 The first commercial version of the Periflux laser Doppler flowmeter invented by Gert Nilsson *et al.* [82]. This instrument used two detectors and a differential detection method to suppress laser and fiber mode noise common to both detectors. (Source: Gert Nilsson, Wheelsbridge AB.)

The system demonstrated by Holloway and Watkins included fiber-optics for light delivery and collection, as well as a photodiode in place of the more cumbersome photomultiplier tube used by Stern. They evaluated their new instrument against the 133Xe clearance technique and were able to measure the effect of injection trauma, which manifests itself as a transient elevation in local blood perfusion due to either the fear or pain of an injection. This effect was suspected for some time, but no other method was capable of directly measuring it and following its time course faithfully.

Watkins and Holloway, later described their instrument in more technical detail [80], identified the modal noise caused by the He–Ne laser as a major developmental problem and found that measurement was limited to 50% of the observation time. The presence of more than one spectral line in the laser output may cause beat frequencies to occur on the photodiode, similar to those produced by Doppler-shifted light. This problem was overcome by Nilsson *et al.* [81] who proposed a dual photodetection system in which the noise common to both detectors could be rejected. The Doppler signal is not affected as the photons arriving at each detector are completely independent and random. Later that year, Nilsson *et al.* [82] presented a further development, incorporating the algorithm developed by Bonner and Nossal [83]. This remains the only signal processing algorithm with a sound theoretical base and has found favor amongst most researchers and manufacturers.

The instruments developed by Holloway and Watkins [77] and Nilsson *et al.* [81] were soon commercially available (Figures 1.10 and 1.11). An early comparison by Fischer *et al.* [84] demonstrated a good correlation between the instruments as well as with microvascular blood flow. Clinical trials were undertaken in many areas and, while good results were often produced, widespread application has eluded the technique. One reason given by clinicians is that the lack of absolute units makes interpretation of the data from different patients difficult. However, the measurand (i.e., microvascular blood flow) is poorly predictable at any given tissue site and time. The assessment of sufficiency of perfusion must, therefore, be based on its variation in response to an appropriate physiological stimulus. Diagnostic differences in microcirculatory response have been consistently reported where a ratiometric (percentage change) analysis has been employed. This invariably involves the comparison of a stimulated value to a resting level.

Clinical trials of these improved instruments exposed the problem of motion artifact noise, which occurs when the modes in which light passes through the fiber are disturbed by movement of the cable, resulting in small losses of light from the core into the cladding. This phenomenon manifests itself in intensity fluctuations at the photodetector similar to the laser Doppler beat frequency. One analytical study demonstrated that the range of frequencies produced is 0–3.5 kHz [85] and that the magnitude can be much larger than the perfusion-related Doppler signal. This problem was accentuated by the fact that the larger-core fibers translated the movement to the tissue, giving rise to tissue-related Doppler shifting.

Further technological improvements facilitated the use smaller fiber-optic cables, a wider range of probes encompassing new application areas, and less noisy semiconductor laser diodes. This led to an increased number of instruments being made available throughout the 1980s. Smaller diameter fibers reduce sensitivity to motion artifact in three ways. First, the smaller core produces fewer modes. Second, the optical beating will be more efficient if there is a reduced spread of paths traveled by the light collected. Last, less of the movement will be transmitted to the probe head.

The use of laser diodes in LDPMs was reported by de Mul *et al.* [86] with the diode laser source and detection integrated in the probe head. This eliminated the need for fiber-optic cables and is insensitive to noise contributions from voluntary motion. The wavelength of the diodes commonly used (780 nm) has further advantages of deeper penetration and reduced dependence on skin color. Also, because the absorption of oxidized and deoxygenated hemoglobin is almost equal at this wavelength, any dependence on oxygen saturation is eliminated. The choice of laser wavelengths is confined (largely by commercial availability) to He–Ne red (632.8 nm) and near-infrared laser diodes (780 nm). The He–Ne system is important for historical reasons as the first instruments were built using these lasers; however, laser diodes are now used in virtually all instruments sold. A greater understanding of both the laser Doppler signal and the associated noise allowed us to develop instruments that can process the entire bandwidth of interest with excellent signal-to-noise performance.

The first European Laser Doppler Users meeting was held in Oxford in 1991. By that time, Becker and Vestweber were able to review 356 publications chosen from almost 1000 studies, and many of Europe's microcirculation experts were now studying its potential in skin, nasal mucosa, liver, kidney, inner ear, and bones and teeth and in disease states such as hypertension and diabetes. Several groups, including the dermatology department in Oxford were examining phenomena such as postural vasoconstriction or the effects of smoking [79, 87]. Before this technology, they had used thermography in a number of publications on skin blood flow. With laser Dopplers, testing the effects of drugs such as prostaglandin E1 on Raynaud's syndrome was being introduced. There were warnings that the technique would be discredited unless better standardized. Already in 1991, automatic scanning with multipoint laser Doppler flux recordings were being introduced [88], and Stringini and Ryan [89] used the technique for wound healing studies.

Perhaps the most remarkable feature of the microcirculation is its enormous temporal and spatial heterogeneity. This has given rise to the introduction of a multichannel instrument and the laser Doppler perfusion imager (LDPI). The multichannel array provides for the spatial assessment of blood flow without the loss of temporal resolution. This facilitates the continuous and real-time measurements of the effects of vasoactive stimuli on different compartments of the same organ or interorgan comparisons. It can be particularly useful in disciplines in which it is necessary to control the blood supply on a regional basis. One example is the use of pharmaceuticals to restrict the blood supply to the tumoral area without affecting local normal tissue. By simultaneously monitoring the perfusion at microregional sites within and in the locus of the tumor during infusion of such agents, immediate information is given as to the selectivity and severity of the drug's effect [90]. Similar, but more graphic information, may be obtained using the LDPI [91] where the entire area of interest is visible and blood flow variations are expected to occur over a much longer time course (Figure 1.12).

The laser Doppler technique is cost effective and easy to use. It is possibly this advantage that has paradoxically become a stumbling block to more universal use of the instrument, because it is quite possible to use the instrument with little knowledge of what is being measured and how. The main laser Doppler

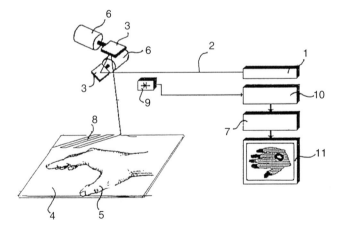

Figure 1.12 First laser Doppler perfusion imager version. (1) Laser, (2) laser beam, (3) mirrors, (4) underlay, (5) living tissue, (6) stepper motors, (7) PC, (8) scanning pattern, (9) photodetector, (10) pre-amp and A/D, (11) Perfusion image. (Source: From patent application 1989.)

developers cooperated in an European Commission-sponsored concerted action (CA) to provide a greater means of comparison of results between active groups, through the establishment of internationally standardized protocols. This CA published a report setting out the principles and practice of the laser Doppler perfusion monitoring and imaging [92]. The continuous, real-time nature of laser Doppler provides an excellent means of following an occlusion and reactive hyperemia and vasomotion (from 0.001 to ~10 Hz) including that mediated by heartbeat, breathing, myogenic, and endothelial function [93]. Mike Stern declared that "We know of no comparable method of demonstrating these microvascular reflexes" [79]. However, since then, a related technique based on an analysis of the speckles in backscattered laser light (laser speckle perfusion imaging, LSPI) and another based on diffuse reflectance spectroscopy, tissue viability imaging (TiVi) [94], have been shown to similarly follow these microvascular reactions.

As the angles in LDP are more or less random and a wide range of velocities are present in the microcirculation, a continuous Doppler frequency spectrum is produced. It is interesting to note that a similar result can be achieved by considering the scattering particle to be a moving reflector of light. The reflected light will interfere with the reference beam, and the resultant intensity will vary with the difference in optical path between the two beams. The number of interference fringes to pass the detector in time is related to the speed of the moving cells. Each time the mirror (cell) moves through a distance equal to half the wavelength of the light, the detector "sees" an interference fringe pass. That is, a fluctuation in light intensity is recorded. Variations in speckle contrast will then be dependent on the velocity distribution of the scatterers. Therefore, this velocity can be determined using a measurement of the statistical behavior of the speckles over time. This is similar to the reading given by a laser Doppler measurement, and in fact, it has been demonstrated that Doppler and time-varying speckle are two methods of arriving at the same result [95].

An exciting new idea first formulated by Takuo Aoyagi in 1972 in a patent filed by the Nikon Kohden Corporation, Japan, was to become the basis for continuous *in vivo* arterial oxygen saturation. This novel concept, which used the fact that light transmission in human tissue varies with arterial pulsations, to isolate the relative absorption of red and infrared light by arterial blood was later published by Nakajima *et al.* [96]. They postulated that the cardiac synchronous variations in the light intensity reaching the detector were entirely attributable to blood volume changes in the small arteries and arterioles "seen" by the probe. Therefore, comparing only the pulsating portion of the red and infrared signals should yield absorption data for arterial blood alone, the absorption of venous blood and other tissues being constant or slowly varying. This filtering mechanism was of tremendous benefit in the area of critical care medicine because the oxygen status of the blood supply rather than that of the mixed vascular bed could be measured. This is a parameter that is subject to reasonably precise regulation in the normal healthy individual at rest (~95–97% saturation) but may suddenly reduce to dangerous levels in the critically ill. In smokers, the maximal value can be only 84% due to a COHb of 15% [97].

The clinical significance of this instrument, particularly for anesthesiology, was realized by William New, himself an anesthesiologist at Stanford University. New developed and marketed a pulse oximeter (Nellcor N100) primarily for monitoring oxygen saturation in patients under anesthesia. Because of the tremendous importance of the technique, more than 20 manufacturers now produce pulse oximeters. Widespread use has, however, led to significant criticism of the technique in certain clinical situations. The instrument was shown to be unreliable in conditions of low perfusion (at the site of measurement, normally the finger), subject movement or shivering, the presence of abnormal hemoglobins (hemoglobin bound to molecules other than oxygen), and even the presence of interfering contaminants such as nail polish in the light path. However, despite these criticisms, the use of a pulse oximeter was firmly established as a "standard of care" in every operating room and intensive care unit in the developed world [98]. The pulse oximeter is a triumph of noninvasive biophotonic monitoring with an elegant technical solution to a real clinical need and enormous commercial success. A comprehensive review of the principles and practice of pulse oximetry was published by Moyle in 1994 [99].

The advent of ultrasound to indicate the relative density of the dermis shed light on the water content of the upper dermis. It was observed that it was increased by venous congestion and relieved by elevation [100]. A series of publications from the laboratory of Serup in Denmark followed.

While the technology allowing frame-by-frame analysis of red cell flow separated by plasma gaps had improved the accuracy of velocity measurements, interpretation of flow and capillary shapes was slow to take into account normal variation in the population. In the 1920s, a single capillary alteration in shape might be correlated with a wide range of diseases, including disturbances in mental health. From the 1970s Bosley working with Gibson, Maricq working with her collaborators, as well as Ryan tried to introduce controls and population surveys as comparisons for problems such as Raynaud's syndrome in which there is vasospasm on even slight cooling or from the use of vibrating industrial tools.

Optical techniques such as illuminating a tissue at a wavelength at which hemoglobin absorbs maximally, thus increasing the contrast of the blood vessels, and adding fluorescing agents to the plasma helped to further show up the full content of the flowing blood up to the vessel wall. This work was led by Konrad Messmer and others, resulting in a technique called orthogonal polarization spectral imaging (OPS). This used a high absorbing, Isobestic point of hemoglobin to enhance contrast in the microcirculation and orthogonal polarizers on the light source and camera. This had the effect of flooding the tissue bed with diffuse light and, as described by Messmer, creating an apparent light source 1 mm below the surface. Technical development is continued now by Can Ince and coworkers (Chapter 2), and several clinical applications have been explored by Jean-Louis Vincent, Daniel de Backer, and others (Chapter 3).

Two- and three-dimensional techniques are the mainstay of this book, so only a brief introduction is required here. Perfusion imagers have recently been reviewed by O'Doherty *et al.* [94]. A brief description is provided in the following paragraphs.

In the 1990s, groups led by Gert Nilsson at Linköping and Tim Essex at Newcastle upon Tyne extended laser Doppler to an imaging technique [91, 101, 102] by raster scanning the laser and detector 15–20 cm above the surface. This gave rise to at least two commercial LDPIs currently marketed by Perimed and Moor Instruments. Most of the instruments are sold for clinical research purposes, and although it has been used for almost every conceivable application involving the microcirculation, it appears that burn depth assessment [103] is the only FDA-approved diagnostic use of LDPI.

The LDPI approach raises challenges, particularly in temporal resolution (due to the raster scanning) and in coping with the speckle nature of images where the light source is a laser. Normally, the number of speckles is dependent solely on the detector configuration. However, the LDPI systems use a large area detector collecting as much light as practical from the illuminated spot on the tissue surface. The spot itself then determines the effective area of detection and is dependent on the tissue properties. It is perhaps because of this and the high variability in surface reflections that most manufacturers have moved to normalize the laser Doppler signal by DC light intensity rather than by the square of the DC light intensity (Chapter 6).

LSPI takes advantage of the speckled nature of laser-illuminated images and specifically the blurring of speckle caused by moving scatterers (red blood cells) to extract an alternate measure of perfusion (cf. Chapter 8). Essentially, when the shutter speed or integration time of the camera is ~10 ms, a greater number and speed of red blood cells in the tissue under study will provide greater blurring. Since it is unnecessary to capture the full laser Doppler spectrum (requiring >25 000 fps), the technical requirements for full-field speckle imagers are much lower than for LDPI. Thus, with uniform illumination of the tissue with an appropriate laser and a standard video rate camera, full-field images of flow-related speckle can be obtained.

Optimal integration time varies from 1 ms for faster flow to 20 ms where the flow in smallest vessels (with slower flow) is being studied [104, 105]. Issues such as the need to know the flow range *a priori* and the fact that the theoretical basis is not as rigorous have meant that laser speckle has a much slower uptake than LDPI. However, later work by Thompson, Dunn and Boas, Duncan shows that the use of multiple integration times may provide a more solid basis for measurement and more reliable perfusion images.

The early demonstrations of speckle imaging for blood flow were in the eye (retinal artery) [106]. With more advanced image processing, Briers and others were able to measure the speckle blurring directly and produce false color maps of the microcirculation in many tissues. LSPIs are much less sensitive to deeper (>200 µm) perfusion, whereas LDPI is sensitive to flow at depths up to approximately 1 mm [107] (Chapter 8). Full-field laser Doppler imaging has become possible with the advent of fast CMOS cameras, and it has been implemented by the groups led by Steenbergen in Twente and Lasser in Lausanne. Currently, the number of pixels and the bandwidth of signal acquired are limited by available cameras as well as high-speed data transfer and signal processing challenges.

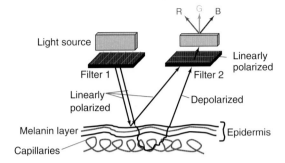

Figure 1.13 Schematic showing the operating principle of subsurface spectroscopic imaging.

Furthermore, there remains the challenge of motion artifact since the Doppler signal due to movement of the living subject is entangled with the blood perfusion signal. A diffuse reflectance technique called *"tissue viability imaging"* was developed to avoid this motion artifact (Figure 1.13). It produces two-dimensional images of the concentration of red cells using an RGB camera to pick out the spectral signature of hemoglobin. Crossed polarizers are used to select only light that has penetrated more than a few hundred microns within the tissue, reducing the influence of surface reflections and melanin [108].

1.7
3D and 4D Tomographic Methods

Microcirculation is of course a three-dimensional structure, and as such, a comprehensive understanding requires a means to study it in three dimensions. Since it is also functional, a fourth dimension, that is, time, is also important. Recently, technological developments have allowed the exploration of the microcirculation in all its exquisite glory and function over time. These include confocal (fluorescence) microscopy, multiphoton microscopy, photoacoustic imaging, and functional optical coherence tomography. Since the first two involve the injection of fluorescent dyes, they have limited potential for application in humans. We compare OCT and fluorescence microscopy in Chapter 13. Photoacoustic tomography and microscopy has enjoyed enormous interest since a seminal paper by Lihong Wang *et al.* (St. Louis) in 2003 [109]. It takes advantage of the diffuse nature of light in tissue to deliver energy to the deep blood vessels even if there is a larger upper vessel in the direct path. The light energy is absorbed preferentially by blood if a suitable wavelength is used (e.g., 560 nm) and, if a suitable short pulse releases an ultrasound pressure wave, which is not scattered in the return path. Since the speed of sound is 1 million times smaller than that of light, the locations of absorbers within the tissue can easily be determined by back projection (Chapter 12). Using this method, many exquisite 3D images of the microvascular architecture have been produced in mouse brain and ear. More recently, the first images were obtained from monkey

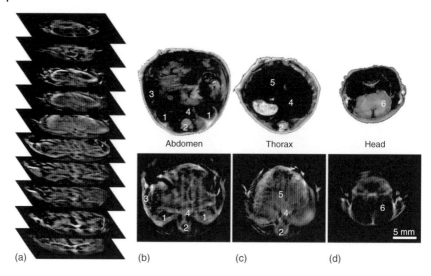

(a) (b) (c) (d)

Figure 1.14 (a–e) Whole body mouse imaging using multi-spectral photoacoustic tomography [111].

brain and the human palm. Zharov and Galanzha have developed methods for tagging, tracking, and destroying tumor cells [110]. Limitations of the technique include the requirement for physical contact (e.g., water or gel). Although it is possible to interferometrically measure the perturbations arriving at the surface, it is quite challenging since these vibrations are of the order of a few nanometers. Penetration and signal to noise require low frequencies, whereas high resolution requires higher frequencies of ultrasound. These factors combine to dictate a depth resolution of 200 pixels. Depths of 30 mm have already been demonstrated and 50–70 mm is theoretically possible (Chapter 12). Ntziachristos and coworkers [111] have advanced multispectral photoacoustic imaging to facilitate whole body mouse scanning in <30 min without water immersion (Figure 1.14).

Perhaps the greatest and most exciting current activity is in 3D and 4D imaging of the microcirculation based on OCT. In contrast to the other techniques, OCT throws away all scattered photons, using an interferometric scheme to select only ballistic photons. This allows a three-dimensional image of the structure to be built up based on the intensity variations due to refractive index variations in the tissue layers. First attempts to add the microvascular architecture were based on the Doppler effect, although this was necessarily weak since the heterodyne mixing efficiency is determined by the coherence between the source and reference beams. Furthermore, it is dependent on the angle between photon and the velocity vector. Since the feeding network of vessels under the papillary loops is generally horizontal, it is almost impossible to detect any flow in that region, and the papillary loops at 5 μm themselves are below the resolution of most OCT systems. A closely related alternative is to determine the velocity from the phase shift, and this is much more sensitive to small Doppler shifts. Most "Doppler" OCT systems now operate on this basis.

Ruikang Wang and coworkers introduced a spatial modulation in the interferogram to separate structure from moving scatterers within the tissue. Originally, this was achieved using a scanning mirror in the reference arm, but more recently, the inherent modulation due to blood flow has been used. Several groups have developed methods to take advantage of speckle variance, which is higher in blood vessels than in static tissues. Variance measures how much the speckle intensity varies over say 10 frames, and this can produce good separation of flowing blood from static tissue. Finally, Martin Leahy's team in Galway have developed a scheme based on dense scanning (separation ∼one-fifth of the resolution of the OCT system) where a simple cross-correlation between two adjacent frames will give excellent separation of structure and flow. The simplicity of this technique facilitates high-speed processing, enabling 4D imaging of microvascular architecture and function. It has been shown to produce high-quality images in humans [112] and brings clinical microcirculation imaging within reach (Figure 1.15).

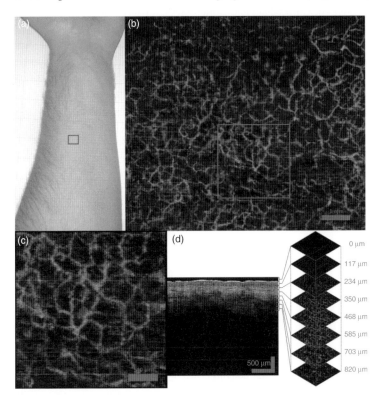

Figure 1.15 (a–d) Correlation mapping OCT. 2D correlation map of sequential frames average correlation value for a square grid of 7 × 7 pixels. The decorrelated (bright) volume contains moving blood cells. The volume shown dark is the region without blood perfusion. Structure and function are automatically coregistered since they are reconstructed from the same original dataset. Using a simple algorithm such as correlation mapping OCT (cmOCT) makes it possible to do 4D imaging at clinically relevant speeds and depths.

1.8
Nonoptical Microcirculation Imaging

For completeness, this text provides three chapters on nonoptical techniques for imaging the microcirculation. These include high-frequency ultrasound, micro-CT, and NMR. Ultrasound is tremendously important for its success in preclinical studies and has advantages of an established clinical follow-up method combining depth with reasonable (circa 100 µm) resolution. Substantial progress in this area has been made by Stuart Foster at the University of Toronto and others (Chapter 15). However, ultrasound requires physical contact with the tissue and bone eliminates the signal, except at very low (1 MHz) frequencies. Perhaps, the gold standard for accurate determination of the 3D architecture of the microcirculation is micro-CT since it has the lowest potential for distortion of any of the methods presented. Unfortunately, it requires the use of ionizing radiation and usually lethal doses of contrast agents. Nonetheless, it could provide a useful tool for comparison and validation of other methods to aid clinical deployment. NMR advancement, especially the exploration of cognitive function using fMRI, has yielded great insights, linking perfusion or oxygen saturation blood oxygenation level-dependent (BOLD) contrast variations in specific locations to specific actions or functions. It does not have the resolution to see individual microvessels, but is sensitive to bulk microcirculatory perfusion. It has great advantages of depth penetration, especially through bone, but is limited in resolution and cost.

There are several other techniques used to probe the microcirculation, which do not yet deserve a Chapter in this book, but we will mention some of them here. Positron emission tomography (PET) simultaneously detects the two gamma photons produced in opposite directions when positrons from the injected radiopharmaceutical annihilate with an electron. 3D reconstructions with ∼2 mm resolution can show blood perfusion, oxygenation, and glucose metabolism by using different chemical agents. The radioisotopes must be used within a couple of hours of their production in a cyclotron, severely limiting the location of PET facilities.

Single photon emission computed tomography (SPECT) uses a gamma camera to make multiple projections of photons from an injected radionuclide to produce a 3D dataset. Unfortunately, the resolution of SPECT is limited to ∼1 cm, so like MRI and PET, its use is limited to bulk microcirculatory perfusion.

1.9
Panel Discussions and International Convergence

In recent years, international efforts have been made to better understand the techniques available for studying the microcirculation. One such initiative takes place at the Photonics West BiOS meeting in San Francisco each year, where a panel of experts report the progress of their technique and debate the merits of the various approaches with questions and input from the audience. Similarly, the Microcirculation Societies meet to discuss the new insights they have gained as

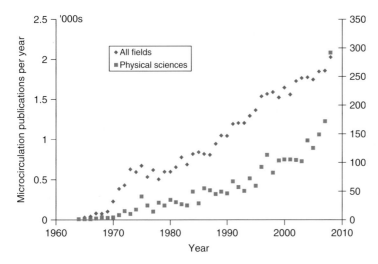

Figure 1.16 The evolution of microcirculation papers published since the 1960s. Television and recording technology enabled videomicroscopy. In the 1980s completion from several companies brought robust laser Doppler instruments to the clinicians. The fraction of the total publications reporting advancements in the instrumentation has risen from circa 5 to 15%. This may be largely due to the arrival of 3D and 4D microcirculation imaging using mainly OCT and photoacoustics.

a result of these new techniques. In recent years, there has been an enormous increase in the publication activity around new techniques for microcirculation imaging (Figure 1.16), and it is inevitable that these new techniques will accelerate the understanding of the microcirculation once again. The evolution of papers on microcirculation published since the 1960s shows the impact of several inventions. The advent of TV in the late 1960s facilitated videomicroscopy and the measurement of speed from the frame rate. Laser Doppler, although invented in 1974, really began to impact publications only in the late 1980s as many robust laser Doppler instruments came on the market. If we only look at the physical sciences journals, we find a striking increase in publications from 2007. Indeed, the percentage of the total publications relating, one assumes, to instrumental improvements has risen from circa 5–15%. This may be largely due to the arrival of 3D and 4D microcirculation imaging using mainly OCT and photoacoustics.

In the following chapters, the many approaches to microcirculation imaging are discussed. Ultimately, the choice of technique will depend on the application site, the research question, cost, and convenience.

References

1. Zweifach, B.W. (1995) in *Clinically Applied Microcirculation Research*, Chapter 9 (eds J.J. Barker, G.L. Anderson, and M.D. Menger), CRC Press, Boca Raton, pp. 129–138.

2. Ryan, T.J. (1965) A new technique for studying the microcirculation of the skin. *J. Roy. Microsc. Soc.*, **84**, 230.

3. Ryan, T.J. (1967) in *In Vivo Techniques in Histology* (ed. G.H. Bourne),

Williams & Wilkins, London, pp. 192–202.

4. Newton, I. (1671) A Letter of Mr. Isaac Newton, Professor of the Mathematics in the University of Cambridge; Containing His New Theory about Light and Colors: Sent by the Author to the Publisher from Cambridge, Febr. 6. 1671/72; in Order to be Communicated to the R. Society. *Phil. Trans. Roy. Soc. Lond.*, **6** (69-80): 3075–3087. doi: 10.1098/rstl.1671.0072.

5. Doppler, J.C. (1842) Ueber das farbige Licht der Doppelsterne und einiger anderer Gestirne des Himmels (On the coloured light from double stars and some Heavenly Bodies). *Treatises R. Bohemian Soc. Sci. Ser. V (Abh. Konigl. Bohm. Ges. Wiss.)*, **3**, 465.

6. Fulton, G.P. (1979) 25th Anniversary Essay 1974–1979, The founding of the Microcirculatory Society, Pamphlet of Microcirculatory Society inc., New York. Reprinted *Anat. Rec.*, **120**, 241–356 and *Angiology*, **6**, 281–358.

7. Bessis, M. and Delpechi, G. (1981) Discovery of the red blood cell with notes on priorities and credits of discoveries, past, present and future. *Blood Cells*, **7**, 447–480.

8. Van Leeuwenhoek, A. (1673) A Specimen of some observations made by a Microscope, contrived by Mr Leewenhoeck in Holland lately communicated by Dr Regnerus de Graaf. *Philos. Trans. R. Soc. Lond., Ser. A*, **8** (94), 6037–6038.

9. Singer, C. (1922) *The Discovery of the Circulation of the Blood*, G. Bell and Sons Ltd., London.

10. Malpighi, M. (1683) *De pulmonibus* (Two letters (1930) translated by Young J). *Proc. R. Soc. Med.*, **23**, 1–11.

11. Spalteholz, W. (1893) Die Veiteilung der blutgefässe inder haut. His. *Arch. Anat. Entwicklungsgesch. Physiol.*, 1–54.

12. Sandison, J.C. (1924) A new method for the microscope study of living growing tissues by the introduction of a transparent chamber in the rabbits ear. *Anat. Rec.*, **28**, 281.

13. Sandison, J.C. (1928) Observations on the growth of blood vessels as seen in the transparent chamber introduced in the rabbit's ear. *Am. J. Anat.*, **41**, 475–496.

14. Clark, E.R. and Clark, E.L. (1939) Microscopic observations on the growth of blood capillaries in the living animal. *Am. J. Anat.*, **64**, 251–301.

15. Clark, E.R. and Clark, E.L. (1935) Observations on changes in blood vascular endothelium in the living animal. *Am. J. Anat.*, **57**, 385–438.

16. Sanders, A.G. and Shubik, P.A. (1964) A transparent window for use in the Syrian hamster. *Isr. J. Exp. Med.*, **11**, 118a.

17. Nishioka, K. and Ryan, T.J. (1972) The influence of the epidermis and other tissues on blood vessel growth in the hamster cheek pouch. *J. Invest. Dermatol.*, **58**, 33–45.

18. Starling, E.H. (1896) On the absorption of fluids from the connective tissue spaces. *J. Physiol. (Lond.)*, **19**, 312–326.

19. Krogh, A. (1922) *The Anatomy and Physiology of Capillaries*, Silliman Memorial Lectures, Yale University Press New Haven, CT, pp. 1–276.

20. Knisely, M.H. (1936) A method of illuminating living structures for microscopic study. *Anat. Rec.*, **64**, 499.

21. Knisely, M.H., Bloch, E.H., Eliot, T.S., and Warner, W. (1947) Sludged blood. *Science*, **106**, 431.

22. Bloch, E.H. (abstracts), (1954) Conference on microcirculatory physiology and pathology: techniques for the microscopic study of small blood vessels and blood flow. *Anat. Rec.*, **120**, 241–358.

23. Monro, P.A.G. (1967) 4th European conference on microcirculation at Cambridge. *Bibl. Anat.*, **9**, 1–458.

24. Monro, P.A.G. (1984) *The Early History of the British Microcirculation Society 1963–1984*, Anglo-German Foundation for the Study of Industrial Society.

25. Florey, H. (1962) *General Pathology*, 3rd edn, Lloyd-Luke Medical Books, Ltd, London.

26. Casley-Smith, J.R. (1995) in *Clinically Applied Microcirculation Research*, Chapter 31 (eds J.J. Barker, G.L. Anderson, and M.D. Menger), CRC Press, Boca Raton, pp. 419–434.

27. Lighthill, M.J. (1968) Motion in narrow capillaries from the standpoint of lubrication theory. *Biorheology*, **5**, 245–252.

28. Monro, P.A.G. (1969) A point source Xenon flash suitable for (cine-) photomicrography of living tissue (Demonstration). 19th September at Royal College of Physicians and Surgeons Glasgow. *http://www.microcirculation.org.uk/*. Accessed 2011.

29. Slaaf, D.W., Tangelder, G.J., Oude, E.G., Brink, M.G.A., and Reneman, R.S. (1995) in *Clinically Applied Microcirculation Research*, Chapter 29 (eds J.J. Barker, G.L. Anderson, and M.D. Menger), CRC Press, Boca Raton, pp. 391–405.

30. Montagna, W. and Ellis, R. (1961) *Advances in the Biology of the Skin*, Blood Vessels and Circulation, Vol. 2, Pergamon Press, Oxford, p. 1–156.

31. Palade, G.E. (1953) The fine structure of blood capillaries. *J. Appl. Physiol.*, **24**, 1424.

32. Hibbs, R.G., Burch, G.E., and Phillips, J.H. (1958) The fine structure of the small blood vessels of normal human dermis and subcutis. *Am. Heart J.*, **56**, 662.

33. Lombard, W.P. (1912) The blood pressure in the arterioles, capillaries and small veins of the human skin. *Am. J. Physiol.*, **29**, 335.

34. Gilje, O. (1953) Capillary microscopy in the diagnosis of skin diseases. *Acta Derm. Venereol.*, **33**, 303.

35. Davis, M.J. and Lorincz, A.L. (1957) An improved technic for capillary microscopy of the skin. *J. Invest. Dermatol.*, **28**, 283.

36. Kanan, M.W. and Ryan, T.J. (1976) in *Microvascular Injury*, Major Problems in Dermatology, Vol. 7, Lloyd Luke Medical, London, pp. 195–220.

37. Lewis, T. (1927) *The Blood Vessels of the Human Skin and their Responses*, Shaw and Sons, pp. 1–322.

38. Ryan, T.J. (1970) in *Blood Vessels of the Skin Special Supplement*, British Journal Dermatology, Vol. **82** (Suppl. 5) (ed. T.J. Ryan), HK Lewis & Co Ltd London, pp. 74–76.

39. Ryan, T.J. (1973) in *Physiology and Pathophysiology of the Skin*, vol. 2, Chapter 16–21 (ed. A. Jarrett), Academic Press, London, p. 638.

40. Ryan, T.J. (1978) in *The Physiology and Pathophysiology of the Skin*, vol. 5, 2nd edn (ed. A. Jarrett), Academic Press, London, pp. 1755–1780.

41. Ryan, T.J. (1976) *Microvascular Injury*, Major Problems in Dermatology, Vol. 7, Lloyd Luke Medical, London, p. 416.

42. Zweifach, B.W. (1961) *Functional Behaviour of the Microcirculation*, Charles C Thomas, Springfield, IL.

43. Trueta, J. (1965) 14 communications and 8 demonstrations. *Biorheology*, **3**, 223–231.

44. Royal Postgraduate Medical School (1967) 14 communications and 7 demonstrations. *Biorheology*, **5**, 85–93.

45. Ashton, N. (1973) Symposium on microcirculation of the eye. *Biorheology*, **10**, 490–499.

46. Ryan, T.J. (2005) in *The Tower of the Winds. A Biography of an Observatory* (eds I. Loudon and J. Burley), Green College, pp. 134–144.

47. Cherry, G.W., Bert Myers, M., Ardran, G., and Ryan, T.J. (1979) The effects of gravity on delayed and transplanted tubed flaps. *Plast. Reconstr. Surg.*, **64**, 156–162.

48. Perera, P., Kurban, A.K., and Ryan, T.J. (1970) The development of the cutaneous microvascular system in the newborn. *Br. J. Dermatol.*, **82** (Suppl. 5), 86–91.

49. Mayer, K.M. (1921) Observations on the capillaries of the normal infant. *Am. J. Dis. Child.*, **22**, 381–387.

50. Ryan, T.J. (1966) The microcirculation of the skin in old age. *Gerontol. Clin.*, **8**, 327–337.

51. Ryan, T.J. (2004) The ageing of the blood supply and the lymphatic drainage of the skin. *Micron*, **35**, 161–171.

52. Kulka, J.P. (1966) Vascular derangement in rheumatoid arthritis, in *Modern Trends in Rheumatology* (ed. A.G.S. Hill), Butterworths, London.

53. Kuwabara, T. and Cogan, D.G. (1960) Studies of retinal patterns. *Arch. Ophthal.*, **64**, 904–911.

54. Ryan, T.J. and Copeman, P.W.M. (1969) Microvascular pattern and blood stasis in skin diseases. *Br. J. Dermatol.*, **81**, 563–573.

55. Hall, M. (1836) Article on hibernation, in *Todd's Cyclopaedia of Anatomy and Physiology*, vol. **II** (ed. R.B. Todd), Longman, London.

56. Paget, J. (1850) Lectures on Inflammation. *Lond. Med. Gaz.*, **45**, 965.

57. Jones, T.W. (1852) Discovery that the veins of the bats wing(which are furnished with valves)are endowed with rhythmical contractility and that outward flow of blood is accelerated by each contraction. *Philos. Trans. R. Soc. London, Ser. A*, **142**, 131, Part 1.

58. Nicoll, P.A. and Webb, R.L. (1946) Blood circulation in the subcutaneous tissue of the living bat's wing. *Ann. N. Y. Acad. Sci.*, **46**, 697.

59. Wiedeman, M.P. (1965) in *In Vivo Techniques in Histology* (ed. G.H. Bourne), Williams & Wilkins, London. pp. 137–148, 162–180.

60. Dintenfass, L. (1985) *Blood Vessels Hyperviscosity and Hypervisosaemia*, Kluwer, p. 172.

61. Maricq, H.R. (1986) Comparison of quantitative and semi-quantitative estimates of nailfold capillary abnormalities in scleroderma spectrum of disorders. *Microvasc. Res.*, **32**, 271.

62. Bosley, P.G.H.J. and Gibson, W.C. (1964) Photomicrographic studies on the nail bed capillary networks in patients who are mentally ill. *Bibl. Anat.*, **4**, 595–616.

63. Davis, E. and Landau, J. (1966) *Clinical Capillary Microscopy*, Charles C Thomas, Springfield, IL.

64. Ryan, T.J. (1969) The epidermis and its blood supply in venous disorders of the leg. *Trans. St. Johns Hosp. Derm. Soc. (London)*, **55**, 51–63.

65. Fagrell, B. and Bollinger, A. (1995) in *Clinically Applied Microcirculation Research*, Chapter 11 (eds J.J. Barker, G.L. Anderson, and M.D., Menger), CRC Press, Boca Raton, pp. 149–160.

66. Xiu, R.-J. (1993) Physiology in traditional medicine. Abstracts of the first Asian Congress for Microcirculation.

67. Intaglietta, M. and Messmer, K. (1995) in *Clinically Applied Microcirculation Research* (eds J.J. Barker, G.L. Anderson, and M.D. Menger), CRC Press, Boca Raton, pp. 139–148.

68. Tsuchiya, M. and Oda, M. (1987) Recent advances in organ microcirculation research. *Int. Angiol.*, **6**, 253.

69. Grayson, W. and Zingg, W. (1975) Fiendel, *Proceedings 1st World Congress of Microcirculation*, Plenum, New York.

70. Tsuchiya, M. *et al.* (eds) (1987) Wayland in Microcirculation, an Update: Proceedings of the Fourth World Congress for Microcirculation, Tokyo, Japan, July 26–30, 1987.

71. Thune, P., Ryan, T.J., Powell, S.M., and Ellis, J.P. (1976) The cutaneous reactions to kallikrein prostaglandin and thurfyl nicotinate in chronic urticaria and the effect of polyphoretin phosphate. *Acta Derm. Venereol.*, **56**, 217–221.

72. Turner, R.H., Kurban, A.K., and Ryan, T.J. (1969) Inhibition of fibrinolysis by human epidermis. *Nature*, **223**, 841–842.

73. Ryan, T.J., Nishioka, K., and Dawber, R.P.R. (1971) Epithelial-endothelial interactions in the control of inflammation through fibrinolysis. *Br. J. Dermatol.*, **84**, 501–515.

74. Chambers, D.R. and Monro, P.A.G. (1969) *Techniques Used in the Study of Microcirculation*, British Microcirculation Society.

75. Ryan, T.J., Jolles, B., and Holti, G. (1972) in *Methods in Microcirculation Studies* (ed. H.K. Lewis), British Microcirculation Society.

76. Barnhill, R.L. and Ryan, T.J. (1983) Biochemical modulation of angiogenesis in the chorioallantoic membrane of the chick embryo. *J. Invest. Dermatol.*, **81**, 485–488.

77. Holloway, G.A. and Watkins, D.W. (1977) Laser Doppler measurement of cutaneous blood flow. *J. Invest. Dermatol.*, **69**, 306–309.

78. Oberg, P.A., Tenland, T., and Nilsson, G.E. (1984) Laser- Doppler flowmetry – a non-invasive and continuous method for blood flow evaluation in microvascular studies. *Acta Med. Scand. Suppl.*, **687**, 17–24.

79. Tanner, R.M., Cherry, G.W., Hale, C., and Ryan, T.J. (1989) Impaired hyperaemic response in the microcirculation in patients with venous leg ulcers. *Br. J. Derm. (Suppl.)*, **121**, 45–46.

80. Watkins, D. and Holloway, G.A. (1978) An instrument to measure cutaneous blood flow using the Doppler shift of laser light. *IEEE Trans. Biomed. Eng.*, *BME*, **25**, 28–33.

81. Nilsson, G.E., Tenland, T., and Oberg, P.A. (1980) A new instrument for continuous measurement of tissue blood flow by light beating spectroscopy. *IEEE Trans.*, *BME*, **27**, 12–19.

82. Nilsson, G.E., Tenland, T., and Oberg, P.A. (1980) Evaluation of a laser Doppler flowmeter for measurement of tissue blood flow. *IEEE Trans.*, *BME*, **27**, 597–604.

83. Bonner, R. and Nossal, R. (1981) Model for laser Doppler measurements of blood flow in tissue. *Appl. Opt.*, **20**, 2097–2107.

84. Fischer, J.C., Parker, P.M., and Shaw, W.W. (1983) Comparison of two laser Doppler flowmeters for the monitoring of dermal blood flow. *Microsurgery*, **4**, 164–170.

85. Newson, T.P., Obeid, A.N., Wolton, R.S., Boggett, D., and Rolfe, P. (1987) Laser Doppler velocimetry: the problem of movement artefact. *J. Biomed. Eng.*, **9**, 169–172.

86. de Mul, F.F.M., van Spijker, J., van der Plas, D., Greve, J., Aarndoudse, J.G., and Smits, T.M. (1984) Mini laser Doppler (blood) flow monitor with diode laser source and detection integrated in the probe. *Appl. Opt.*, **23**, 2970–2973.

87. Doblhoff-Brown, D., Cherry, G.W., Kokko, T., Khoo, L., and Ryan, T.J. (1991) Abnormal postural vasconstriction in patients with venous insufficiency. *Int. J. Microcirc., Clin. Exp.*, **10**, 389 (abstract).

88. Svedman, C., Cherry, G.W., and Ryan, T.J. (1998) The veno-arteriolar reflex in venous leg ulcer patients studies

by laser Doppler imaging. *Acta Derm. Venereol. (Stockh)*, **78**, 258–261.

89. Stringini, L. and Ryan, T.J. (1996) in *Skin Ageing and Photoageing*, vol. **14** (ed. A. Ledo), Elsevier, pp. 197–206.

90. Hill, S.A., Pigott, K.H., Saunders, M.I., Powell, M.E.B., Arnold, S., Obeid, A., Ward, G., Leahy, M., Hoskin, P.J., and Chaplin, D.J. (1996) Microregional blood flow in murine and human tumours assessed using laser Doppler microprobes. *Br. J. Cancer*, **74**, 260–263.

91. Wardell, K., Braverman, I.M., Silverman, D.G., and Nilsson, G.E. (1993) Spatial heterogeneity in normal skin perfusion recorded with laser doppler imaging and flowmetry. *Microvasc. Res.*, **48**, 26–38.

92. Leahy, M.J., de Mul, F.F.M., Nilsson, G.E., and Maniewski, R. (1999) Principles and practice of the laser Doppler perfusion technique. *Eur. Soc. Eng. Med. Technol. Health Care*, **7**, 143–162.

93. Rossi, M., Carpi, A., Galetta, F., Franzoni, F., and Santoro, G. (2008) Skin vasomotion investigation: a useful tool for clinical evaluation of microvascular endothelial function? *Biomed. Pharmacother.*, **62**, 541–545.

94. O'Doherty, J., McNamara, P., Clancy, N.T., Enfield, J.G., and Leahy, M.J. (2009) Comparison of instruments for investigation of microcirculatory blood flow and red blood cell concentration. *J. Biomed. Opt.*, **14** (3).

95. Briers, J.D. (1996) Laser Doppler and time-varying speckle: a reconciliation. *J. Opt. Soc. Am. A*, **13**, 345–350.

96. Nakajima, S., Hirai, Y., Takase, H., Kuse, A., Aoyagi, T., Kishi, M., and Yamaguchi, K. (1975) Performances of new pulse wave earpiece oximeter. *Resp. Circ.*, **23**, 41–45.

97. Zander, R. (1991) in *The Oxygen Status of Arterial Human Blood* (eds R. Zander and F. Mertzlufft), Karger, Basel, pp. 1–13.

98. Kelleher, J.F. (1989) Pulse oximetry. *J. Clin. Monit.*, **5**, 37–62.

99. Moyle, J.T.B. (1994) in *Pulse Oximetry* (eds C.E.W. Hahn and A.P. Adams), BMJ Publishing Group, London.

100. Hu, D., Phan, T.T., Cherry, G.W., and Ryan, T.J. (1998) Dermal oedema assessed by high frequency ultrasound in venous leg ulcers. *Br. J. Dermatol.*, **138**, 815–820.

101. Essex, T.J.H. and Byrne, P.O. (1991) A laser Doppler scanner for imaging blood flow in skin. *J. Biomed. Eng.*, **13**, 189–194.

102. Nilsson, G.E., Jakobsson, A., and Wårdell, K. (1989) Imaging of tissue blood flow by coherent light scattering. Proceedings of the IEEE 11th Annual EMBS Conference, Seattle, November 9–12.

103. Monstrey, S., Hoeksema, H., Verbelen, J., Pirayesh, A., and Blondeel, P. (2008) Assessment of burn depth and burn wound healing potential. *Burns*, **34**, 761–769.

104. Boas, D.A. and Dunn, A.K. (2010) Laser speckle contrast imaging in biomedical optics. *J. Biomed. Opt.*, **15** (1), 011109.

105. Yuan, S., Devor, A., Boas, D.A., and Dunn, A.K. (2005) Determination of optimal exposure time for imaging of blood flow changes with laser speckle contrast imaging. *Appl. Opt.*, **44** (10), 1823–1830.

106. Briers, J.D. and Fercher, A.F. (1982) Retinal blood-flow visualization by means of laser speckle photography. *Invest. Ophthalmol. Vis. Sci.*, **22** (2), 255–259.

107. Briers, J.D. and Webster, S. (1996) Laser speckle contrast analysis (LASCA): a nonscanning, full-field technique for monitoring capillary blood flow. *J. Biomed. Opt.*, **1**, 174–179.

108. O'Doherty, J., Nilsson, G.E., Henricson, J., Sjöberg, F., and Leahy, M.J. (2007) Sub-epidermal imaging by polarised light rejection for assessment of microvascular patency. *Skin Res. Technol.*, **13** (4), 472–484.

109. Wang, X. *et al.* (2003) Non-invasive laser-induced photoacoustic tomography for structural and functional imaging of the brain in vivo. *Nat. Biotechnol.*, **21** (7), 803–806.

110. Galanzha, E.I., Shashkov, E.V., Kelly, T., Kim, J.-W., Yang, L., and Zharov, V.P. (2009) In vivo magnetic enrichment and multiplex photoacoustic detection of circulating tumour cells. *Nat. Nanotechnol.*, **4** (12), 855–860.

111. Razansky, D., Buehler, A., and Ntziachristos, V. (2011) Volumetric real-time multispectral optoacoustic tomography of biomarkers. *Nat. Protoc.*, **6** (8), 1121–1129.

112. Enfield, J., Jonathan, E., and Leahy, M.J. (2011) In vivo imaging of the microcirculation of the volar forearm using correlation mapping optical coherence tomography (OCT). *Biomed. Opt. Express*, **2** (5), 1184–1193.

2
Sidestream Dark-Field (SDF) Video Microscopy for Clinical Imaging of the Microcirculation

Dan M. J. Milstein, Rick Bezemer, and Can Ince

2.1
Introduction

As part of the circulatory system, the microcirculation (i.e., blood vessels <100 μm in diameter) is the site where hormones, gases (such as O_2 and CO_2), nutrients, water, and waste products are exchanged between the blood and tissue cells. Microcirculation consists of an intertwined network of arterioles, capillaries, postcapillary venules, and short vascular segments known as *arteriovenous shunts*. The maintenance of proper microcirculatory perfusion is attributed to the arterioles, which regulate vascular resistance and in so doing, regulate capillary blood flow. Endothelial cells lining the vascular lumen are sensitive to hemodynamic changes and can perceive changes in vascular transmural pressure, shear stress, and pO_2 [1–3]. Adjustments in vascular tone are attributed to endothelial cells signaling circular smooth muscle cells, which alternately contract and relax depending on the metabolic needs of a particular tissue. Smooth muscle cell contractions increase blood pressure and vascular resistance and redistribute arteriolar and capillary blood flow; thus, microvascular resistance is determined by factors affecting either vascular (e.g., angioarchitecture, diameter, length) or rheological (e.g., hematocrit, viscosity, and wall shear stress) parameters. The exchange of blood constituents occurs principally through discontinuities or pores along the capillary wall (endothelial) junctions. Capillary networks and microvascular attributes in each organ system are directly related to the functional role performed by an organ as a whole. To this end, the amount of functional capillaries may be related to the metabolic or functional requirements of an organ or tissue compartment.

In 1661, Marcello Malpighi (1628–1694) used a microscope to investigate a frog lung and discovered for the first time, long, thin-walled tubes linking arteries and veins, which he termed *capillaries*. The discovery of capillaries and their surrounding arteriolar and venular components marks the start of early microcirculation investigation. Microscopes have since then evolved from a simple single-lens apparatus into elaborate complex instruments, enabling detailed observations of the microcirculation with flowing red blood cells (RBCs). The first reports on intravital microscopy (IVM) for the study of tissue microcirculation and cellular interactions

Microcirculation Imaging, First Edition. Edited by Martin J. Leahy.
© 2012 Wiley-VCH Verlag GmbH & Co. KGaA. Published 2012 by Wiley-VCH Verlag GmbH & Co. KGaA.

date back to 1839 [4]. Intravital microcirculation research has traditionally been done using tissue transillumination techniques, often requiring fluorescent contrast agents, with invasive tissue sample preparations for *in vivo* observations. In 1971, Sherman *et al.* [5] reported for the first time a new method employing an incident dark-field illumination technique for IVM, which improved the *in vivo* study of solid organ subsurface microcirculation. They described the technique as capable of providing depth in the imaging field with a three-dimensional quality in the observed sample of interest. Although incident dark-field illumination has improved the imaging of tissue microvascular networks, a substantially large amount of tissue surface reflections have still accounted for weaknesses in the technique. With the introduction of a versatile incident illuminator in combination with a polarizer and analyzer, Slaaf *et al.* [6] have eliminated a substantial amount of tissue surface reflection, improving the image quality of the technique. Microcirculation images generated using this approach resulted in intraluminal RBCs appearing as dark circulating structures flowing on a light background. An important development that led to the clinical applicability of the techniques described by Sherman *et al.* [5] and Slaaf *et al.* [6] was the implementation of these optical modalities into handheld microscopy instruments. This clinically applicable, portable, handheld imaging system overcame the remaining technical impracticalities of IVM (i.e., the need for contrast enhancement agents and the bulky setup) and became known as orthogonal polarization spectral (OPS) imaging [7]. Figure 2.1 illustrates schematic diagrams of both the OPS and dark-field imaging techniques.

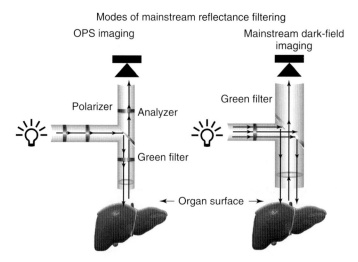

Figure 2.1 OPS imaging and mainstream dark-field imaging as used in combination in the clinical OPS devices. (Cytoscan® by Cytometrics.)

OPS imaging has enabled first-time observations and investigations on exposed organ and tissue surface microcirculation in clinical research at the patient's bedside. Since the introduction of OPS imaging, numerous clinical studies have been undertaken on various organ and tissue compartments, brain [8, 9], conjunctiva [10], oral cavity (i.e., gingiva and sublingual mucosa) [11–17], intestines [18–20], liver [21], nail fold [22], pancreas [23, 24], rectum [25, 26], skin [27–31], and vaginal mucosa [32], directed at elucidating the clinical significance of the role of microcirculation in both health and disease. An important clinical breakthrough, using OPS imaging, was realized when sublingual microcirculation during sepsis, septic shock, and resuscitation revealed altered microcirculation perfusion and hemodynamic properties at the patient bedside, providing more sensitive information about patient outcome than conventional clinical parameters such as systemic hemodynamics and oxygen-derived variables [13, 15, 33, 34]. Additional applications of OPS imaging include clinical investigations on microcirculatory dysfunction in severe malaria [35], the progress of wound healing [36, 37], the effects of blood transfusion [38], and the microcirculatory characteristics of oral squamous cell carcinoma [39].

OPS imaging operates by epi-illuminating the tissue, embedding the microcirculation with polarized green light [7, 40]. Backscattered, depolarized light is projected onto a charge-coupled device (CCD) camera after it passes an analyzer (i.e., a polarizer orthogonally oriented with respect to the incident polarization). The light reflected by the tissue surface, which is not depolarized, is blocked by this analyzer. By eliminating reflected light and imaging only backscattered light, subsurface structures, such as microcirculation, can be observed. The use of green light (548 nm wavelength) ensures sufficient optical absorption by the (de)oxyhemoglobin-containing RBCs as opposed to lack of absorption by the tissue embedding the microcirculation, hence creating contrast (i.e., RBCs are visualized as dark circulating structures on a light background). Although incorporated into the OPS imaging system, it is not a commonly known fact that a dark-field imaging modality is used in these instruments, which is primarily responsible for the image quality of the OPS imaging device (commercialized by Cytometrics under the name of Cytoscan®). Despite major contributions to the field of intravital microcirculation imaging, OPS still harbors several shortcomings such as suboptimal capillary imaging due to motion-induced image blurring and the need for an external high-power light source.

Driven by the success of OPS imaging, a novel imaging system, called sidestream dark-field (SDF) imaging, was developed with the aim of improving microcirculation image quality and eliminating the need of an external light source for illumination. Much in the same way that OPS operates, SDF imaging employs a central light guide equipped with concentrically placed light-emitting diodes (LEDs) to provide SDF illumination (Figure 2.2). The lens system in the core of the light guide is optically isolated from the illuminating outer ring, preventing microcirculation images from contamination by tissue surface reflections. Light from the illuminating outer core of the SDF probe, penetrates the tissue of interest and illuminates the tissue-embedded microcirculation by scattering. The LEDs

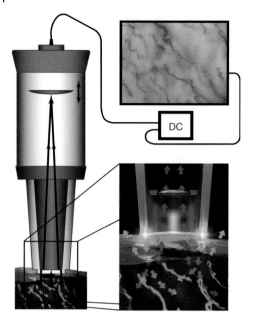

Figure 2.2 The working principles of sidestream dark-field (SDF) imaging.

emit green light with a wavelength of 530 nm, which was chosen to correspond to an isosbestic point in the absorption spectra of (de)oxyhemoglobin (i.e., at $\lambda = 530$ nm, $\mu_{a,\text{deoxyHb}} = \mu_{a,\text{oxyHb}} = 205\,\text{cm}^{-1}$) to ensure optimal optical absorption by hemoglobin (Hb) in circulating RBCs independent of the Hb oxygenation state. The imaging output on a monitor portrays RBCs flowing as dark moving globules against a white/grayish background. Imaging optimization correcting for motion-induced hemodynamic blurring (i.e., flowing RBCs) has been resolved by synchronizing the LED light pulse illumination with the CCD camera frame rate, resulting in intravital stroboscopy using short illumination intervals (13 ms). SDF imaging has the benefit of low-power LED illumination. This enables battery and (portable) computer operation for ambulatory and on-site (emergency) applications, where high mobility is of great importance.

2.2
Quantifying the Functional State of the Microcirculation

The nutritive perfusion of an organ or tissue is dependent on the number and anatomical distribution of the capillaries and the blood flow within these conduits. There are two main parameters that describe the ability of the microcirculation to transport oxygen to the tissues by the Hb-carrying RBCs: functional capillary density (FCD) and microcirculatory flow. The density of perfused vessels identifies the proximity of functional capillaries to the tissue parenchymal cells (e.g., facilitating better diffusion of oxygen) and the flow in the vessels identifies the convection of oxygen in the microcirculation. A parameter universally evaluated to quantify the quality of tissue perfusion is FCD. *FCD is defined as the total length of RBC-perfused capillaries per observation area* and is usually performed using a computer-assisted video analysis software package. Microcirculation research has demonstrated the impact of disease (sepsis, heart failure, and cardiogenic shock) and interventions (various surgical procedures, blood transfusion, and pharmacotherapeutic) in influencing alterations in tissue FCD. Although computer-assisted quantification of blood vessel length is required to calculate FCD in tissues with irregular microvascular patterns (e.g., sublingual microcirculation), in other tissues (e.g., gingival, labial, and buccal mucosa) consisting of regular microvascular patterns, FCD can be calculated as the number of repetitive structures (i.e., hairpin-shaped capillary loops) per observation area; thus simplifying quantification of FCD without the aid of specialized software. De Backer and coworkers [13] introduced a semiquantitative method of measuring FCD from OPS images by looking specifically at microcirculatory alterations in septic patients. Their scoring method is based on the principle that the density of the vessels is proportional to the total number of vessels crossing arbitrary lines. By drawing a grid with three equidistant horizontal and vertical lines and superimposing it onto a screen portraying the video images of sublingual microcirculation, vessel density by volume was calculated as the number of vessels crossing the lines divided by the total length of the grid lines. Once the total number of crossing vessels has been determined, perfusion can be evaluated by the eye as being present (flow), absent (no flow), or intermittent (i.e., no flow at least 50% of the time). Using vessel density and flow characteristics, the proportion of perfused vessels (PPV (%)) can be calculated using the following formula: 100 × (total number of vessels − (no flow + intermittent flow))/total number of vessels. Finally, an estimate of FCD, defined as perfused vessel density (PVD), can be calculated by multiplying the vessel density by the PPV.

Microcirculation flow and flow patterns have been measured by a semiquantitative scoring method known as the microvascular flow index (MFI). MFI scoring essentially relies on determining the overall predominant flow type in microcirculation images. On the basis of blood flow characteristics of the microcirculation observed in the tissue of interest, a classification system using numerical coding was developed: 0, no flow; 1, intermittent flow; 2, sluggish flow; and 3, continuous flow. To determine the MFI, microcirculatory images are divided into four quadrants and blood flow assessments are categorized on the basis of vessel diameters into small (10–25 μm), medium (26–50 μm), and large (51–100 μm) microvessels. Subsequently, the flow properties of each vessel type are averaged to represent information about each vessel in the microcirculatory images. In a validation study by Boerma *et al.* [41], a good intrarater and interrater reproducibility for MFI scoring in both sublingual and stomal (i.e., gut villi in ileostomy and crypts in colostomy) microcirculation was reported in patients with abdominal sepsis. A more quantifiable method for determining capillary RBC flow dynamics was introduced by Ellis *et al.* [42]. Their method of assessing RBC flow dynamics consisted of an image

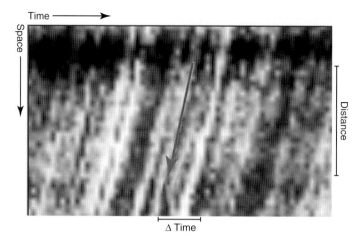

Figure 2.3 An original space–time diagram used for determining microvascular red blood cell velocities. The red arrow traces a dark band representing the instantaneous velocity of a single RBC.

analysis approach using space–time diagrams to quantify convective parameters. In space–time images (Figure 2.3), the temporal and spatial heterogeneities of RBC velocity and cell column densities can be evaluated. In these graphs plotting distance (*y*-axis) against time (*x*-axis), the kinetics of flowing RBCs is represented by dark diagonal bands separated by light diagonal bands coinciding with plasma gaps. Although this technique can provide a more detailed and quantifiable way of determining RBC velocities in individual capillaries, it requires time-consuming manual techniques for analysis. Recently, this method has been integrated into an automated analysis program and is discussed in more detail later.

2.3
Microcirculatory Image Acquisition

2.3.1
SDF Instrument

The SDF imaging instrument is housed in a small cylindrical body with the objective lens probe projecting outward from one end of the cylindrical encasement (Figure 2.4). The SDF probe is fitted with a 5× objective lens system, as is the OPS device. The SDF power pack has a video connector output, which in turn can be directly connected to a computer screen or television monitor. The SDF focusing mechanism functions by adjusting a large dial situated at the opposite end of the cylindrical encasement. The mechanism operates by axial translation of the CCD chip with respect to the fixed lens system at the tip of the SDF probe. Before applying the SDF probe to the surface of the tissue of interest,

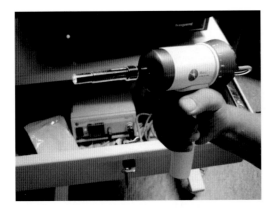

Figure 2.4 Photograph of the SDF imaging device
illustrating the cylindrical encasement and the objective lens
probe covered with a sterile disposable cap.

a protective sterile disposable cap is securely attached around the probe. Once
the probe has been positioned exactly perpendicular on the tissue surface,
alterations in microcirculation perfusion must be avoided by eliminating
pressure-induced artifacts; this is achieved by gently pulling the probe back until
contact is lost and then slowly advancing to the point at which contact is regained
with the microcirculation in proper focus [43].

In a validation study comparing SDF and OPS imaging [44], both nail fold
and sublingual microcirculatory areas were imaged from the same locations
and compared. Moreover, imaging quality was also determined by employing a
specially developed image quality quantification system based on blood vessel
contrast with respect to the surrounding tissue by evaluating cross-sectional
grayscale histograms. Nail fold capillary diameters and RBC velocities yielded equal
quantitative results when measured by both techniques. Sublingual venular image
quality also showed comparable results between the two techniques. However,
capillary imaging quality and contrast was significantly better using the SDF
technique (Figure 2.5). Moreover, SDF images also depicted increased resolvability
in the granularity of flowing RBC columns in venules in comparison to OPS
images. The results of the validation study confirm the validity of SDF imaging for
the assessment of microcirculation geometry and intravascular blood flow kinetics.

Several image acquisition key points have been identified to achieve improved
image acquisition [43], including imaging of at least five sites per organ or tissue
region, avoidance of pressure-induced artifacts, elimination of secretions (such as
excess saliva), proper focus and contrast adjustments, and optimal recording quality.
The intrinsic heterogeneity or variability of the microcirculation dictates that at
least five adjacent sites should be imaged to accurately quantify the microcirculation
in a region of interest. However, when analyzing the images, some clips may be
unsuitable for analysis and should be discarded. It was concluded that at least three
image sites could produce reliable quantification, although if possible, five sites
should be obtained for evaluation. Capillaries and venules may be very sensitive

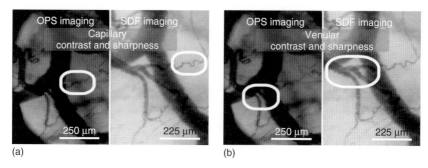

Figure 2.5 Comparison of the same sublingual microcirculation location using OPS imaging and SDF imaging. Panels (a) and (b) illustrate the improved imaging quality of the microvasculature using the SDF technique when compared with that using OPS. (Reprinted from Goedhart *et al.* [44] with permission.)

to pressure applied by the probe and can result in collapsed microvasculature; by gently retracting and advancing the imaging probe on the tissue surface, these artifacts can be avoided [45, 46]. Furthermore, reduction of excess secretions or extravasated blood is recommended and can be performed by gentle cleaning of the lens surface or the area of interest.

In combination with the above-mentioned recommendations for proper image acquisitions, several technical issues should be addressed. Images should be captured and stored as DV-AVI files, which can enable the investigator to perform frame-by-frame image analysis if necessary. Accordingly, it is recommended to record at least 20 s per image site.

2.4
Automated Microcirculation Image Analysis

The analysis of microcirculation video recordings can be lengthy, and for reasons of practicality, a specially designed automated vascular analysis (AVA) software package was developed [47]. Once acquired and digitized, microcirculation images must be (semi)quantified to evaluate (alterations in) the functionality of the microcirculation to distinguish between health and disease and to assess the effects of therapeutic interventions. As mentioned previously, several scoring systems have been developed for measurement and calculation of microcirculatory functionality determinants, such as capillary density and perfusion. To objectify microvascular image analysis while minimizing user input, specialized software packages have been developed. CapImage was, for a long time, the only commercially available software program for the analysis of microcirculation images. CapImage provided a quantitative method for the estimation of blood vessel diameter, length, and RBC velocity [42]; yet, vessel segment selection and vessel geometry determination were done manually by superimposed line drawing on vessels, requiring a large degree of user interaction, which was very time consuming and increased observer bias significantly. In a validation study comparing a new analysis software, CapiScope, with CapImage, comparable results for vessel geometry and RBC velocities were obtained [48]. Although both these software programs enabled semiautomated analysis of microcirculatory blood flow from consecutive images, the analysis was restricted to straight vessel segments.

More recently, Dobbe *et al.* developed a novel software package for microcirculation analysis, known as *automated vascular analysis* [47]. This software automatically determines vessel center lines in both straight and curved vessel segments (a process known as *skeletonization*), in order to measure vessel geometry and RBC velocities. The first step in microcirculatory analysis procedure is image sequence stabilization, performed using 2D cross-correlation. In the next step, by time-averaging an image sequence, interruptions in capillary blood flow (e.g., plasma gaps and/or leukocytes) are filled in, which enhances capillary geometry detection. Blood vessel center lines are subsequently determined automatically by a method previously described by Steger [49]. The technique detects each center line pixel in blood vessels as the point at which the steepness in the grayscale intensity profile normal to the center line is maximal. After vessel wall detection and skeletonization, the software automatically cuts vessels at bifurcations for determination of RBC velocities in separate vessel segments. The investigator is allowed to interact with the above-mentioned segmentation process by cutting, deleting, or connecting vessel segments. The novel RBC velocity determination technique, implemented by Dobbe *et al.*, maps the randomly distributed vessel center line pixels onto the equidistant intervals of the space–time diagram using linear interpolation [47]. RBC velocity can then be determined by automatic detection or manual detection of the slope of the line structure in the space–time diagram [42]. Using this new programed algorithm, the software is able to automatically estimate the orientation and velocity of RBC flow.

The AVA software was validated using video simulations of microvessels with known diameters and RBC velocities [47]. The simulation movie was also analyzed with CapiScope using default factory settings, as recommended by the software manufacture. In addition, to illustrate clinical utility, sublingual SDF recordings were acquired from a healthy volunteer and from a patient intraoperatively during cardiac luxation (i.e., a procedure used during heart surgery involving lifting and repositioning of the heart, which results in a direct decrease in cardiac output) while undergoing open-heart surgery. The results demonstrated a close agreement between the two software packages for vessel diameters and lengths. However, using AVA, vessel density measurements (i.e., total vessel length (μm)/field of view (μm^2)) were performed in 67% of the time needed using CapiScope. Moreover, determination of vessel diameter distribution took ~4 h with CapiScope versus 10 min using AVA. RBC velocity analysis using AVA was done manually and was very accurate (i.e., with a standard deviation of 4% in the range of 2.5–1000 μm s^{-1}); assessment of blood velocity in all vessels within the recording was performed in ~10% of the time required using CapiScope. Automated velocity assessment with AVA in simulated blood vessels was 95% accurate for velocities of up to

$750\,\mu\mathrm{m\,s^{-1}}$. Validation and comparison of the two software has also shown that CapiScope was unable to measure velocities below $50\,\mathrm{pixels\,s^{-1}}$ ($<35\,\mu\mathrm{m\,s^{-1}}$) and produced relatively large errors for higher velocities [47].

Dobbe *et al.* [47] have initiated the first step toward automated RBC velocity assessment in curved vessels. Compared to CapiScope, AVA increases accuracy and reduces user interaction and analysis time radically. However, visual inspection of the results of microcirculation images superimposed onto each other and their possible interactions during selected phases in the analysis remains necessary. It is important to realize when analyzing microcirculatory images that software-mediated image stabilization implies a minor reduction in image size and, thus, in microvascular geometry and RBC kinetics. Furthermore, different video display standards (e.g., NTSC and PAL) use dimensions that may affect the presentation of the microcirculatory image on a screen. Future OPS and SDF research should be aimed at improving image quality, enhancing video frame rate and resolution, and reducing illumination intervals (i.e., $<13\,\mathrm{ms}$), to improve software-based microcirculatory image analysis of vessel geometry and RBC velocity.

2.5
International Consensus on Microcirculation Image Acquisition and Analysis

As stated in Section 2.1, microcirculatory alterations may play an important role in the development of (multiple) organ failure in critically ill patients, especially in severe sepsis and septic shock. The rapid development of image acquisition technology and systematic (semi)quantitative analytical scoring methods has led to great variations in image acquisition and analysis among medical research centers investigating the microcirculation. These variations in analytical results, in conjunction with the analysis-mediated conclusions on microcirculation function, have led to the organization of a round table conference in November 2007, aiming to achieve a consensus on microcirculatory image acquisition and analysis to standardize the clinical assessment of the microcirculation.

In the consensus report [43], it was concluded that, due to the heterogeneous nature of the microcirculation, ideally, five sites of an organ must be imaged and analyzed to draw reliable conclusions on microcirculation functionality. The recommended optical magnification for human sublingual microcirculation is $5\times$, given that the heterogeneity of the microcirculation cannot be taken into account when using higher magnification. An important aspect of microcirculatory image acquisition, which applies for both OPS and SDF imaging, is prevention of pressure-induced artifacts. Pressure on the microvasculature can alter perfusion and thereby result in unreliable analysis and conclusions about the microcirculation. During the consensus meeting, it was concluded that venular flow should always be continuous rather than stopped or intermittent and that (patho)physiologically induced microcirculatory alterations occur mainly at the capillary level. Thus, it was determined that venular perfusion was a good indicator for the presence of pressure artifacts. Trzeciak *et al.* [45] recently proposed a standard operating procedure for microcirculation image acquisition, serving as a guide for prevention of pressure-induced artifacts. Briefly, the imaging probe should be advanced to the microvasculature until flow is partially obstructed. Then, the probe should be carefully withdrawn until contact with the tissue of interest is lost. Finally, the probe should be advanced once again to the point at which contact with the tissue of interest is regained. By recording continuously during this procedure, adequate images for analysis can be included and extracted from the digital videotape segment obtained from the tissue of interest.

In oral medicine, this technique is particularly important since the capillaries in the gingiva are highly prone to rapid vascular collapse when positioning the imaging probe for measurements. As a consequence, since the SDF device relies on Hb in circulating RBCs for contrast imaging, no microcirculation can be observed. In a recent study by Milstein *et al.* [46], the assessment of cytostatic-based polychemotherapy on rabbit maxillary gingival perfusion was performed with the SDF imaging device mounted on a micromanipulator. Using a setup with a micromanipulator easily enabled fine control of probe positioning and the acquisition of stable microcirculation images on the gingival mucosa without obstructing gingival microvascular perfusion.

When analyzing SDF images, one should first identify the capillary microvessels, which are vessels with a diameter ≤ 25 µm. Geometrical and perfusion analysis will mainly be performed on these conduits, since they are the primary determinants of tissue perfusion. In the round table consensus meeting [43], three parameters were agreed upon, which comprehensively describe microcirculatory alterations as seen in sepsis: (i) PVD [13], representing an estimate of the FCD; (ii) MFI [41], providing information about the mean flow properties present; and (iii) the perfusion heterogeneity [45], derived from the MFI calculation as a crucial parameter for identifying the oxygen extracting capabilities of the tissue embedding the microcirculation.

PVD provides an accurate estimate of microcirculatory FCD. The advantage of the PVD score is that it accounts for most variables involved in tissue perfusion, including vascular density and PPV. A disadvantage, however, is that RBC velocities cannot be accounted for in continuously perfused capillaries. MFI scoring is relatively simple to perform; however, the score does not provide any information on the FCD and is discontinuous. A change from 1 to 0 might have different implications than say a change from 2 to 1; this complicates the interpretation of the MFI score. The consensus is that all index parameters (PVD, PPV, and MFI) should be measured to comprehensively describe the functional state of the microcirculation. In addition, to distinguish between perfused and nonperfused microvessels, the MFI score, provided that flow is homogeneously distributed within the imaged video segment, can differentiate between flow types, hence providing more detailed information on perfusion dynamics. Although PPV does not distinguish between flow types, it does provide information on flow heterogeneity within the imaged microvasculature. Trzeciak *et al.* [45] investigated early sublingual microcirculatory perfusion derangements in patients with severe sepsis and septic shock. They semiquantified the MFI in five imaged sites and calculated a flow heterogeneity index (HetIndex), defined as the highest site flow velocity minus the lowest site flow velocity, divided by the mean flow velocity across all five sublingual sites. Patients with sepsis had more heterogeneous blood flow when compared to their control group. The results of this study showed that nonsurviving patients had a more heterogeneous flow distribution than surviving patients. Hence, flow velocity, capillary density, and flow heterogeneity could independently contribute to the risk of organ dysfunction in sepsis.

In summary, scoring should include a vascular density index (PVD and PPV), a capillary perfusion index (MFI), and a HetIndex to describe tissue perfusion dynamics. It is important to emphasize, however, that these scoring systems have been developed and validated for identifying and quantifying microcirculatory networks as they pertain to human sublingual microcirculation during sepsis and septic shock scenarios. For scoring microcirculatory alterations during other disease states, although applicable, it is recommended that each parameter be validated first for each particular condition.

2.6
Future Prospects

In the future, technological improvements in microcirculatory imaging will be realized with the incorporation of more advanced camera technology with improvements in image resolution and video frame rates. This will enable RBC velocity measurements in high flow vessels (e.g., $>1000 \, \mu m \, s^{-1}$) with more accurate vessel geometry determination. Technological modifications in conjunction with fully automated analytical software with advanced built-in microcirculatory scoring systems will lead to rapid and more exact determination of microcirculatory functionality in both clinical and experimental settings. To this end, future research should also be dedicated to the precise role of vessel diameter and RBC velocity as they relate to oxygen delivery to tissue parenchymal cells. Efforts have already been made to assess microcirculation MFI in critically ill patients on-site (patient bedside) in a (near) real-time point-of-care (POC) setting [50]. The results from that study indicated a good correlation between bedside-derived POC MFI scores and conventional offline analysis. However, on-site microcirculatory measurements of vessel length, diameter, and RBC velocity would be more difficult to realize, since images must be stabilized and time averaged to obtain the desired parameters. Another point of concern for OPS and SDF imaging is to eliminate pressure artifacts related to application of the SDF probe onto organ and tissue surfaces [40, 45]. Lindert *et al.* [40] has engineered a suction device that can be placed around an OPS probe. Suction applied via small perforations in the device prevented the OPS probe from applying pressure onto the tissue and subsequently reduced movement during microcirculatory image acquisition. Recently, a similar suction device, the image acquisition stabilizer (IAS), was developed and clinically validated for SDF imaging [51]. The IAS can be directly attached around the tip of the SDF probe disposable plastic cap. Using the IAS increased the yield of analyzable microcirculatory images by reducing both image drifting and the force necessary to prevent pressure artifacts, resulting in prolonged stable image recordings. Moreover, the results also showed that there was no significant difference in blood flow in small, medium, or large blood vessels in comparison to data acquisitions without the IAS.

Another clinically favorable feature enhancing intravital microvascular research would be a microcirculatory oxygenation imaging modality directly implemented into a handheld device. Such an imaging modality would provide images of the microcirculation, in which oxygenation in each pixel is expressed in false colors (e.g., blue to red representing 0–100% blood oxygenation) [52]. This technique could allow on-site assessment of microcirculatory tissue oxygenation, which would be of use especially in emergency medicine, where quick assessment of microcirculatory functionality is desired.

2.7
Conclusion

Microcirculatory image acquisition and analysis has advanced considerably since the discovery of the capillary in the late seventeenth century. The introduction of intravital SDF imaging and the new AVA software has significantly improved microcirculation assessment, bringing the clinician ever closer to real-time diagnostics at the microvascular level. The consensus on microcirculatory image acquisition and analysis has furthermore standardized OPS and SDF protocols to enable the comparison of microcirculatory alterations among different studies. With technological advancements, conclusions based on the analysis of the microcirculation have eased the transition from bench to bedside, enabling the clinician to rapidly distinguish between health and disease and to evaluate the impact of therapeutic interventions at the bedside.

References

1. Davies, P.F. (1995) Flow-mediated endothelial mechanotransduction. *Physiol. Rev.*, **75**, 519–560.

2. Bevan, J.A. and Laher, I. (1991) Pressure and flow-dependent vascular tone. *FASEB J.*, **5**, 2267–2273.

3. Paternotte, E., Gaucher, C., Labrude, P., Stoltz, J.F., and Menu, P. (2008) Review: behaviour of endothelial cells faced with hypoxia. *Biomed. Mater. Eng.*, **18**, 295–299.

4. Wagner, R. (1839) *Erläuterungstafeln zur Physiologie und Entwicklungsgeschichte*, Leopold Voss, Leipzig.

5. Sherman, H., Klausner, S., and Cook, W.A. (1971) Incident dark-field illumination: a new method for microcirculatory study. *Angiology*, **22**, 295–303.

6. Slaaf, D.W., Tangelder, G.J., Reneman, R.S., Jager, K., and Bollinger, A. (1987) A versatile incident illuminator for intravital microscopy. *Int. J. Microcirc. Clin. Exp.*, **6**, 391–397.

7. Groner, W., Winkelman, J.W., Harris, A.G. *et al.* (1999) Orthogonal polarization spectral imaging: a new method for study of the microcirculation. *Nat. Med.*, **5**, 1209–1212.

8. Mathura, K.R., Bouma, G.J., and Ince, C. (2001) Abnormal microcirculation in brain tumours during surgery. *Lancet*, **358**, 1698–1699.

9. Pennings, F.A., Bouma, G.J., and Ince, C. (2004) Direct observation of the human cerebral microcirculation during aneurysm surgery reveals increased arteriolar contractility. *Stroke*, **35**, 1284–1288.

10. Schaser, K.D., Settmacher, U., Puhl, G. et al. (2003) Noninvasive analysis of conjunctival microcirculation during carotid artery surgery reveals microvascular evidence of collateral compensation and stenosis-dependent adaptation. *J. Vasc. Surg.*, **37**, 789–797.

11. Lindeboom, J.A., Mathura, K.R., Harkisoen, S., van den Akker, H.P., and Ince, C. (2005) Effect of smoking on the gingival capillary density: assessment of gingival capillary density with orthogonal polarization spectral imaging. *J. Clin. Periodontol.*, **32**, 1208–1212.

12. Lindeboom, J.A., Mathura, K.R., Ramsoekh, D. et al. (2006) The assessment of the gingival capillary density with orthogonal spectral polarization (OPS) imaging. *Arch. Oral Biol.*, **51**, 697–702.

13. De Backer, D., Creteur, J., Preiser, J.C., Dubois, M.J., and Vincent, J.L. (2002) Microvascular blood flow is altered in patients with sepsis. *Am. J. Respir. Crit. Care Med.*, **166**, 98–104.

14. De Backer, D., Creteur, J., Dubois, M.J., Sakr, Y., and Vincent, J.L. (2004) Microvascular alterations in patients with acute severe heart failure and cardiogenic shock. *Am. Heart J.*, **147**, 91–99.

15. Sakr, Y., Dubois, M.J., De Backer, D., Creteur, J., and Vincent, J.L. (2004) Persistent microcirculatory alterations are associated with organ failure and death in patients with septic shock. *Crit. Care Med.*, **32**, 1825–1831.

16. Dubois, M.J., De Backer, D., Creteur, J., Anane, S., and Vincent, J.L. (2003) Effect of vasopressin on sublingual microcirculation in a patient with distributive shock. *Intensive Care Med.*, **29**, 1020–1023.

17. Erol-Yilmaz, A., Atasever, B., Mathura, K. et al. (2007) Cardiac resynchronization improves microcirculation. *J. Card. Fail.*, **13**, 95–99.

18. Siegemund, M., Stegenga, M.E., Mathura, K. et al. (1999) Changes in the porcine microcirculation of the ileum after supra-mesenteric aortic cross-clamping. *Intensive Care Med.*, **25** (Suppl. 1), S10 (abstract).

19. Tugtekin, I.F., Radermacher, P., Theisen, M. et al. (2001) Increased ileal-mucosal-arterial PCO2 gap is associated with impaired villus microcirculation in endotoxic pigs. *Intensive Care Med.*, **27**, 757–766.

20. Boerma, E.C., van der Voort, V., Spronk, P.E., and Ince, C. (2007) Relationship between sublingual and intestinal microcirculatory perfusion in patients with abdominal sepsis. *Crit. Care Med.*, **35**, 1055–1060.

21. Langer, S., Harris, A.G., Biberthaler, P., von Dobschuetz, E., and Messmer, K. (2001) Orthogonal polarization spectral imaging as a tool for the assessment of hepatic microcirculation: a validation study. *Transplantation*, **71**, 1249–1256.

22. Mathura, K.R., Vollebregt, K.C., Boer, K., de Graaff, J.C., Ubbink, D.T., and Ince, C. (2001) Comparison of OPS imaging and conventional capillary microscopy to study the human microcirculation. *J. Appl. Physiol.*, **91**, 74–78.

23. von Dobschuetz, E., Biberthaler, P., Mussack, T., Langer, S., Messmer, K., and Hoffmann, T. (2003) Noninvasive in vivo assessment of the pancreatic microcirculation: orthogonal polarization spectral imaging. *Pancreas*, **26**, 139–143.

24. Schaser, K.D., Puhl, G., Vollmar, B. et al. (2005) In vivo imaging of human pancreatic microcirculation and pancreatic tissue injury in clinical pancreas transplantation. *Am. J. Transplant.*, **5**, 341–350.

25. Mathura, K.R., Alic, L., van Deventer, S., and Ince, C. (2000) The rectal microcirculation observed during inflammatory bowel disease using OPS imaging. *J. Vasc. Res.*, **37** (S1), 40 (abstract).

26. Biberthaler, P., Langer, S., Luchting, B., Khandoga, A., and Messmer, K. (2001) In vivo assessment of colon microcirculation: comparison of the new OPS imaging technique with intravital microscopy. *Eur. J. Med. Res.*, **6**, 525–534.

27. Vollebregt, K.C., Boer, K., Mathura, K.R., de Graaff, J.C., Ubbink, D.T., and Ince, C. (2001) Impaired vascular function in women with pre-eclampsia observed with orthogonal polarisation spectral imaging. *Br. J. Obstet. Gynaecol.*, **108**, 1148–1153.

28. Langer, S., Biberthaler, P., Harris, A.G., Steinau, H.U., and Messmer, K. (2001) In vivo monitoring of microvessels in skin flaps: introduction of a novel technique. *Microsurgery*, **21**, 317–324.

29. Langer, S., Hatz, R., Harris, A.G., Hernandez-Richter, T., Maiwald, G., and Messmer, K. (2001) Assessing the microcirculation in a burn wound by use of OPS imaging. *Eur. J. Med. Res.*, **6**, 231–234.

30. Genzel-Boroviczeny, O., Strotgen, J., Harris, A.G., Messmer, K., and Christ, F. (2002) Orthogonal polarization spectral imaging (OPS): a novel method to measure the microcirculation in term and preterm infants transcutaneously. *Pediatr. Res.*, **51**, 386–391.

31. Kroth, J., Weidlich, K., Hiedl, S., Nubaum, C., Christ, F., and Genzel-Boroviczeny, O. (2008) Functional vessel density in the first month of life in preterm neonates. *Pediatr. Res.*, **64**, 567–571.

32. Van den Oever, H.L., Dzoljic, M., Ince, C., Hollmann, M.W., and Mokken, F.C. (2006) Orthogonal polarization spectral imaging of the microcirculation during acute hypervolemic hemodilution and epidural lidocaine injection. *Anesth. Analg.*, **103**, 484–487.

33. Spronk, P.E., Ince, C., Gardien, M.J., Mathura, K.R., Oudemans-van Straaten, H.M., and Zandstra, D.F. (2002) Nitroglycerin in septic shock after intravascular volume resuscitation. *Lancet*, **360**, 1395–1396.

34. Ince, C. (2005) The microcirculation is the motor of sepsis. *Crit. Care*, **9** (Suppl. 4), S13–S19.

35. Dondorp, A.M., Ince, C., Charunwatthana, P. *et al.* (2008) Direct in vivo assessment of microcirculatory dysfunction in severe falciparum malaria. *J. Infect. Dis.*, **197**, 79–84.

36. Lindeboom, J.A., Mathura, K.R., Aartman, I.H., Kroon, F.H., Milstein, D.M., and Ince, C. (2007) Influence of the application of platelet-enriched plasma in oral mucosal wound healing. *Clin. Oral Implants Res.*, **18**, 133–139.

37. Milstein, D.M., Mathura, K.R., Lindeboom, J.A., Ramsoekh, D., Lindeboom, R., and Ince, C. (2009) The temporal course of mucoperiosteal flap revascularization at guided bone regeneration-treated implant sites: a pilot study. *J. Clin. Periodontol.*, **36**, 892–897.

38. Genzel-Boroviczeny, O., Christ, F., and Glas, V. (2004) Blood transfusion increases functional capillary density in the skin of anemic preterm infants. *Pediatr. Res.*, **56**, 751–755.

39. Lindeboom, J.A., Mathura, K.R., and Ince, C. (2006) Orthogonal polarization spectral (OPS) imaging and topographical characteristics of oral squamous cell carcinoma. *Oral Oncol.*, **42**, 581–585.

40. Lindert, J., Werner, J., Redlin, M., Kuppe, H., Habazettl, H., and Pries, A.R. (2002) OPS imaging of human microcirculation: a short technical report. *J. Vasc. Res.*, **39**, 368–372.

41. Boerma, E.C., Mathura, K.R., van der Voort, V., Spronk, P.E., and Ince, C. (2005) Quantifying bedside-derived imaging of microcirculatory abnormalities in septic patients: a prospective validation study. *Crit. Care*, **9**, R601–R606.

42. Ellis, C.G., Ellsworth, M.L., Pittman, R.N., and Burgess, W.L. (1992) Application of image analysis for evaluation of red blood cell dynamics in capillaries. *Microvasc. Res.*, **44**, 214–225.

43. De Backer, D., Hollenberg, S., Boerma, C. *et al.* (2007) How to evaluate the microcirculation: report of a round table conference. *Crit. Care*, **11**, R101.

44. Goedhart, P.T., Khalilzada, M., Bezemer, R., Merza, J., and Ince, C. (2007) Sidestream Dark Field (SDF) imaging: a novel stroboscopic LED ring-based imaging modality for clinical assessment

of the microcirculation. *Opt. Express*, **15**, 15101–15114.

45. Trzeciak, S., Dellinger, R.P., Parrillo, J.E. *et al.* (2007) Early microcirculatory perfusion derangements in patients with severe sepsis and septic shock: relationship to hemodynamics, oxygen transport, and survival. *Ann. Emerg. Med.*, **49**, 88–98.

46. Milstein, D.M., Bezemer, R., Lindeboom, J.A., and Ince, C. (2009) The acute effects of CMF-based chemotherapy on maxillary periodontal microcirculation. *Cancer Chemother. Pharmacol.*, **64**, 1047–1052.

47. Dobbe, J.G., Streekstra, G.J., Atasever, B., van Zijderveld, R., and Ince, C. (2008) Measurement of functional microcirculatory geometry and velocity distributions using automated image analysis. *Med. Biol. Eng. Comput.*, **46**, 659–670.

48. Schaudig, S., Dadasch, B, Kellam, K.R., and Christ, F., (2001) Validation of an analysis software for OPS-imaging used in humans. Proceedings of the 7th World Congress for Microcirculation, 2001.

49. Steger, C. (1998) An unbiased detector of curvilinear structures. *IEEE Trans. Pattern Anal. Mach. Intell.*, **20**, 113–125.

50. Arnold, R.C., Parrillo, J.E., Phillip, D.R. *et al.* (2009) Point-of-care assessment of microvascular blood flow in critically ill patients. *Intensive Care Med.*, **35**, 1761–1766.

51. Balestra, G.M., Bezemer, R., Boerma, E.C. *et al.* (2010) Improvement of Sidestream Dark Field Imaging with an Image Acquisition Stabilizer. *BMC Med. Imaging*, **10**, 15.

52. Styp-Rekowska, B., Disassa, N.M., Reglin, B. *et al.* (2007) An imaging spectroscopy approach for measurement of oxygen saturation and hematocrit during intravital microscopy. *Microcirculation*, **14**, 207–221.

3
Clinical Applications of SDF Videomicroscopy

Daniel De Backer and Jean-Louis Vincent

3.1
Introduction

In recent years, microcirculatory alterations have been increasingly implicated in the development of organ dysfunction, failure, and death in critically ill patients. Until recently, adequacy of tissue perfusion has been assumed from systemic measures including blood pressure, cardiac output, and mixed venous oxygen saturation and from laboratory variables such as blood lactate concentrations. However, resuscitation aimed only at normalizing these macrocirculatory parameters may be insufficient to improve perfusion and oxygenation at the microcirculatory level. The development of techniques with which the microcirculation can be directly visualized at the bedside has provided us with the opportunity to study regional blood flow in health and disease [1]. Alterations in microcirculatory blood flow have been identified in several disease processes, and studies are beginning to evaluate the clinical implications of these changes and the effects that currently used therapies have on them. In Chapter 2, Dr Ince detailed the historical and technical development of the orthogonal polarization spectral (OPS) and sidestream dark-field (SDF) imaging techniques. In this chapter, we discuss results from clinical studies using these instruments. Most of the data are from studies that have monitored the microcirculation in the sublingual area, so this is assumed throughout the chapter unless otherwise stated.

3.2
Microcirculatory Alterations Visualized with OPS/SDF Imaging

3.2.1
In Sepsis

In healthy volunteers, a single daily dose of lipopolysaccharide (LPS) was associated with decreased flow in medium and large microvessels as visualized with SDF after just 2 h, in association with increased cytokine levels [2]. However, by day 5,

Microcirculation Imaging, First Edition. Edited by Martin J. Leahy.
© 2012 Wiley-VCH Verlag GmbH & Co. KGaA. Published 2012 by Wiley-VCH Verlag GmbH & Co. KGaA.

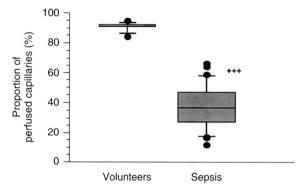

Figure 3.1 Capillary perfusion in patients with severe sepsis and healthy volunteers. $^{+++}p < 0.001$ versus volunteers. (From Ref. [3] with permission.)

the cytokine response and microcirculatory alterations were absent, suggesting that a degree of immune tolerance had developed. Using OPS, we demonstrated decreased capillary density and a reduced proportion of perfused capillaries in 50 patients with severe sepsis and septic shock compared to healthy volunteers or ICU control patients (Figure 3.1) [3]. Heterogeneity of blood flow was also increased in patients with sepsis. Importantly, these changes were unrelated to global hemodynamic or oxygenation parameters and were more severe in nonsurvivors than in survivors [3]. Since our original report in 2002 [3], at least 15 trials have reported similar findings in adult patients with sepsis [4–18] and several have noted that these changes occur early in the course of sepsis. Using SDF imaging, Spanos *et al.* [17] reported that for small vessels ($<20\,\mu$m), the microvascular flow index, the heterogeneity index, and the proportion of perfused vessels were already lower in patients with sepsis and severe sepsis within 6 h of diagnosis compared to healthy volunteers. Importantly, the microcirculatory alterations improve over time in survivors, but not in nonsurvivors, suggesting a role of the microcirculation in outcome and a potential place for microcirculatory monitoring to follow the effects of therapeutic interventions (see later). In this context, using OPS imaging to monitor the sublingual microcirculation on the day of onset of septic shock and each day until resolution of shock, Sakr *et al.* [5] noted that the proportion of perfused small vessels improved over time in survivors but not in nonsurvivors. Moreover, despite similar hemodynamic and oxygenation profiles and use of vasopressors at the end of shock, patients dying from multiple organ failure after the resolution of shock had a lower percentage of perfused small vessels than survivors (57.4% (46.6–64.9%) vs 79.3% (67.2–83.2%); $p = 0.02$).

3.2.2
In Severe Heart Failure and Cardiogenic Shock

Microcirculatory alterations have also been reported in patients with severe heart failure and cardiogenic shock. In 40 patients with severe heart failure, including

31 with cardiogenic shock, the proportion of perfused small vessels was reduced compared to ICU control patients examined the day before cardiac surgery (63% (46–65%) in heart failure and 49% (38–64%) in cardiogenic shock vs 92% (90–93%) in ICU controls, $p < 0.001$) [19]. Again, these alterations were greater in patients who did not survive. Jung *et al.* similarly reported reduced microvascular perfusion in patients with cardiogenic shock when compared to those without it, associated with an increase in blood lactate levels [20].

3.2.3
During and after Cardiac Arrest

During cardiac arrest, it is expected that the microcirculation would be impaired. In a patient with prolonged cardiac arrest in hypothermic conditions, Elbers *et al.* [21] observed that cardiopulmonary resuscitation (CPR) was able to provide some microvascular perfusion, which disappeared during brief interruptions of CPR. In patients who survived after CPR, Donadello *et al.* [22] reported severe microvascular alterations, which returned towards normal after a few days. Another interesting observation was made during aortic cross-clamping: even though cardiac output stops abruptly, the sublingual microcirculation is preserved for ~20 s, first stopping in capillaries and then in larger vessels [23]. This time interval during which microvascular perfusion is preserved after cardiac output is stopped is likely related to the time required for arterial pressure to drop to mean systemic pressure, suggesting that perfusion pressure is a more important determinant of microvascular perfusion than cardiac output.

3.2.4
In Surgery

3.2.4.1 Cardiac Surgery
Using sublingual OPS, Bauer *et al.* [24] reported that functional capillary density was reduced during cardiopulmonary bypass (CPB), returning to normal 1 h after discontinuation of CPB. Similarly, den Uil *et al.* [25] observed, using SDF imaging, that decreases in microvascular flow index occurred during CPB, irrespective of changes in systemic blood pressure; again, these changes returned to normal once the CPB was discontinued. We investigated the microcirculatory changes in 15 patients undergoing cardiac surgery (9 with and 6 without CPB) and compared them to 7 patients undergoing thyroidectomy [26]. The proportion of perfused vessels was similar in all three groups at baseline and decreased similarly after induction of anesthesia; it decreased further during CPB. Immediately after surgery, alterations were more severe in CPB patients than in patients undergoing off-pump surgery and had already normalized in the thyroidectomy patients ($p = 0.0005$ vs cardiac surgery). In both cardiac surgery groups, these microcirculatory alterations decreased with time but persisted at 24 h. The severity

of microvascular alterations correlated with peak lactate levels after cardiac surgery ($y = 11.5 - 0.15x$; $r^2 = 0.65$; $p < 0.05$) and with severity of organ dysfunction after surgery but was not related to global hemodynamic variables. Atasever *et al.* [27] reported that CPB was associated with a 43% decrease in functional capillary density and that off-pump surgery was associated with reduced capillary blood flow. Interestingly, in patients undergoing CPB, there were no differences in microcirculatory parameters when pulsatile perfusion was used compared to when nonpulsatile flow was used [28], although pulsatile flow is often promoted as having more beneficial effects on the microcirculation [29].

3.2.4.2 Noncardiac Surgery

Anesthesia can in itself induce some microvascular alterations, but these are usually transient. In our study discussed above, patients undergoing thyroid surgery and those undergoing cardiac surgery developed similar modest microcirculatory alterations after induction of anesthesia, which rapidly disappeared in the patients undergoing thyroid surgery [26]. Similarly, in healthy women given propofol for anesthesia for transvaginal oocyte retrieval, a 17% decrease in the density of perfused capillaries was observed, which had resolved by 3 h after the propofol infusion [30]. In 25 patients undergoing major abdominal surgery, Jhanji *et al.* [31] reported that the small vessel microvascular flow index and the proportion and density of perfused small vessels were lower in patients who developed complications after surgery than in those who did not.

Recently, Snoeijs *et al.* [32] investigated the renal microcirculation in kidneys from donors after cardiac death, which inevitably undergo some degree of ischemic injury, and in living donor kidneys, in which the ischemic injury is minimal. The peritubular capillaries of the donor kidneys were visualized by SDF during transplant surgery. Capillary blood flow during the early reperfusion phase was markedly reduced in the kidneys from donors after cardiac death compared to the living donor kidneys. The authors suggested that these findings can help in encouraging the development of interventions to increase microvascular perfusion and thus improve early graft function and enable expansion of the currently limited donor pool with kidneys that have suffered prolonged ischemia. Moreover, such findings could also apply to other conditions associated with ischemia including stroke, liver resection, and acute myocardial infarction. OPS has also been used to assess microcirculatory changes in other transplanted organs, including the liver and pancreas [33, 34].

3.2.5
Subarachnoid Hemorrhage

In patients with subarachnoid hemorrhage (SAH), OPS imaging applied to the cerebral cortex showed initially decreased capillary density, which increased during aneurysm surgery [35]. Microvasospasms could also be observed, which were not apparent with other imaging modalities.

3.2.6
Dermatology

The microcirculation is disturbed in various diseases affecting the skin, and monitoring of microcirculatory changes could be used for diagnosis and to monitor treatments. OPS imaging has been used to give information about burn wound depth [36], and Virgini-Magalhaes *et al.* [37] suggested that OPS was useful for evaluating the microangiopathy of chronic venous insufficiency. OPS has also been used to assess and describe the microcirculatory changes present in skin cancers [38] and to identify the early microcirculatory changes present in the oral mucositis associated with high-dose chemotherapy in patients with hematological malignancies [39]. Other suggested dermatological conditions in which OPS/SDF imaging could play a role in diagnosis and prognostication include leprosy and psoriasis [40], but further study is needed to develop fully the potential of this technique in these fields.

3.2.7
Oncology

In a case report, Meinders and Elbers [41] reported that the microcirculation was severely impaired in a patient with acute leukemia. These alterations were related to leukostasis and disappeared when the white blood cell count was decreased by chemotherapy. However, chemotherapy in itself may also induce some microvascular alterations. The sublingual microcirculation has been shown to be altered in patients with myeloma receiving melphalan chemotherapy, and these alterations could at least in part be attributed to the toxicity of chemo-therapy [39].

3.2.8
Cirrhosis

The microcirculation has been shown to be altered in patients with decompensated cirrhosis but not in patients with cirrhosis with similar severity but not undergoing acute decompensation [42]. As infections often trigger cirrhosis decompensation, it is difficult to ensure from this report that these alterations were not related to an underlying infection, even though the authors were unable to document infections in these patients.

3.2.9
Pediatric Use

SDF is an excellent tool to evaluate the microcirculation in newborns. Even though the sublingual area is difficult to evaluate in children (small size, need for cooperation), the skin, particularly of the axilla or head, is easy to examine: the epidermis is of very limited thickness and hairs are scarce, so excellent visualization is often obtained. It has been shown that preterm infants often present microvascular alterations that term infants do not share. Genzel-Boroviczeny *et al.* [43] reported that there were no differences in vessel density or diameter between term and preterm babies, but that red blood cell velocity increased as the hematocrit decreased in preterm infants. Top *et al.* [44] made similar observations in the buccal mucosa. These alterations were improved by red blood cell transfusions [45] and by increasing the incubator temperature [46]. Weidlich and colleagues [47] suggested that intraindividual changes in functional small vessel density could be used as a marker of infection in preterm infants.

Infants suffering from severe respiratory failure present severe alterations in sublingual microcirculation compared to same-aged controls; interestingly, these alterations improved when these infants were placed on extracorporeal membrane oxygenation (ECMO) [48]. Finally, Top and colleagues [49] performed daily measurements (up to three days) in pediatric patients suffering from severe sepsis and reported that nonsurvivors had persistent microcirculatory alterations, whereas microcirculatory changes rapidly improved in survivors, confirming in pediatric sepsis the data observed by Sakr *et al.* in adults [5].

3.3
Response of Microcirculatory Variables to Therapeutic Interventions

Various therapeutic interventions have been demonstrated to influence microcirculatory changes, notably in patients with severe sepsis. Trzeciak *et al.* [12] used SDF to assess the microcirculation in patients with sepsis undergoing early goal-directed resuscitation, consisting of intravenous volume expansion, vasopressors, inotropes, and blood products in a stepwise manner to achieve predefined quantitative end points of resuscitation derived from invasive hemodynamic monitoring. In patients whose organ dysfunction resolved with resuscitation, as defined by decreasing sequential organ failure assessment (SOFA) scores, 88% had an increased microcirculatory flow index compared to only 47% of those whose SOFA scores did not improve. We have recently observed that early fluid administration could improve the microcirculation, while later fluid loading may be less beneficial [16]; these effects were not related to the type of solution used. As reported in earlier studies, microcirculatory changes were correlated to changes in blood lactate levels (Figure 3.2) but not to changes in global hemodynamic variables such as cardiac index and mean arterial pressure. In a small study of 20 patients with severe sepsis undergoing early goal-directed therapy, Dubin *et al.* [50] suggested that hydroxyethyl starch solutions may have more beneficial effects on the microcirculation than normal saline solutions. In one study, blood transfusions were shown to influence microcirculatory parameters in patients with sepsis with altered capillary perfusion before the transfusion [11]. In patients undergoing cardiac surgery, blood transfusion was associated with increased microcirculatory density as assessed by SDF imaging [51]. Simultaneous spectrophotometry showed that microcirculatory hemoglobin concentration and hemoglobin oxygen saturation were also increased.

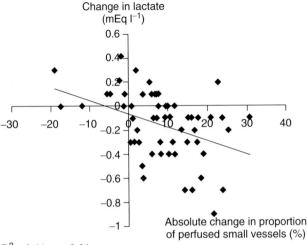

$R^2 = 0.41, p < 0.01$

Figure 3.2 Relationship between changes in proportion of perfused small vessels and changes in lactate levels. Change in lactate $= -0.011$, change in proportion of perfused vessels $= 0.064$, $R^2 = 0.41$, and $p = 0.0012$. (From Ref. [16] with permission.)

In preterm infants, blood transfusion was reported to improve functional capillary density assessed by OPS imaging through the skin of the upper arm [45].

Dobutamine has been shown to improve capillary perfusion but with marked individual variation [6]. Recently, Morelli *et al.* [52] suggested that levosimendan (0.2 µg kg^{-1} min^{-1}) had more beneficial effects on the sublingual microcirculation compared to a standard dose of dobutamine (5 µg kg^{-1} min^{-1}). Several groups have reported no changes in microvascular variables during increases in norepinephrine dose to achieve increases in arterial pressure [13, 53]. It should be noted that many of these trials reported a high heterogeneity in the response to the intervention, attributed either to the timing of the intervention [16] or to the underlying state of the microcirculation before any intervention [11, 13], with an improvement in patients with the most severe microcirculatory alterations at baseline and lack of change or even worsening of the microcirculation in patients with an initially better-preserved microcirculation.

As the microcirculatory changes in sepsis are characterized by a decreased number of vessels and increased heterogeneity, recruitment of microcirculatory units using vasodilatory agents may be an option to improve microcirculatory flow. In an early study, Spronk *et al.* [4] reported that infusion of 0.5 mg of nitroglycerin increased microvascular flow in patients with septic shock, and we reported that topically applied acetylcholine corrected microvascular alterations in patients with sepsis [3]. However, in a recent, randomized controlled trial of 70 patients with septic shock, administration of 2 mg h^{-1} nitroglycerin after protocolized resuscitation had no effect on the microcirculation [15], although it may be that the resuscitation in these patients was so effective at restoring the microcirculation that no further improvement could be visualized [54]. In patients with acute heart failure, den Uil *et al.* [55] demonstrated that a low dose of nitroglycerin (33 µg min^{-1}) significantly improved the microcirculation, although there was some variability in the response to nitroglycerin among patients. In a subsequent study, the same group used incremental doses of nitroglycerin (up to 133 µg min^{-1}) and reported that nitroglycerin increased tissue perfusion in all patients in a dose-dependent manner [56]. Taken together, these data suggest that nitroglycerin may improve the microcirculation, but the variability in effective dose and in response suggests that this drug should not be administered without further evaluating its effects.

Hydrocortisone (HC) is frequently used in patients with septic shock despite conflicting evidence regarding its benefits [57]. In 20 patients with septic shock, Buchele and colleagues [14] reported that administration of moderate doses of HC (50 mg per 6 h) was associated with an early and consistent improvement in capillary perfusion (Figure 3.3), independent of the response to an adrenocorticotropic hormone (ACTH) test; the changes in microvascular perfusion were not related to changes in arterial pressure. Although consistent, the magnitude of these changes was relatively limited and risks associated with HC may outweigh its beneficial effects on the microcirculation.

The administration of drotrecogin alfa (activated) has been demonstrated to improve survival in patients with severe sepsis [58], although the exact mechanisms of action are unclear. In 20 patients with severe sepsis who received drotrecogin alfa (activated), the proportion of perfused capillaries increased already at 4 h (from 64% (51–80%) to 84% (71–88%), $p < 0.01$); these changes were not seen in patients who were not treated with the drug because of contraindications [6]. The improvement in microvascular blood flow was associated with a more rapid resolution of hyperlactatemia, and interestingly, at the end of the drug infusion, microvascular perfusion decreased transiently.

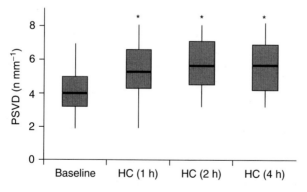

Figure 3.3 Evolution of perfused small vessel density (PSVD) over time after administration of 50 mg per 6 h hydrocortisone (HC) in patients with septic shock (***$p < 0.05$ compared with baseline). (From Ref. [14] with permission.)

Several recent publications have also investigated the effect of extracorporeal support devices on microcirculatory perfusion in patients with cardiogenic shock. Using SDF imaging, intra-aortic balloon counterpulsation, mechanical support devices, and ECMO were shown to increase sublingual microcirculatory flow in patients with cardiogenic shock [59–61]. Interestingly, weaning from an intra-aortic balloon pump (IABP), when no longer deemed necessary, was accompanied by a moderate improvement in the sublingual microcirculation [62], suggesting that it is not the device or the intervention in itself that improves the microcirculation but rather its timely implementation and, perhaps, the decrease in the release of endogenous vasoconstrictive substances. Cardiac resynchronization therapy has also been reported to improve the microcirculation in patients with heart failure [63], and as already mentioned, ECMO improved the microcirculation in neonates with severe respiratory infection [48].

3.4
Perspective

Is SDF the ideal tool to monitor the microcirculation? Microcirculatory alterations in critically ill patients are characterized by heterogeneity within the investigated area (vessels without any flow or with intermittent flow in close vicinity to well-perfused vessels), and heterogeneity is a crucial determinant of tissue oxygenation [64, 65]. In addition, it is also important to realize that therapeutic interventions should aim at recruiting the microcirculation more than just pushing more flow into already perfused vessels. Hence, direct visualization of the microcirculation with SDF appears to be the technique of choice as it allows this heterogeneity of perfusion to be detected at the bedside, something that other techniques may be unable to do. Unfortunately, direct visualization of the microcirculation is restricted to a few easily accessible organs, such as the sublingual area, and requires specific skills of the investigator both for image acquisition and for image analysis. Finally, SDF may not be applied in all patients, as it requires safe access to the sublingual area (sedation or collaboration) and is not feasible during noninvasive mechanical ventilation.

As we have seen, microvascular alterations frequently occur in critically ill patients, especially in sepsis. These microvascular alterations have been associated with severity of organ dysfunction and outcome and are often present when global hemodynamic parameters appear normal. Various interventions have been shown to improve microcirculatory flow, but whether monitoring the microcirculation and titrating such therapies according to microcirculatory response could be associated with improved outcomes has not yet been studied. In the study by Trzeciak et al. [12], when the early goal-directed resuscitation protocol led to improved organ dysfunction scores, 88% of patients had increased microcirculatory flow compared to 47% of those who had no improvement in their organ function. Importantly, there were no associated differences in global hemodynamics, suggesting that targeting the microcirculation, rather than the macrocirculation as is currently done, could be beneficial in patients with sepsis. Nevertheless, the microcirculation is fed by the macrocirculation, and without adequate global hemodynamics, the microcirculation will never operate in an optimal manner. Microcirculatory data cannot be taken in isolation and should be used to complement the full clinical assessment.

Further studies are needed to demonstrate that targeting the microcirculation can indeed improve outcomes, and until the results of such studies are available, it would seem reasonable to ensure that the global hemodynamic status is optimized before attempting to intervene at the microcirculatory level. Clearly, this is just the beginning for microcirculatory research, and the potential clinical applications are enormous. Results of more studies focusing on the impact of interventions that are known to improve outcomes on the microcirculation and using microcirculatory monitoring to guide therapy in different patients groups and conditions are eagerly awaited.

References

1. De Backer, D., Ospina-Tascon, G., Salgado, D., Favory, R., Creteur, J., and Vincent, J.L. (2010) Monitoring the microcirculation in the critically ill patient: current methods and future approaches. *Intensive Care Med.*, **36**, 1813–1825.

2. Draisma, A., Bemelmans, R., van der Hoeven, J.G., Spronk, P., and Pickkers, P. (2009) Microcirculation and vascular reactivity during endotoxemia and endotoxin tolerance in humans. *Shock*, **31**, 581–585.

3. De Backer, D., Creteur, J., Preiser, J.C., Dubois, M.J., and Vincent, J.L. (2002) Microvascular blood flow is altered in patients with sepsis. *Am. J. Respir. Crit. Care Med.*, **166**, 98–104.

4. Spronk, P.E., Ince, C., Gardien, M.J., Mathura, K.R., Oudemans-van Straaten, H.M., and Zandstra, D.F. (2002) Nitroglycerin in septic shock after intravascular volume resuscitation. *Lancet*, **360**, 1395–1396.

5. Sakr, Y., Dubois, M.J., De Backer, D., Creteur, J., and Vincent, J.L. (2004) Persistent microcirculatory alterations are associated with organ failure and death in patients with septic shock. *Crit. Care Med.*, **32**, 1825–1831.

6. De Backer, D., Creteur, J., Dubois, M.J., Sakr, Y., Koch, M., Verdant, C., and Vincent, J.L. (2006) The effects of

dobutamine on microcirculatory alterations in patients with septic shock are independent of its systemic effects. *Crit. Care Med.*, **34**, 403–408.

7. De Backer, D., Verdant, C., Chierego, M., Koch, M., Gullo, A., and Vincent, J.L. (2006) Effects of drotrecogin alfa activated on microcirculatory alterations in patients with severe sepsis. *Crit. Care Med.*, **34**, 1918–1924.

8. Creteur, J., De Backer, D., Sakr, Y., Koch, M., and Vincent, J.L. (2006) Sublingual capnometry tracks microcirculatory changes in septic patients. *Intensive Care Med.*, **32**, 516–523.

9. Boerma, E.C., van der Voort, P.H., Spronk, P.E., and Ince, C. (2007) Relationship between sublingual and intestinal microcirculatory perfusion in patients with abdominal sepsis. *Crit. Care Med.*, **35**, 1055–1060.

10. Trzeciak, S., Dellinger, R.P., Parrillo, J.E., Guglielmi, M., Bajaj, J., Abate, N.L., Arnold, R.C., Colilla, S., Zanotti, S., and Hollenberg, S.M. (2007) Early microcirculatory perfusion derangements in patients with severe sepsis and septic shock: relationship to hemodynamics, oxygen transport, and survival. *Ann. Emerg. Med.*, **49**, 88–98.

11. Sakr, Y., Chierego, M., Piagnerelli, M., Verdant, C., Dubois, M.J., Koch, M., Creteur, J., Gullo, A., Vincent, J.L., and

De Backer, D. (2007) Microvascular response to red blood cell transfusion in patients with severe sepsis. *Crit. Care Med.*, **35**, 1639–1644.

12. Trzeciak, S., McCoy, J.V., Phillip, D.R., Arnold, R.C., Rizzuto, M., Abate, N.L., Shapiro, N.I., Parrillo, J.E., and Hollenberg, S.M. (2008) Early increases in microcirculatory perfusion during protocol-directed resuscitation are associated with reduced multi-organ failure at 24 h in patients with sepsis. *Intensive Care Med.*, **34**, 2210–2217.

13. Dubin, A., Pozo, M.O., Casabella, C.A., Palizas, F., Murias, G., Moseinco, M.C., Kanoore, E.V., Palizas, F. Jr., Estenssoro, E., and Ince, C. (2009) Increasing arterial blood pressure with norepinephrine does not improve microcirculatory blood flow: a prospective study. *Crit. Care*, **13**, R92.

14. Buchele, G.L., Silva, E., Ospina-Tascon, G.A., Vincent, J.L., and De Backer, D. (2009) Effects of hydrocortisone on microcirculatory alterations in patients with septic shock. *Crit. Care Med.*, **37**, 1341–1347.

15. Boerma, E.C., Koopmans, M., Konijn, A., Kaiferova, K., Bakker, A.J., van Roon, E.N., Buter, H., Bruins, N., Egbers, P.H., Gerritsen, R.T., Koetsier, P.M., Kingma, W.P., Kuiper, M.A., and Ince, C. (2010) Effects of nitroglycerin on sublingual microcirculatory blood flow in patients with severe sepsis/septic shock after a strict resuscitation protocol: a double-blind randomized placebo controlled trial. *Crit. Care Med.*, **38**, 93–100.

16. Ospina-Tascon, G., Neves, A.P., Occhipinti, G., Donadello, K., Buchele, G., Simion, D., Chierego, M.L., Silva, T.O., Fonseca, A., Vincent, J.L., and De Backer, D. (2010) Effects of fluids on microvascular perfusion in patients with severe sepsis. *Intensive Care Med.*, **36**, 949–955.

17. Spanos, A., Jhanji, S., Vivian-Smith, A., Harris, T., and Pearse, R.M. (2010) Early microvascular changes in sepsis and severe sepsis. *Shock*, **33**, 387–391.

18. Pottecher, J., Deruddre, S., Teboul, J.L., Georger, J.F., Laplace, C., Benhamou, D., Vicaut, E., and Duranteau, J. (2010) Both passive leg raising and intravascular volume expansion improve sublingual microcirculatory perfusion in severe sepsis and septic shock patients. *Intensive Care Med.*, **36**, 1867–1874.

19. De Backer, D., Creteur, J., Dubois, M.J., Sakr, Y., and Vincent, J.L. (2004) Microvascular alterations in patients with acute severe heart failure and cardiogenic shock. *Am. Heart J.*, **147**, 91–99.

20. Jung, C., Ferrari, M., Rodiger, C., Fritzenwanger, M., Goebel, B., Lauten, A., Pfeifer, R., and Figulla, H.R. (2009) Evaluation of the sublingual microcirculation in cardiogenic shock. *Clin. Hemorheol. Microcirc.*, **42**, 141–148.

21. Elbers, P.W., Craenen, A.J., Driessen, A., Stehouwer, M.C., Munsterman, L., Prins, M., van Iterson, M., Bruins, P., and Ince, C. (2010) Imaging the human microcirculation during cardiopulmonary resuscitation in a hypothermic victim of submersion trauma. *Resuscitation*, **81**, 123–125.

22. Donadello, K., Favory, R., Salgado, D., Creteur, J., De Backer, D., Gottin, L., Vincent, J.L., and Taccone, F.S. (2010) Microcirculatory alterations after cardiac arrest: a pilot study. *Intensive Care Med.*, **36**, S179 (abstract).

23. Elbers, P.W., Ozdemir, A., Heijmen, R.H., Heeren, J., van Iterson, M., van Dongen, E.P., and Ince, C. (2010) Microvascular hemodynamics in human hypothermic circulatory arrest and selective antegrade cerebral perfusion. *Crit. Care Med.*, **38**, 1548–1553.

24. Bauer, A., Kofler, S., Thiel, M., Eifert, S., and Christ, F. (2007) Monitoring of the sublingual microcirculation in cardiac surgery using orthogonal polarization spectral imaging: preliminary results. *Anesthesiology*, **107**, 939–945.

25. den Uil, C.A., Lagrand, W.K., Spronk, P.E., van Domburg, R.T., Hofland, J., Luthen, C., Brugts, J.J., van der Ent, M., and Simoons, M.L. (2008) Impaired sublingual microvascular perfusion during surgery with cardiopulmonary bypass: a pilot study. *J. Thorac. Cardiovasc. Surg.*, **136**, 129–134.

26. De Backer, D., Dubois, M.J., Schmartz, D., Koch, M., Ducart, A., Barvais, L.,

and Vincent, J.L. (2009) Microcirculatory alterations in cardiac surgery: effects of cardiopulmonary bypass and anesthesia. *Ann. Thorac. Surg.*, **88**, 1396–1403.

27. Atasever, B., Boer, C., Goedhart, P., Biervliet, J., Seyffert, J., Speekenbrink, R., Schwarte, L., De Mol, B., and Ince, C. (2011) Distinct alterations in sublingual microcirculatory blood flow and hemoglobin oxygenation in on-pump and off-pump coronary artery bypass graft surgery. *J. Cardiothorac. Vasc. Anesth.*, **25**, 784–790.

28. Elbers, P.W., Wijbenga, J., Solinger, F., Yilmaz, A., van Iterson, M., van Dongen, E.P., and Ince, C. (2011) Direct observation of the human microcirculation during cardiopulmonary bypass: effects of pulsatile perfusion. *J. Cardiothorac. Vasc. Anesth.*, **25**, 250–255.

29. Ji, B. and Undar, A. (2006) An evaluation of the benefits of pulsatile versus nonpulsatile perfusion during cardiopulmonary bypass procedures in pediatric and adult cardiac patients. *ASAIO J.*, **52**, 357–361.

30. Koch, M., De Backer, D., Vincent, J.L., Barvais, L., Hennart, D., and Schmartz, D. (2008) Effects of propofol on human microcirculation. *Br. J. Anaesth.*, **101**, 473–478.

31. Jhanji, S., Lee, C., Watson, D., Hinds, C., and Pearse, R.M. (2009) Microvascular flow and tissue oxygenation after major abdominal surgery: association with post-operative complications. *Intensive Care Med.*, **35**, 671–677.

32. Snoeijs, M.G., Vink, H., Voesten, N., Christiaans, M.H., Daemen, J.W., Peppelenbosch, A.G., Tordoir, J.H., Peutz-Kootstra, C.J., Buurman, W.A., Schurink, G.W., and van Heurn, L.W. (2010) Acute ischemic injury to the renal microvasculature in human kidney transplantation. *Am. J. Physiol. Renal Physiol.*, **299**, F1134–F1140.

33. Puhl, G., Schaser, K.D., Pust, D., Kohler, K., Vollmar, B., Menger, M.D., Neuhaus, P., and Settmacher, U. (2005) Initial hepatic microcirculation correlates with early graft function in human orthotopic liver transplantation. *Liver Transpl.*, **11**, 555–563.

34. Schaser, K.D., Puhl, G., Vollmar, B., Menger, M.D., Stover, J.F., Kohler, K., Neuhaus, P., and Settmacher, U. (2005) In vivo imaging of human pancreatic microcirculation and pancreatic tissue injury in clinical pancreas transplantation. *Am. J. Transplant.*, **5**, 341–350.

35. Uhl, E., Lehmberg, J., Steiger, H.J., and Messmer, K. (2003) Intraoperative detection of early microvasospasm in patients with subarachnoid hemorrhage by using orthogonal polarization spectral imaging. *Neurosurgery*, **52**, 1307–1315.

36. Goertz, O., Ring, A., Kohlinger, A., Daigeler, A., Andree, C., Steinau, H.U., and Langer, S. (2010) Orthogonal polarization spectral imaging: a tool for assessing burn depths? *Ann. Plast. Surg.*, **64**, 217–221.

37. Virgini-Magalhães, C.E., Porto, C.L., Fernandes, F.F., Dorigo, D.M., Bottino, D.A., and Bouskela, E. (2006) Use of microcirculatory parameters to evaluate chronic venous insufficiency. *J. Vasc. Surg.*, **43**, 1037–1044.

38. Lindeboom, J.A., Mathura, K.R., and Ince, C. (2006) Orthogonal polarization spectral (OPS) imaging and topographical characteristics of oral squamous cell carcinoma. *Oral Oncol.*, **42**, 581–585.

39. Milstein, D.M., te Boome, L.C., Cheung, Y.W., Lindeboom, J.A., van den Akker, H.P., Biemond, B.J., and Ince, C. (2010) Use of sidestream dark-field (SDF) imaging for assessing the effects of high-dose melphalan and autologous stem cell transplantation on oral mucosal microcirculation in myeloma patients. *Oral Surg. Oral Med. Oral Pathol. Oral Radiol. Endod.*, **109**, 91–97.

40. Treu, C.M., Lupi, O., Bottino, D.A., and Bouskela, E. (2011) Sidestream dark field imaging: the evolution of real-time visualization of cutaneous microcirculation and its potential application in dermatology. *Arch. Dermatol. Res.*, **303**, 69–78.

41. Meinders, A.J. and Elbers, P.W. (2009) Images in clinical medicine: leukocytosis and sublingual microvascular blood flow. *N. Engl. J. Med.*, **360**, e9.

42. Sheikh, M.Y., Javed, U., Singh, J., Choudhury, J., Deen, O., Dhah, K., and Peterson, M.W. (2009) Bedside

sublingual video imaging of microcirculation in assessing bacterial infection in cirrhosis. *Dig. Dis. Sci.*, **54**, 2706–2711.

43. Genzel-Boroviczeny, O., Strotgen, J., Harris, A.G., Messmer, K., and Christ, F. (2002) Orthogonal polarization spectral imaging (OPS): a novel method to measure the microcirculation in term and preterm infants transcutaneously. *Pediatr. Res.*, **51**, 386–391.

44. Top, A.P., van Dijk, M., van Velzen, J.E., Ince, C., and Tibboel, D. (2011) Functional capillary density decreases after the first week of life in term neonates. *Neonatology*, **99**, 73–77.

45. Genzel-Boroviczeny, O., Christ, F., and Glas, V. (2004) Blood transfusion increases functional capillary density in the skin of anemic preterm infants. *Pediatr. Res.*, **56**, 751–755.

46. Genzel-Boroviczeny, O., Seidl, T., Rieger-Fackeldey, E., Abicht, J., and Christ, F. (2007) Impaired microvascular perfusion improves with increased incubator temperature in preterm infants. *Pediatr. Res.*, **61**, 239–242.

47. Weidlich, K., Kroth, J., Nussbaum, C., Hiedl, S., Bauer, A., Christ, F., and Genzel-Boroviczeny, O. (2009) Changes in microcirculation as early markers for infection in preterm infants--an observational prospective study. *Pediatr. Res.*, **66**, 461–465.

48. Top, A.P., Ince, C., van Dijk, M., and Tibboel, D. (2009) Changes in buccal microcirculation following extracorporeal membrane oxygenation in term neonates with severe respiratory failure. *Crit. Care Med.*, **37**, 1121–1124.

49. Top, A.P., Ince, C., de Meij, N., van Dijk, M., and Tibboel, D. (2011) Persistent low microcirculatory vessel density in nonsurvivors of sepsis in pediatric intensive care. *Crit. Care Med.*, **39**, 8–13.

50. Dubin, A., Pozo, M.O., Casabella, C.A., Murias, G., Palizas, F., Moseinco, M.C., Kanoore, E.V., Palizas, F. Jr., Estenssoro, E., and Ince, C. (2010) Comparison of 6% hydroxyethyl starch 130/0.4 and saline solution for resuscitation of the microcirculation during the early goal-directed therapy of septic patients. *J. Crit. Care*, **25**, 659–658.

51. Yuruk, K., Almac, E., Bezemer, R., Goedhart, P., De Mol, B., and Ince, C. (2011) Blood transfusions recruit the microcirculation during cardiac surgery. *Transfusion.*, **51**, 961–967.

52. Morelli, A., Donati, A., Ertmer, C., Rehberg, S., Lange, M., Orecchioni, A., Cecchini, V., Landoni, G., Pelaia, P., Pietropaoli, P., Van Aken, H., Teboul, J.L., Ince, C., and Westphal, M. (2010) Levosimendan for resuscitating the microcirculation in patients with septic shock: a randomized controlled study. *Crit. Care*, **14**, R232.

53. Jhanji, S., Stirling, S., Patel, N., Hinds, C.J., and Pearse, R.M. (2009) The effect of increasing doses of norepinephrine on tissue oxygenation and microvascular flow in patients with septic shock. *Crit. Care Med.*, **37**, 1961–1966.

54. Favory, R., Salgado, D., Vincent, J.L., and De Backer, D. (2010) Can normal be more normal than normal? *Crit. Care Med.*, **38**, 737–738.

55. den Uil, C.A., Lagrand, W.K., Spronk, P.E., van der Ent, M., Jewbali, L.S., Brugts, J.J., Ince, C., and Simoons, M.L. (2009) Low-dose nitroglycerin improves microcirculation in hospitalized patients with acute heart failure. *Eur. J. Heart Fail.*, **11**, 386–390.

56. den Uil, C.A., Caliskan, K., Lagrand, W.K., van der Ent, M., Jewbali, L.S., van Kuijk, J.P., Spronk, P.E., and Simoons, M.L. (2009) Dose-dependent benefit of nitroglycerin on microcirculation of patients with severe heart failure. *Intensive Care Med.*, **35**, 1893–1899.

57. Vincent, J.L. (2008) Steroids in sepsis: another swing of the pendulum in our clinical trials. *Crit. Care*, **12**, 141.

58. Bernard, G.R., Vincent, J.L., Laterre, P.F., LaRosa, S.P., Dhainaut, J.F., Lopez-Rodriguez, A., Steingrub, J.S., Garber, G.E., Helterbrand, J.D., Ely, E.W., and Fisher, C.J. Jr. (2001) Efficacy and safety of recombinant human activated protein C for severe sepsis. *N. Engl. J. Med.*, **344**, 699–709.

59. Jung, C., Lauten, A., Rodiger, C., Krizanic, F., Figulla, H.R., and Ferrari, M. (2009) Effect of intra-aortic balloon

pump support on microcirculation during high-risk percutaneous intervention. *Perfusion*, **24**, 417–421.

60. Jung, C., Rodiger, C., Fritzenwanger, M., Schumm, J., Lauten, A., Figulla, H.R., and Ferrari, M. (2009) Acute microflow changes after stop and restart of intra-aortic balloon pump in cardiogenic shock. *Clin. Res. Cardiol.*, **98**, 469–475.

61. den Uil, C.A., Maat, A.P., Lagrand, W.K., van der Ent, M., Jewbali, L.S., van Thiel, R.J., Spronk, P.E., and Simoons, M.L. (2009) Mechanical circulatory support devices improve tissue perfusion in patients with end-stage heart failure or cardiogenic shock. *J. Heart Lung Transplant.*, **28**, 906–911.

62. Munsterman, L.D., Elbers, P.W., Ozdemir, A., van Dongen, E.P., van Iterson, M., and Ince, C. (2010) Withdrawing intra-aortic balloon pump support paradoxically improves microvascular flow. *Crit. Care*, **14**, R161.

63. Erol-Yilmaz, A., Atasever, B., Mathura, K., Lindeboom, J., Wilde, A., Ince, C., and Tukkie, R. (2007) Cardiac resynchronization improves microcirculation. *J. Card. Fail.*, **13**, 95–99.

64. Ellis, C.G., Bateman, R.M., Sharpe, M.D., Sibbald, W.J., and Gill, R. (2002) Effect of a maldistribution of microvascular blood flow on capillary $O(2)$ extraction in sepsis. *Am. J. Physiol. Heart Circ. Physiol.*, **282**, H156–H164.

65. Goldman, D., Bateman, R.M., and Ellis, C.G. (2006) Effect of decreased O2 supply on skeletal muscle oxygenation and O2 consumption during sepsis: role of heterogeneous capillary spacing and blood flow. *Am. J. Physiol. Heart Circ. Physiol.*, **290**, H2277–H2285.

4
Laser Doppler Flowmetry

Ingemar Fredriksson, Marcus Larsson, and Tomas Strömberg

Laser Doppler flowmetry (LDF) is based on the Doppler frequency shift that occurs when coherent light is scattered by a moving object. The magnitude of the frequency shift is determined from the optical beating that occurs when shifted and nonshifted coherent light are mixed. In 1961, Forrester [1] described how this photoelectric mixing could be used as a spectroscopic tool. In 1964, Cummins *et al.* [2] showed experimentally that the frequency content of the optical beating, as derived from a scattering fluid, depended on the velocity of the moving scatterers. The first successful *in vivo* measurements on moving red blood cells (RBCs) were conducted in 1975 by Stern [3]. Soon thereafter, the first fiberoptic LDF system was presented by Holloway and Watkins [4], and it was improved by Nilsson *et al.* [5]. The theory and its implementations were further improved during the early 1980s [5–7], and the first imaging system (LDPI, laser Doppler perfusion imaging, in contrast to single point systems LDPM, laser Doppler perfusion monitoring) was presented in 1989 by Nilsson *et al.* [8]; see also [9, 10]. Since then, the technique has evolved into commercial products for noninvasive assessment of temporal and spatial variations in the tissue perfusion.

Over the years, LDF has become a well-established technique for measuring microcirculatory blood flow. Noninvasive assessment is achieved using either probe-based systems (LDPM) or imaging systems (LDPI). Even though the conventional LDF perfusion measure is in arbitrary units, the technique has been applied as a research tool in diverse areas such as assessment of ulcers [11, 12], burns [13, 14], and wound healing [15–17]; irritant and allergy patch testing [18–20]; diabetic microangiopathy assessment [21–23]; quantifying microcirculatory disorders [24–26]; skin tumor characterization [27]; amputation level determination [28, 29]; neurosurgery [30]; and dentistry [31, 32], among many others.

4.1
Theory

In LDF, the frequency content of light that has been backscattered from tissue is analyzed to retrieve information about the blood flow in the microcirculation. In the following sections, the basic principles and theories to understand how this is achieved is presented. This includes how moving RBCs cause scattered light to become Doppler shifted (see Section 4.1.1) and how these Doppler shifts can be quantified by analyzing the fluctuating detector current generated by the beating speckle pattern that is formed on the photodetector by the backscattered light (see Section 4.1.2). These frequency shifts are conventionally summarized into a single perfusion value that scales to the tissue fraction and velocity of the moving RBCs in the examined tissue volume (see Section 4.2).

4.1.1
The Single Doppler Shift

When light is emitted, reflected, scattered, or detected by a moving object a frequency shift will occur. This so called Doppler effect was first described by Johan Christian Doppler in 1842 [33]. In LDF, this effect causes light that passes through a perfused tissue to become Doppler shifted when being scattered by moving RBCs.

Consider the position r_{RBC} of a RBC moving with velocity v, located at r_0 at time $t = 0$, then $r_{RBC} = vt + r_0$. An electromagnetic wave in direction k (the circular wave number; $k = |k| = 2\pi/\lambda$ (rad m^{-1}), where λ is the wavelength), can be expressed as

$$E(k,r) = E_0 \exp(-j(\omega t - kr))$$

An electromagnetic wave impinging the RBC is then

$$
\begin{aligned}
E(k_i, r_{RBC}) &= E_0 \exp\left(-j\left(\omega t - k_i r_{RBC}\right)\right) \\
&= E_0 \exp\left(-j\left(\omega t - k_i\left(vt + r_0\right)\right)\right) \\
&= E_0 \exp\left(-j\left(\left(\omega - k_i v\right)t - k_i r_0\right)\right)
\end{aligned}
\tag{4.1}
$$

When the light is scattered in direction k_s, it will be emitted with frequency $\omega - k_i v$. The scattered electromagnetic wave observed at a point of detection r_D, with r_1 being the vector from the RBC to the detection point ($r_1 = r_D - r_{RBC} = r_D - vt - r_0$), can therefore be expressed as

$$E(k_s, r_D) = E_0 \exp\left(-j\left(\left(\omega - k_i v\right)t - k_i r_0 - k_s\left(r_D - vt - r_0\right)\right)\right)$$

$$= E_0 \exp\left(-j\left(\left(\omega - \underbrace{(k_i - k_s)\,v}_{q}\right)t - \underbrace{(k_i - k_s)\,r_0}_{\psi_0} - \underbrace{k_s r_D}_{\psi_D}\right)\right)$$

$$= E_0 \exp\left(-j\left(\left(\omega - \underbrace{qv}_{\Delta\omega}\right)t - \psi_0 - \psi_D\right)\right)
\tag{4.2}$$

where the scattering vector is denoted as q; $q = k_i - k_s$. For a scattering angle θ and an angle φ between q and v (Figure 4.1), a single Doppler shift, expressed in angular frequency, is given by

$$\Delta\omega = qv = 4\pi\frac{v}{\lambda}\sin\frac{\theta}{2}\cos\phi.
\tag{4.3}$$

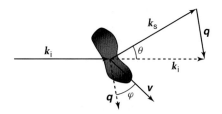

Figure 4.1 Incident (k_i) and scattering wave propagation vectors (k_s), the velocity vector (v), the scattering vector (q), and the angles involved in a single scattering event causing a Doppler shift.

4.1.2
The Doppler Power Spectrum

All light, non-Doppler-shifted, single shifted, and multiple shifted, that impinges the detector will interfere (under the assumption of equal polarization direction). When the light is coherent, the interference gives rise to a speckle pattern, and due to the small frequency differences within the light, caused by the Doppler shifts, this speckle pattern will move and change intensity rhythmically – known as light beating. The beating causes amplitude variations in the detector current, which can be analyzed by its power spectral density, the Doppler power spectrum, $P_D(f)$. This section, based on the theoretical work by Forrester [1] and Cummins and Swinney [35], extended by Larsson [36] and Fredriksson [37], shows the relationship between individual Doppler shifts and the Doppler power spectrum. Parts of this section have already been presented in [38].

Consider light originating from a laser source, which is backscattered from tissue and impinges on the tip of an optical fiber or emerges from a small spot on a tissue surface. Some of this light has retained its laser frequency, while some has undergone small frequency changes because of Doppler shifts. The phase of the light can be assumed to be random because of the various optical path lengths in the medium and the fact that the differences in optical path length are generally much larger than the wavelength of the light. For simplicity, consider this light as being electrical (E) field sources on the fiber tip or tissue surface, with the frequency and phase as given above, emitting E-fields in all directions. At the surface of a detector positioned some distance away from these E-field sources, a beating speckle pattern will form from the superposition of all E-fields. A 10 ms sequence of such a simulated speckle pattern is shown in Figure 4.2. The simulation was based on 10 000 E-fields with frequencies $\beta = \beta_L \pm 2.5$ kHz ($\beta =$ optical frequency), where $\beta_L \approx 3.8 \times 10^{14}$ Hz (780 nm), and random phase. The E-fields were distributed on a 0.125 mm in diameter fiber tip and moved with a velocity up to 2.5 mm s^{-1}. The speckle pattern formed on a 1×1 mm detector surface placed 5 cm away from the fiber tip is shown.

The theoretical derivation of the Doppler power spectrum starts by considering the light that impinges the detector. This light has a frequency content described by the optical Doppler spectrum $G(\beta)$, created from the individual Doppler shifts,

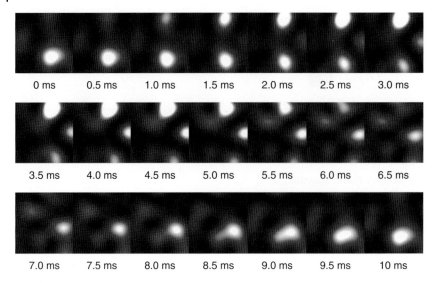

| 0 ms | 0.5 ms | 1.0 ms | 1.5 ms | 2.0 ms | 2.5 ms | 3.0 ms |

| 3.5 ms | 4.0 ms | 4.5 ms | 5.0 ms | 5.5 ms | 6.0 ms | 6.5 ms |

| 7.0 ms | 7.5 ms | 8.0 ms | 8.5 ms | 9.0 ms | 9.5 ms | 10 ms |

Figure 4.2 A 10 ms sequence of a simulated speckle pattern on a 1×1 mm detector surface placed 5 cm away from a 0.125 mm diameter fiber tip.

normalized so that

$$\int_0^\infty G_c(\beta)d\beta = i_{\mathrm{DC,c}} \tag{4.4}$$

where $i_{\mathrm{DC,c}}$ is the average current generated by the detector, under the assumption that the light is spatially coherent over the detector. Dividing the optical Doppler spectrum into frequency intervals, the E-field of the light on the detector in the mth interval can be expressed as a function of time t as

$$E_m(t) = \sqrt{G_m \Delta\beta} \exp\left(j\left(2\pi\,\Delta\beta mt + \varphi_m\right)\right) \tag{4.5}$$

where $G_m\Delta\beta = G_c(\beta_m)\Delta\beta$ is the intensity of the mth frequency interval and ϕ_m is a random phase. The generated detector current can be expressed by summing over all frequencies

$$
\begin{aligned}
i_c(t) &= E(t)E(t)^* \\
&= \Delta\beta \sum_{m=0}^{\infty} \left(\sqrt{G_m} \exp\left(j\left(2\pi\,\Delta\beta mt + \varphi_m\right)\right)\right) \\
&\quad \times \sum_{m=0}^{\infty} \left(\sqrt{G_m} \exp\left(-j\left(2\pi\,\Delta\beta mt + \varphi_m\right)\right)\right) \\
&= \Delta\beta \sum_{m=0}^{\infty}\sum_{n=0}^{\infty} \left(\sqrt{G_m G_n} \exp\left(j\left(2\pi\left(m-n\right)\Delta\beta t + \left(\varphi_m - \varphi_n\right)\right)\right)\right)
\end{aligned} \tag{4.6}
$$

where $*$ denotes the complex conjugate.

A double sum over n and m can be rewritten as $\sum_{m,n} = \sum_{m<n} + \sum_{m=n} + \sum_{m>n}$. Applying this to Eq. (4.6) and reordering m and n in the third term gives us

$$
i_c(t) = \Delta\beta \left[\sum_{m=0}^{\infty} G_m \right.
$$

$$
+ \sum_{m=0}^{\infty} \sum_{n=m+1}^{\infty} \left(\sqrt{G_m G_n} \left(\exp\left(j\left(2\pi\left(m-n \right)\Delta\beta t + \left(\varphi_m - \varphi_n \right) \right) \right) \right) \right.
$$

$$
\left. + \exp\left(-j\left(2\pi\left(m-n \right)\Delta\beta t + \left(\varphi_m - \varphi_n \right) \right) \right) \right]
$$

$$
= \underbrace{\Delta\beta \sum_{m=0}^{\infty} G_m}_{i_{DC,c}} + \underbrace{2\Delta\beta \sum_{m=0}^{\infty} \sum_{n=m+1}^{\infty} \left(\sqrt{G_m G_n} \cos\left(2\pi\left(m-n \right)\Delta\beta t + \left(\varphi_m - \varphi_n \right) \right) \right)}_{i_{AC,c}}
$$

$$
\tag{4.7}
$$

By letting $\Delta\beta \to 0$ and changing the sum to an integral, the first term in the resulting expression is identified as $i_{DC,c}$ (Eq. (4.4)). The second term varies over time and is denoted $i_{AC,c}$. By introducing $b = n - m$ and $\psi_{m,b} = \varphi_{m+b} - \varphi_m$, $i_{AC,c}$ can be written as

$$
i_{AC,c}(t) = 2\Delta\beta \sum_{m=0}^{\infty} \sum_{b=1}^{\infty} \left(\sqrt{G_m G_{m+b}} \cos\left(2\pi b\Delta\beta t + \psi_{m,b} \right) \right) \tag{4.8}
$$

Now, let $i_{ac,c}$ be a function of $b\Delta\beta$ and t, that is, dropping the sum over b in Eq. (4.8)

$$
i_{AC,c}(b\Delta\beta, t) = 2\Delta\beta \sum_{m=0}^{\infty} \left(\sqrt{G_m G_{m+b}} \cos\left(2\pi b\Delta\beta t + \psi_{m,b} \right) \right) \tag{4.9}
$$

Before continuing, $f = b\Delta\beta$ is also introduced (note that $n > m$ which leads to $b > 0$ and $f > 0$, and that generally $f \ll \beta$). The power spectral density of the time-varying part of the detector current, $P_{D,c}(f)$, is calculated from $i_{AC,c}(f, t) = i_{AC,c}(b\Delta\beta, t)$ as

$$
P_{D,c}(f) = \frac{\langle i_{AC,c}(f, t)^2 \rangle}{\Delta\beta}
$$

$$
= 4\Delta\beta \left\langle \left[\sum_{m=0}^{\infty} \left(\sqrt{G_m G_{m+b}} \cos\left(2\pi f t + \psi_{m,b} \right) \right) \right]^2 \right\rangle
$$

$$
= 4\Delta\beta \left[\sum_{m=0}^{\infty} \left(G_m G_{m+b} \left\langle \cos^2\left(2\pi f t + \psi_{m,b} \right) \right\rangle \right) \right.
$$

$$
\left. + \sum_{m=0}^{\infty} \sum_{\substack{n=0 \\ n\neq m}}^{\infty} \left(\sqrt{G_m G_{m+b} G_n G_{n+b}} \left\langle \cos\left(2\pi f t + \psi_{m,b} \right) \cos\left(2\pi f t + \psi_{n,b} \right) \right\rangle \right) \right]
$$

$$
= 4\Delta\beta \sum_{m=0}^{\infty} \left(G_m G_{m+b} \left\langle \cos^2\left(2\pi f t + \psi_{m,b} \right) \right\rangle \right)
$$

$$+2\Delta\beta\sum_{\substack{m=0 \\ n\neq m}}^{\infty}\sum_{n=0}^{\infty}\left(\sqrt{G_m G_{m+b} G_n G_{n+b}}\left\langle\cos\left(4\pi ft + \psi_{m,b} + \psi_{n,b}\right)\right\rangle\right)$$

$$+2\Delta\beta\sum_{\substack{m=0 \\ n\neq m}}^{\infty}\sum_{n=0}^{\infty}\left(\sqrt{G_m G_{m+b} G_n G_{n+b}}\left\langle\cos\left(\psi_{m,b} - \psi_{n,b}\right)\right\rangle\right) \qquad (4.10)$$

where $\langle\ldots\rangle$ is the time average. The time averages for the three cosine terms are

$$\left\langle\cos^2\left(2\pi ft + \psi_{m,b}\right)\right\rangle = \frac{1}{2}$$
$$\left\langle\cos\left(4\pi ft + \psi_{m,b} + \psi_{n,b}\right)\right\rangle = 0$$
$$\left\langle\cos\left(\psi_{m,b} - \psi_{n,b}\right)\right\rangle = \cos\left(\psi_{m,b} - \psi_{n,b}\right) \qquad (4.11)$$

and $P_{D,c}(f)$ can thus be rewritten as

$$P_{D,c}(f) = 2\Delta\beta\sum_{m=0}^{\infty}\left(G_m G_{m+b}\right)$$

$$+2\Delta\beta\sum_{\substack{m=0 \\ n\neq m}}^{\infty}\sum_{n=0}^{\infty}\left(\sqrt{G_m G_{m+b} G_n G_{n+b}}\cos\left(\psi_{m,b} - \psi_{n,b}\right)\right) \qquad (4.12)$$

The second term does not equal zero for any individual frequency. However, the term averages to zero over any small frequency interval, that is, over any small interval in b.[1] Therefore we ignore that term and write $P_{D,c}(f)$ as

$$P_{D,c}(f) = 2\Delta\beta\sum_{m=0}^{\infty}\left(G_m G_{m+b}\right) = 2\sum_{m=0}^{\infty}\left(G_c\left(\beta_m\right) G_c\left(\beta_m + f\right)\Delta\beta\right) \qquad (4.13)$$

By letting $\Delta\beta \to 0$, we can rewrite the sum to an integral

$$P_{D,c}(f) = 2\int_0^{\infty} G_c(\beta) G_c(\beta + f) d\beta = 2\left(G_c * G_c\right)(f) \qquad (4.14)$$

where $*$ denotes the cross-correlation (note that $G_c(\beta) = 0$ for $\beta < 0$). As stated above, f is >0 in this derivation, and therefore $P_{D,c}(f)$ is extended for f so that

$$P_{D,c}(f) = \begin{cases} 2\left(G_c * G_c\right)(f) & \text{for} \quad f > 0 \\ 0 & \text{for} \quad f \leq 0 \end{cases} \qquad (4.15)$$

The assumption of spatial coherence over the whole detector can be relaxed as suggested below. Any given point on the detector is highly correlated with points within a certain area around the point. This area is called a *coherence area* A_c, and the size of A_c can be predicted on the basis of the wavelength of the light λ_L,

---

1) This statement has been validated by numerically calculating the term over various intervals in b for random phases ϕ_m, $B_m = 1$ for all m, and $\Delta\beta = 1/N$ where N was finite.

and the solid angle Ω between the area of illumination and each point on the detector [39]

$$A_c \approx \frac{\lambda_L^2}{\Omega} \tag{4.16}$$

Since the distance D between the detector and the fiber tip or the surface area on the tissue from which the backscattered light illuminates the detector is usually much larger than the radius r of the fiber tip or the tissue area, the solid angle can be approximated to

$$\Omega \approx \frac{\pi r^2}{D^2} \tag{4.17}$$

In total

$$n_c = \frac{A_{det}}{A_c} \tag{4.18}$$

coherence areas fit on the detector, which for the case of the simulated setup used for Figure 4.2 gives $n_c \approx 8$. Each coherence area can be considered as an independent realization of the same stochastic process, and $i_{DC,c}$, $i_{AC,c}$, and $P_{D,c}(f)$ derived above are thus valid for each single coherence area. The static current generated over the whole detector is simply summarized as

$$i_{DC} = \sum_{n_c} i_{DC,c} = n_c i_{DC,c}, \tag{4.19}$$

whereas, due to the random phases between the various $i_{AC,c}$, the time-varying part of the whole detector is summarized as

$$i_{AC} = \sum_{n_c} i_{AC,c} = \sqrt{n_c} i_{AC,c} \tag{4.20}$$

In analogy with Eq. (4.4), the optical Doppler spectrum $G(\beta)$ over the whole detector is normalized so that

$$\int_0^\infty G(\beta)d\beta = i_{DC} \tag{4.21}$$

It then follows from Eqs. (4.4), (4.19), and (4.21) that

$$G(\beta) = n_c G_c(\beta) \tag{4.22}$$

and then it follows, by combining Eqs. (4.10), (4.11), (4.20), and (4.22), that the Doppler power spectrum generated by the whole detector is expressed as

$$P_D(f) = \begin{cases} \frac{2}{n_c}(G*G)(f) & \text{for} \quad f > 0 \\ 0 & \text{for} \quad f \leq 0 \end{cases} \tag{4.23}$$

In Figure 4.3, the effect of an increased velocity (panel a) and an increased RBC tissue fraction (panel b) on the Doppler power spectrum is shown. It can be seen that an increased velocity broadens the spectrum, whereas an increased RBC tissue fraction first increases the power for all frequencies > 0 Hz, and for high tissue fractions, also causes a significant broadening because of multiple Doppler shifts.

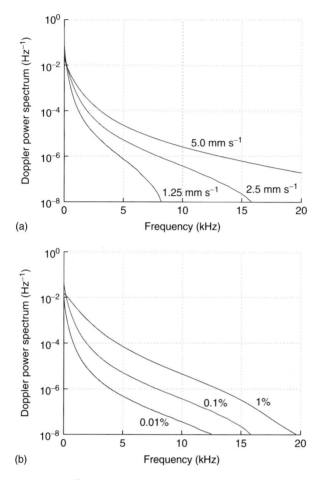

(a)

(b)

Figure 4.3 Effect on the Doppler power spectrum for increased velocity (a) and increased RBC tissue fraction (b).

These spectra are based on Monte Carlo simulations of a static homogeneous medium with $\mu_a = 0.1\,\text{mm}^{-1}$, $\mu_s = 13\,\text{mm}^{-1}$, and $g = 0.85$ containing RBCs in blood (435 g RBC per l blood, hematocrit (HCT) = 42%) with $\mu_a = 0.5\,\text{mm}^{-1}$, $\mu_s = 222\,\text{mm}^{-1}$, and $g = 0.991$ (a Gegenbauer kernel phase function with $\alpha_{\text{Gk}} = 1.0$ and $g_{\text{Gk}} = 0.948$). The optical Doppler spectra $G(\beta)$ were given by the simulation, and the Doppler power spectra calculated using Eq. (4.13). In Figure 4.3a, the RBC tissue fraction is 0.1 g RBC/100 g tissue (or percentage) and the RBC velocity shown on the x-axis is the mean velocity of a rectangular velocity distribution between zero and twice that mean velocity. In Figure 4.3b, the velocity of the RBCs is evenly distributed between 0 and 5 mm s^{-1}. The fiber separation is 0.25 mm, and both emitting and receiving fibers have a core diameter of 0.125 mm and a numerical aperture (NA) = 0.37.

4.2
Conventional Measures

The conventional perfusion measure is calculated as the first moment of the Doppler power spectrum normalized with i^2_{DC} [7]

$$S_{perf} = \frac{\int_{-\infty}^{\infty} f P_D(f) df}{i^2_{DC}} \tag{4.24}$$

Note that $P_D(f) = 0$ for $f \le 0$ (Eq. (4.15)). Similarly, an RBC tissue fraction estimate is calculated as

$$S_{CMBC} = \frac{\int_{-\infty}^{\infty} P_D(f) df}{i^2_{DC}} \tag{4.25}$$

where CMBC is a commonly used abbreviation for concentration of moving RBCs. The meaning of these measures was first evaluated by Bonner and Nossal [6]. The evaluation in this section is based on Larsson *et al.* [36] and has been partly presented earlier in [38]. A homogeneous medium is assumed.

First, Beer–Lambert's law lets us estimate the fraction of non-Doppler-shifted photons

$$\zeta_0 \approx e^{-\langle d \rangle \zeta_{RBC} \mu_{s,RBC}} \tag{4.26}$$

where $\langle d \rangle$ is the average path length, ζ_{RBC} is the tissue fraction of RBCs, and $\mu_{s,RBC}$ is the scattering coefficient of the RBCs. Since we really have a distribution of path lengths, this is only an approximation that introduces significant errors; but it is enough for the examination in this section. We also define the fraction of Doppler-shifted photons $\zeta_D = 1 - \zeta_0$ and introduce

$$H(\beta) = \frac{G(\beta) \left(1 - \delta \left(\beta - \beta_L\right)\right)}{i_{DC} \zeta_D} \tag{4.27}$$

where δ is Dirac's delta function. Note that $\int_{-\infty}^{\infty} H(\beta) d\beta = 1$. Furthermore, $G(\beta)$ is divided into one non-Doppler-shifted part $G_0(\beta)$ and one Doppler-shifted part $G_D(\beta)$ as in (Eq. (4.4))

$$\begin{cases} G_0(\beta) = i_{DC} \zeta_0 \delta \left(\beta - \beta_L\right) \\ G_D(\beta) = i_{DC} \zeta_D H(\beta) \end{cases} \tag{4.28}$$

By using Eq. (4.23), $P_D(f)$ can then be rewritten as

$$\begin{aligned} P_D(f) &= 2n_c^{-1}(G \star G)(f) \\ &= 2n_c^{-1}\left((G_0 + G_D) \star (G_0 + G_D)\right)(f) \\ &= 2n_c^{-1}\left(\underbrace{(G_0 \star G_0)(f)}_{\text{stationary}} + 2\underbrace{(G_0 \star G_D)(f)}_{\text{heterodyne}} + \underbrace{(G_D \star G_D)(f)}_{\text{homodyne}} \right) \end{aligned} \tag{4.29}$$

for $f > 0$. The stationary, heterodyne, and homodyne terms can be rewritten as

$$(G_0 * G_0)(f) = \int_{-\infty}^{\infty} G_0(\beta)G_0(\beta + f)d\beta$$

$$= i_{DC}^2 \zeta_0^2 \int_{-\infty}^{\infty} \delta(\beta - \beta_L)\delta(\beta - \beta_L + f)\, d\beta$$

$$= i_{DC}^2 \zeta_0^2 \delta(f)$$

$$= 0 \text{ for } f > 0 \qquad (4.30)$$

$$(G_0 * G_D)(f) = \int_{-\infty}^{\infty} G_0(\beta)G_D(\beta + f)d\beta$$

$$= i_{DC}^2 \zeta_0 \zeta_D \int_{-\infty}^{\infty} \delta(\beta - \beta_L)H(\beta + f)d\beta$$

$$= i_{DC}^2 \zeta_0 \zeta_D H(\beta_L + f) \qquad (4.31)$$

$$(G_D * G_D)(f) = \int_{-\infty}^{\infty} G_D(\beta)G_D(\beta + f)d\beta$$

$$= i_{DC}^2 \zeta_D^2 \int_{-\infty}^{\infty} H(\beta)H(\beta + f)d\beta \qquad (4.32)$$

Inserting Eqs. (4.30–4.32) into Eq. (4.29) gives

$$P_D(f) = 2n_c^{-1}i_{DC}^2 \left(2\zeta_0 \zeta_D H(\beta_L + f) + \zeta_D^2 \int_{-\infty}^{\infty} H(\beta)H(\beta + f)d\beta \right) \qquad (4.33)$$

for $f > 0$. Inserting this result into Eq. (4.25) yields

$$s_{CMBC} = \frac{\int_{-\infty}^{\infty} P_D(f)df}{i_{DC}^2}$$

$$= \frac{2i_{DC}^2}{n_c i_{DC}^2} \left(2\zeta_0 \zeta_D \int_{-\infty}^{\infty} H(\beta_L + f)\, df \right.$$

$$\left. + \zeta_D^2 \int_{-\infty}^{\infty} \int_{-\infty}^{\infty} H(\beta)H(\beta + f)d\beta\, df \right)$$

$$= \frac{2}{n_c} \left(2\zeta_0 \zeta_D + \zeta_D^2 \int_{-\infty}^{\infty} H(\beta) \int_{-\infty}^{\infty} H(\beta + f)df\, d\beta \right)$$

$$= \frac{2}{n_c} \left(2\zeta_0 \zeta_D + \zeta_D^2 \int_{-\infty}^{\infty} H(\beta)d\beta \right)$$

$$= \frac{2}{n_c} \left(2\zeta_0 \zeta_D + \zeta_D^2 \right)$$

$$= \frac{2}{n_c} \left(1 - \zeta_0^2 \right)$$

$$\approx \underbrace{\frac{2}{n_c}}_{A} \underbrace{\left(1 - e^{-2\langle d \rangle c_{RBC}\mu_{s,RBC}} \right)}_{B} \qquad (4.34)$$

and similarly when inserted into Eq. (4.24)

$$
s_{\text{perf}} = \frac{\int_{-\infty}^{\infty} f P_D(f) df}{i_{\text{DC}}^2}
$$

$$
= \langle f \rangle \frac{\int_{-\infty}^{\infty} P_D(f) df}{i_{\text{DC}}^2}
$$

$$
\approx \underbrace{\langle f \rangle}_{\mathbb{C}} \ \underbrace{\frac{2}{n_c}}_{\mathbb{A}} \ \underbrace{\left(1 - e^{-2\langle d \rangle c_{\text{RBC}} \mu_{\text{s,RBC}}}\right)}_{\mathbb{B}} \tag{4.35}
$$

where $\langle f \rangle$ is the average frequency of $P_D(f)$. To understand the meaning of s_{CMBC} and s_{perf}, each of the terms $\mathbb{A}$, $\mathbb{B}$, and $\mathbb{C}$ are now analyzed. Term $\mathbb{A}$ is constant as long as n_c is constant, which may not be the case in an LDPI system (see Section 4.3). In practice, i_{AC} and i_{DC} are often processed separately, giving two different amplifications of the signals, which implies that the term $\mathbb{A}$ may rather be $\left(2k_{\text{AC}}^2\right)/\left(n_c k_{\text{DC}}^2\right)$ Term $\mathbb{B}$ can be rewritten using the MacLaurin series expansion of e, that is, $e^x = 1 + x/1! + x^2/2! + \cdots$ For low RBC tissue fractions, $\mathbb{B}$ can thus be approximated to $2\langle d \rangle c_{\text{RBC}} \mu_{\text{s,RBC}}$, which is linear to the RBC tissue fraction. For higher RBC tissue fractions, higher order moments of the MacLaurin series have to be considered, introducing nonlinearities. This leads to an underestimation of the CMBC and perfusion values for higher RBC tissue fractions. Furthermore, the path length generally decreases when the RBC tissue fraction increases [40], making the underestimation even worse.

We know from Eq. (4.1) that the size of each Doppler shift is linearly dependent on the velocity of the moving RBC. Therefore, term C will be linearly dependent on the RMS velocity of RBCs [6], under the assumption that everything else is constant and the bandwidth of the system is wide enough. However, the average frequency increases when the photons are Doppler shifted multiple times, which they are to a greater extent when the RBC tissue fraction is high. This compensates the nonlinearities introduced in term $\mathbb{B}$ to some extent, but not entirely.

In conclusion, CMBC reflects the concentration (tissue fraction) of moving RBCs and the perfusion value reflects the tissue fraction of RBCs times their average velocity. It can also be noted that since s_{CMBC} and s_{perf} are normalized with i_{DC}^2, they are independent of the total detected light intensity. The relationship between the tissue fraction of RBCs in a homogeneous medium and simulated s_{CMBC} and s_{perf} are shown in Figure 4.4. The simulated setup was the same as described at the end of Section 4.1.2. The velocity of the RBCs in the medium was evenly distributed between 0 and 5 mm s^{-1}. In this figure, the nonlinear behavior of not only s_{CMBC} but also s_{perf} becomes evident. It must be emphasized that the nonlinearity is strongly dependent on the geometry and optical properties of the medium and therefore cannot be easily accounted for, as suggested in [7].

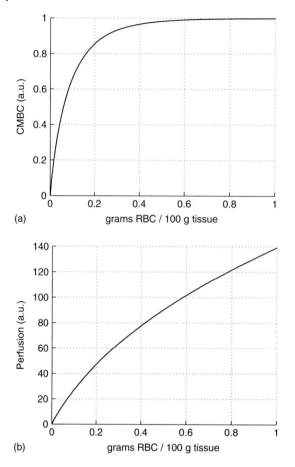

(a)

(b)

Figure 4.4 Relationship between RBC tissue fraction and s_{CMBC} (a) and s_{perf} (b).

4.3
Hardware Realizations

As stated at the beginning of this chapter, both single point (LDPM) and imaging (LDPI) LDF systems exist. In this section, the special characteristics of these systems, as well as a newer type of imaging system based on fast CMOS cameras, are described. Noise reduction and typical calibration procedures are also described.

4.3.1
LDPM

In single point systems, optical fibers are typically used to guide the light from the laser source to the tissue and from the tissue to the detector. Most often, separate fibers are used, but a single fiber can also be used when a very small

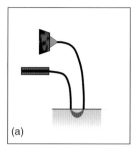 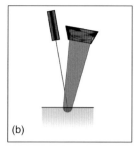 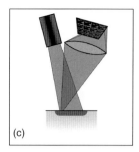

Figure 4.5 Schematic illustrations of the various LDF modalities, LDPM (a), LDPI (b), and CMOS imager (c).

measurement volume is wanted [40]. The most common source–detector distance in probes provided by the two leading manufacturers of LDF instruments (Perimed AB, Järfälla, Sweden, and Moor Instruments Ltd., Axminster, UK) is 0.25 mm. Generally, short source–detector distances have been preferred to limit the measurement depth, to improve signal to noise and to avoid a high degree of multiple Doppler shifts leading to severe nonlinearities in the conventional CMBC and perfusion measures.

In a fiber-based system, the detector fiber illuminates the detector at a certain distance between the fiber tip and the detector (Figure 4.5a). The illuminating angle is constant and determined from the numerical aperture of the fiber, under the reasonable assumption that the light impinging on the fiber has a uniform angle distribution. During these conditions, the number of coherence areas on the detector is constant (Eq. (4.18)), and the DC-squared normalized Doppler power spectrum $P_D(f)/i_{DC}^2$ will only depend on the optical spectrum $G(\beta)$ (Eq. (4.23)).

Another type of LDPM system, not based on fibers, also exists, where the optics and electronics are built on a single probe or chip that is in direct contact with the tissue [41]. These systems are less sensitive to movements and can therefore be used under less-controlled situations, but at low perfusion levels, the signal-to-noise ratio is lower due to the shorter coherence length of the lasers used.

4.3.2
LDPI

In a conventional imaging system (Figure 4.5b), a laser beam is scanned over the tissue of interest to form an image. In each scanning position, the perfusion value is calculated and transformed into a pixel value, and the scanning procedure lasts for a couple of minutes to form an entire image. The detector is typically placed some 20–30 cm above the tissue surface. In some systems, a lens focuses the light on the detector.

The backscattered light from the impinging laser beam escapes the tissue from a spot centered on the point of injection, with a radially decaying intensity. The slope of the decay, and thus the apparent spot size, is strongly dependent on the absorption properties of the tissue. The spot size, by itself, reduces the calculated perfusion value since it affects the solid angle to the detector points. Since an increased RBC tissue fraction increases the total absorption of the tissue and thus reduces the spot size, the increase in the estimated CMBC and perfusion will be underestimated. The effect, which is explained below, is similar for both systems with and without a light-focusing lens in front of the detector [42].

For simplicity, assume that the backscattered light exits the tissue in a homogenous spot. For a system without a lens in front of the detector, the solid angle between the spot and each point on the detector varies with the square of the radius r of the spot (Eq. (4.17)). As given by Eq. (4.35), the perfusion value is inversely proportional to the number of coherence areas n_c, which in turn is linearly dependent on r^2 (Eqs. 4.16–4.18). Therefore, the calculated perfusion value is inversely proportional to r^2 for a system without a lens.

For a system with a light-focusing lens, the solid angle is determined by the dimension and position of the lens and is thus independent of the spot size. However, as the lens focuses the light on the detector, the illuminated part of the detector will directly depend on the size of the spot, under the assumption that the entire spot is imaged on the detector. Therefore, the "active" detector area will depend on r^2 and the calculated perfusion value is inversely proportional to r^2 also for a system with a lens.

4.3.3
CMOS Imager

A conventional LDPI system has the drawbacks that it is slow and that the estimated perfusion value is affected by the spot size of backreflected light. Both these drawbacks are addressed with the new generation of LDPI systems, which are based on fast CMOS cameras [43, 49]. In these systems, the backscattered light is focused on a detector array, where every pixel in the array is used to calculate a perfusion value from the part of the tissue that the pixel sees (Figure 4.5c). By simultaneously illuminating the whole tissue area of interest, the whole image is acquired simultaneously, which is naturally faster than scanning the area point by point. Every pixel in the array also has a constant solid angle (based on the lens), and they can be assumed to be evenly illuminated, so the perfusion value is independent of the spot size.

The major drawback with these systems is that the cameras used are not yet fast enough. A normal Doppler power spectrum has frequency components of significant power up to about 15 kHz. The sample frequency thus has to be at least 30 kHz to collect the entire frequency content of the Doppler signal and avoid aliasing. The system presented in [43] operated with a sampling frequency of only 8 kHz, which will have the effect that when the velocity of the RBCs is increased, a substantial part of the energy in the Doppler power spectrum will exceed 4 kHz and the expected increase in the perfusion value will be underestimated, or the perfusion value may even decrease.

4.3.4
Noise

Various types of noise influence the Doppler power spectrum. Some of this noise originates from variations in background light intensity and common mode noise. To get rid of this latter type of noise, a differential detector technique is often used for i_{AC}, which simply calculates the difference between the light falling on two adjacent detectors. By calculating the difference, common noise is cancelled out, whereas the statistical properties of the two separate realizations of i_{AC} remain [5].

However, other types of noise are not removed by this technique. The amplitude of shot noise, which is a variation in photoelectron emission rate of the detector, is linearly dependent on the total detector current i_{DC}, whereas thermal noise is constant as long as the temperature is held constant [44]. Consequently, an expression of these types of noise can be established

$$P_{noise}\left(f, i_{DC}\right) = k_{noise}(f)i_{DC} + l_{noise}(f) \tag{4.36}$$

where the parameter k_{noise} relates to the shot noise and l_{noise} to the thermal noise.

4.3.5
Calibration

Two different objectives are reached when calibrating an LDF system. First, the noise parameters k_{noise} and l_{noise} in Eq. (4.36) are calculated. This is done by measuring the signal at different DC levels on a static scattering object, that is, an object without any moving scatterers, such as a piece of white plastic. The noise perfusion value is then calculated and subtracted from the measured perfusion values during the normal measurements.

Second, a reference perfusion value is measured. In the Periflux 5000 system (Perimed AB, Järfälla, Sweden), this is achieved by placing the measurement probe in a motility standard such as a beaker containing a certain concentration of polystyrene microspheres diluted in water. Owing to Brownian motion, these microspheres, acting as scatterers, move with a certain velocity distribution, which is dependent on the temperature. Thus, all backscattered light is Doppler shifted, and in the case of the Periflux 5000 system, the perfusion level measured in this setup is set to 250 pu (perfusion units) at 22 °C. Since this is a repeatable procedure, all other perfusion values can be compared. Other systems have similar calibration routines.

A slightly different calibration procedure is presented in [45]. First, the noise spectrum $P_{noise}\left(f, i_{DC}\right)$ is subtracted directly from the Doppler power spectrum $P_D(f)$. Second, the resulting Doppler power spectrum is normalized with the CMBC from the motility measurement, which is calculated as

$$s_{CMBC,mot} = \frac{\int_{-\infty}^{\infty} \left(P_{mot}(f) - P_{noise}\left(i_{DC,mot}, f\right)\right) \, df}{i_{DC,mot}^2} \tag{4.37}$$

Thus, the calibrated Doppler power spectrum is calculated as

$$P_D'(f) = \frac{\left(P_D(f) - P_{noise}\left(i_{DC}, f\right)\right)/i_{DC}^2}{s_{CMBC,mot}} \qquad (4.38)$$

The modification of the second calibration step provides a unity CMBC where all the detected light is Doppler shifted (see Eq. (4.34)). The measured Doppler power spectra can thus be easily compared to simulated spectra. Another positive consequence of this is that the second calibration step can be performed with any scattering liquid in which Brownian motion is present. The calibration is not limited to expensive motility standard that has to be exchanged from time to time, and it is independent of the temperature.

4.3.6
Measurement Depth and Volume

For an accurate physiological interpretation of the perfusion estimate, it is important to have an estimate of the depth or volume that most of the signal originates from. It is common to hear that the measurement volume is about $1\,mm^3$ or the measurement depth is in the order of 1 mm, but depending on system properties as well as optical properties of the measured tissue, blood tissue fraction and flow distribution in the tissue, the actual measurement volume, or measurement depth can vary manifold.

Over the years, only two publications have focused on this problem, namely, Jakobsson and Nilsson 1993 [46] and Fredriksson *et al.* 2009 [40]. In both these publications, an important distinction is made between sampling depth/volume and measurement depth/volume. While the sampling depth/volume reveals where the detected light has been propagating, the measurement depth/volume reveals where the perfusion signal has been affected. Since the perfusion signal is to a major extent only affected by moving RBCs, this is an important distinction and the measurement depth/volume can differ significantly from the sampling depth/volume.

Both the articles mentioned above are based on Monte Carlo simulations. Fredriksson *et al.* accounted for multiple Doppler shifts and speckle effects that affect the measurement depth/volume in LDPI. In Tables 4.1 and 4.2, typical measurement depths for some common laser Doppler wavelengths, source–fiber separations (for LDPM), and beam diameters (for LDPI) are shown for some different tissue types. The measurement depth is defined so that $1 - e^{-1} \approx 63\%$ of the perfusion value originates above that depth. An in depth discussion about how different system parameters, optical properties, and other tissue properties affect the measurement depth and volume as well as further examples on both measurement depth and volume can be found in [40].

Table 4.1 Measurement depth in millimeters for muscle, liver, as well as gray and white matter for the wavelengths 543, 633, and 780 nm.

LDPM fiber separation/LDPI beam Ø (mm)	Muscle			Liver			Gray matter			White matter		
	543	633	780	543	633	780	543	633	780	543	633	780
LDPM 0.0	0.10	0.18	0.19	0.046	0.11	0.13	0.088	0.15	0.16	0.064	0.092	0.099
LDPM 0.25	0.23	0.48	0.55	0.11	0.31	0.40	0.21	0.43	0.48	0.12	0.19	0.20
LDPM 0.50	0.29	0.62	0.73	0.14	0.40	0.52	0.27	0.58	0.64	0.17	0.27	0.28
LDPM 1.2	0.40	0.83	0.96	0.19	0.56	0.71	0.37	0.79	0.86	0.26	0.45	0.46
LDPI 0.5	0.19	0.60	0.79	0.053	0.23	0.53	0.17	0.48	0.68	0.10	0.17	0.20
LDPI 2.0	0.24	0.73	0.92	0.054	0.32	0.66	0.21	0.59	0.81	0.12	0.22	0.26

Table 4.2 Measurement depth in millimeters for skin on index finger pulp and volar side of the forearm both at rest and at 44 °C heat provocation.

LDPM fiber separation/LDPI beam Ø (mm)		Index finger			Forearm unprovoked			Forearm provoked		
		543	633	780	543	633	780	543	633	780
LDPM	0.0	0.31	0.33	0.35	0.43	0.48	0.52	0.52	0.60	0.65
LDPM	0.25	0.32	0.35	0.41	0.44	0.49	0.53	0.53	0.61	0.66
LDPM	0.50	0.34	0.36	0.50	0.45	0.50	0.55	0.54	0.61	0.67
LDPM	1.2	0.40	0.53	0.85	0.50	0.56	0.70	0.58	0.66	0.73
LDPI	0.5	0.33	0.36	0.53	0.44	0.50	0.56	0.53	0.62	0.67
LDPI	2.0	0.34	0.39	0.68	0.46	0.52	0.63	0.55	0.64	0.70

4.4
Monte Carlo and LDF

Although the Doppler effect is a light wave phenomenon, the Monte Carlo technique that is based on the particle representation of light has been used throughout this chapter to quantify the Doppler power spectrum from a simulated medium. This may seem contradictory. However, each individual Doppler shift is calculated using the wave representation of light and the Doppler shift of each photon is then stored as an extra attribute of the photon in the Monte Carlo simulation [34]. The calculation of the Doppler power spectrum is based on the optical Doppler spectrum, which is given from the distribution of photons with different total

Doppler shifts. In summary, the photons in the Monte Carlo simulations behave as information carriers, but both the individual Doppler shifts and the resulting Doppler power spectra are calculated using light wave theory, using input from the information-carrying photons.

It has frequently been shown that Doppler power spectra calculated with the aid of Monte Carlo simulations correlate with *ex vivo* measurements for LDPM [47, 48, 50, 51]. Recently, it has been shown that they correlate well with *in vivo* measurements [37]. For LDPI, on the other hand, speckle effects also have to be considered [40].

References

1. Forrester, A.T. (1961) Photoelectric mixing as a spectroscopic tool. *J. Opt. Soc. Am.*, **51** (3), 253–259.
2. Cummins, H.Z., Knable, N., and Yeh, Y. (1964) Observation of diffusion broadening of Rayleigh scattered light. *Phys. Rev. Lett.*, **12**, 150–153.
3. Stern, M.D. (1975) In vivo evaluation of microcirculation by coherent light scattering. *Nature*, **254** (5495), 56–58.
4. Holloway, G.A. Jr. and Watkins, D.W. (1977) Laser Doppler measurement of cutaneous blood flow. *J. Invest. Dermatol.*, **69** (3), 306–309.
5. Nilsson, G.E., Tenland, T., and Öberg, P.A.A. (1980) A new instrument for continuous measurement of tissue blood flow by light beating spectroscopy. *IEEE Trans. Biomed. Eng.*, **27** (1), 12–19.
6. Bonner, R. and Nossal, R. (1981) Model for laser Doppler measurements of blood flow in tissue. *Appl. Opt.*, **20** (12), 2097–2107.
7. Nilsson, G.E. (1984) Signal processor for laser Doppler tissue flowmeters. *Med. Biol. Eng. Comput.*, **22** (4), 343–348.
8. Nilsson, G.E., Jakobsson, A., and Wårdell, K. (1989) Imaging of tissue blood flow by coherent light scattering. Engineering in Medicine and Biology Society, 1989. Images of the Twenty-First Century. Proceedings of the Annual International Conference of the IEEE Engineering, Vol. 2, pp. 391–392.
9. Essex, T.J.H. and Byrne, P.O. (1991) A laser Doppler scanner for imaging blood-flow in skin. *J. Biomed. Eng.*, **13** (3), 189–194.
10. Wårdell, K., Jakobsson, A., and Nilsson, G.E. (1993) Laser-Doppler perfusion imaging by dynamic light-scattering. *IEEE Trans. Biomed. Eng.*, **40** (4), 309–319.
11. Gschwandtner, M.E. *et al.* (1999) Laser Doppler imaging and capillary microscopy in ischemic ulcers. *Atherosclerosis*, **142** (1), 225–232.
12. Timar-Banu, O. *et al.* (2001) Development of noninvasive and quantitative methodologies for the assessment of chronic ulcers and scars in humans. *Wound Repair Regen.*, **9** (2), 123–132.
13. Barachini, P. *et al.* (2004) Skin blood flow pattern in burns outcomes. *Burns*, **30** (4), 312–316.
14. Holland, A.J.A., Martin, H.C.O., and Cass, D.T. (2002) Laser Doppler imaging prediction of burn wound outcome in children. *Burns*, **28** (1), 11–17.
15. Nayeri, F. *et al.* (2002) Hepatocyte growth factor may accelerate healing in chronic leg ulcers: a pilot study. *J. Dermatolog. Treat.*, **13** (2), 81–86.
16. Uhl, E. *et al.* (2003) Influence of platelet-derived growth factor on micro-circulation during normal and impaired wound healing. *Wound Repair Regen.*, **11** (5), 361–367.
17. Omar, A.A. *et al.* (2004) Treatment of venous leg ulcers with dermagraft(R). *Eur. J. Vasc. Endovasc. Surg.*, **27** (6), 666–672.
18. Johansen, J.D. *et al.* (1998) Allergens in combination have a synergistic effect on the elicitation response: a study of fragrance-sensitized individuals. *Br. J. Dermatol.*, **139** (2), 264–270.

19. Fluhr, J.W. *et al.* (2001) Testing for irritation with a multifactorial approach: comparison of eight non-invasive measuring techniques on five different irritation types. *Br. J. Dermatol.*, **145** (5), 696–703.

20. Aramaki, J. *et al.* (2001) Irritant patch testing with sodium lauryl sulphate: interrelation between concentration and exposure time. *Br. J. Dermatol.*, **145** (5), 704–708.

21. Shapiro, S.A. *et al.* (1998) Normal blood flow response and vasomotion in the diabetic charcot foot. *J. Diabetes Complicat.*, **12** (3), 147–153.

22. Skrha, J. *et al.* (2001) Comparison of laser-Doppler flowmetry with biochemical indicators of endothelial dysfunction related to early microangiopathy in Type 1 diabetic patients. *J. Diabetes Complicat.*, **15** (5), 234–240.

23. Meyer, M.F. *et al.* (2003) Impaired 0.1-Hz vasomotion assessed by laser Doppler anemometry as an early index of peripheral sympathetic neuropathy in diabetes. *Microvasc. Res.*, **65** (2), 88–95.

24. Herrick, A.L. and Clark, S. (1998) Quantifying digital vascular disease in patients with primary Raynaud's phenomenon and systemic sclerosis. *Ann. Rheum. Dis.*, **57** (2), 70–78.

25. Clark, S. *et al.* (1999) xLaser doppler imaging – a new technique for quantifying microcirculatory flow in patients with primary Raynaud's phenomenon and systemic sclerosis. *Microvasc. Res.*, **57** (3), 284–291.

26. Kanetaka, T. *et al.* (2004) Laser Doppler skin perfusion pressure in the assessment of Raynaud's phenomenon. *Eur. J. Vasc. Endovasc. Surg.*, **27** (4), 414–416.

27. Stücker, M. *et al.* (2002) High-resolution laser Doppler perfusion imaging aids in differentiating between benign and malignant melanocytic skin tumours. *Acta Derm. Venereol.*, **82** (1), 25–29.

28. Lantsberg, L. and Goldman, M. (1991) Laser Doppler flowmetry, transcutaneous oxygen tension measurements and Doppler pressure compared in patients undergoing amputation. *Eur. J. Vasc. Surg.*, **5** (2), 195–197.

29. Ray, S.A. *et al.* (1997) The predictive value of laser Doppler fluxmetry and transcutaneous oximetry for clinical outcome in patients undergoing revascularisation for severe leg ischaemia. *Eur. J. Vasc. Endovasc. Surg.*, **13** (1), 54–59.

30. Wårdell, K. *et al.* (2007) Intracerebral microvascular measurements during deep brain stimulation implantation using laser Doppler perfusion monitoring. *Stereotact. Funct. Neurosurg.*, **85** (6), 279–286.

31. Hartmann, A., Azerad, J., and Boucher, Y. (1996) Environmental effects on laser Doppler pulpal blood-flow measurements in man. *Arch. Oral Biol.*, **41** (4), 333–339.

32. Soo-ampon, S. *et al.* (2003) The sources of laser Doppler blood-flow signals recorded from human teeth. *Arch. Oral Biol.*, **48** (5), 353–360.

33. Doppler, J.C. (1842) Über das farbige Licht der Doppelsterne und einiger anderer Gestirne des Himmels [On the coloured light of the double stars and some other stars of the heavens]. *Abh. Konigl. Böhm. Ges. Wiss.*

34. Fredriksson, I., Larsson, M., and Strömberg, T. (2008) Optical microcirculatory skin model: assessed by Monte Carlo simulations paired with in vivo laser doppler flowmetry. *J. Biomed. Opt.*, **13** (1), 014015.

35. Cummins, H.Z. and Swinney, H.L. (1970) in *Progress in Optics* (ed. E. Wolf), North-Holland, Amsterdam, pp. 135–200.

36. Larsson, M. (2004) *Influence of Optical Properties on Laser Doppler Flowmetry*, Linköping University, Linköping, p. xii, 64.

37. Fredriksson, I. (2009) *Quantitative Laser Doppler Flowmetry*, Department of Biomedical Engineering, Linköping University, Linköping.

38. Fredriksson, I., Fors, C., and Johansson, J. (2012) Laser Doppler Flowmetry – A Theoretical Framework. *http://www.imt.liu.se/bit/ldf/ldf.pdf.*

39. Siegman, A.E. (1966) The antenna properties of optical heterodyne receivers. *Proc. IEEE*, **54** (10), 1350–1356.

40. Fredriksson, I., Larsson, M., and Stromberg, T. (2009) Measurement

depth and volume in laser Doppler flowmetry. *Microvasc. Res.*, **78** (1), 4–13.

41. Serov, A.N., Nieland, J., and Oosterbaan, S. *et al.* (2006) Integrated optoelectronic probe including a vertical cavity surface emitting laser for laser Doppler perfusion monitoring. *IEEE Trans. Biomed. Eng.*, **53** (10), 2067–2074.

42. Rajan, V. *et al.* (2006) Speckles in laser Doppler perfusion imaging. *Opt. Lett.*, **31** (4), 468–470.

43. Serov, A. and Lasser, T. (2006) Full-field high-speed laser Doppler imaging system for blood-flow measurements. *Proc. SPIE*, **6080**, 608004, 1–8.

44. Karlsson, M.G.D. (2005) *Movement Artifact Reduction in Laser Doppler Blood Flowmetry: Myocardial Perfusion Applications*, Department of Biomedical Engineering, Linköpings Universitet, Linköping, p. xii, 84.

45. Fredriksson, I., Larsson, M., Salomonsson, F., and Strömberg, T. (2011) Improved calibration procedure for laser Doppler perfusion monitors. in *Proc. SPIE*, 7906.

46. Jakobsson, A. and Nilsson, G.E. (1993) Prediction of sampling depth and photon pathlength in laser Doppler flowmetry. *Med. Biol. Eng. Comput.*, **31** (3), 301–307.

47. de Mul, F.F.M. *et al.* (1995) Laser-Doppler velocimetry and monte-carlo simulations on models for blood perfusion in tissue. *Appl. Opt.*, **34** (28), 6595–6611.

48. Kienle, A. *et al.* (1996) Determination of the scattering coefficient and the anisotropy factor from laser Doppler spectra of liquids including blood. *Appl. Opt.*, **35** (19), 3404–3412.

49. Serov, A.N. *et al.* (2003) Quasi-parallel laser-Doppler perfusion imaging using a CMOS image sensor, *Proc. SPIE*, **5067**, 73–84.

50. Larsson, M., Steenbergen, W., and Strömberg, N.O.T. (2002) Influence of optical properties and fiber separation on laser Doppler flowmetry. *J. Biomed. Opt.*, **7** (2), 236–243.

51. Larsson, M. and Strömberg, N.O.T. (2006) Toward a velocity-resolved microvascular blood flow measure by decomposition of the laser Doppler power spectrum. *J. Biomed. Opt.*, **11** (1), 014024.

5

Toward Assessment of Speed Distribution of Red Blood Cells in Microcirculation

Adam Liebert, Stanislaw Wojtkiewicz, and Roman Maniewski

5.1
Introduction

Laser Doppler flowmetry remains a prospective technique of microcirculation assessment. Despite serious advancements of the instrumentation [1, 2] and successes of clinical tests [3, 4] of the methodology, the laser Doppler systems are mostly used for research applications and not for routine clinical examinations. In recent decades, modern optical, electronic, and fiber optic techniques combined with advanced signal processing were applied in order to provide depth-resolved perfusion assessment [5–8] and imaging of perfusion of large tissue area [9–11] based on the laser Doppler technique. Since the microvasculature is a complex system that depends on multiple physical and physiological factors (such as hematocrit, psychological state of the subject, ambient temperature, humidity, etc.) the procedures for measurement of perfusion need standardization. In most clinical studies, stimulation tests are applied, which allow the changes of the relative signals measured to be obtained. However, even the interindividual repeatability of such measurements carried out in clinical conditions may be rather low because of the influence of the above-mentioned factors. This effect, together with the lack of absolute calibration of the signals, represents obstacles for acceptance of the laser Doppler perfusion assessment technique in clinical practice.

The perfusion assessed by laser Doppler flowmetry represents a product of speed and concentration of the moving red blood cells averaged in the volume interrogated by the photons traveling from the source to the detector [12]. It was shown that the perfusion signal depends on the optical properties of the medium under investigation [13]. It was also proposed that the signal can be normalized by a quantity related to the volume through which the laser light passes. Such a procedure may lead to strict dependence of the signals on perfusion of the tissue [14, 15].

Classical signal processing used in laser Doppler perfusion measurements is based on an evaluation of the first moment of the AC component of the power spectral density of the optical signal remitted from the tissue. It was shown that the first moment is linearly related to the perfusion of the tissue [16]. However, the absolute value of the speed and concentration of the red blood cells remains unknown. The spectrum of the laser Doppler signal contains information on the speed distribution of the particles moving in the volume interrogated by the photons traveling from the source to the detector [17], and this information can be extracted by appropriate processing [18–20]. The processing technique is based on spectral decomposition using the Doppler frequency shift probability distribution obtained for a single Doppler scattering event. Considering a single Doppler scattering event, it can be shown that this probability depends only on distributions of the scattering angle and the angle between direction of the photon and the particle. In consequence, assuming that the last angle is random and the scattering angle probability distribution can be estimated by the Henyey–Greenstein phase function, the Doppler frequency shift probability distribution for a single Doppler scattering event can be calculated by Monte Carlo simulations. It can also be derived analytically, which makes the procedure much faster. The measured laser Doppler spectrum represents superposition of spectra formed by the distribution of Doppler frequency shifts scaled along frequency axis for different speeds of the moving particles. The system of linear equations formed by summing these distributions can be solved in order to assess the distribution of speed of the moving particles. Moreover, a theoretical basis for the evaluation of spectra obtained in a multiple scattering regime was proposed. However, the inverse solution problem becomes ill-posed, and the system of equations is very difficult to solve for the multiple scattering regime. The method of laser Doppler spectrum decomposition was validated using Monte Carlo simulations by generation of laser Doppler spectra for assumed distributions of speed of moving particles. The method was also tested in phantom experiments. Finally, the speed distributions were obtained for red blood cells moving in a microvascular network during venous and arterial occlusion as well as during thermal stimulation of the tissue.

5.2
Theory of Laser Doppler Spectrum Decomposition

5.2.1
Single Doppler Scattering

The theory described below is based on several assumptions that were used previously to show that the laser Doppler perfusion signals are linearly related to the concentration of red blood cells and their speed [16, 21]. The most critical assumption is that the concentration of red blood cells is small and, in consequence, that the probability that a single photon will undergo more than one Doppler scattering event during its travel between source and detector is very small. This assumption leads to the observation that the first moment of the spectrum of the laser Doppler signal is related to the perfusion of the tissue. With this assumption, we consider the spectrum of the laser Doppler signal, which can be measured for a medium filled with particles moving at single speed, but with random direction of movement. The geometry of a single Doppler scattering event is presented in Figure 5.1.

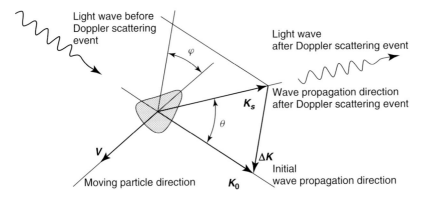

Figure 5.1 Geometry of a laser Doppler scattering event occurring at a moving particle [22].

The frequency shift that is caused by such a scattering event occurring on a particle moving with speed V is expressed by the following formula:

$$\Delta f = \frac{2nV}{\lambda} \sin\left(\frac{\theta}{2}\right) \cos\varphi \tag{5.1}$$

where φ is an angle between directions of the photon and the moving particle, θ is the scattering angle, λ is the wavelength, and n is the refractive index of the medium, assuming that

- the directions of the photons are random
- the particles move in random directions
- particles move with speed V
- photon can undergo only one Doppler shift scattering event

The spectrum of the laser Doppler signal represents a distribution of probability called Doppler shift probability distribution (DSPD). As can be noted from Eq. (5.1), this probability distribution depends only on the distributions of the scattering angle θ and the angle between the direction of the photon and the direction of the particle φ. The first angle depends on anisotropy of the scattering in the medium. Commonly, the light scattering in the tissue is described by a phase function proposed by Henyey and Greenstein for the assessment of scattering angle distribution during light penetration through interstellar clouds [23]. It was reported that this phase function can be used to estimate the scattering angle distribution for living tissues [24]. Actually, for tissue optics, the original Henyey–Greenstein phase functions need a small modification [25–27], that is, multiplication by sine of scattering angle θ

$$f_\Theta(\theta) = \frac{\left(1 - g^2\right) \sin\theta}{2\left(1 + g^2 - 2g\cos\theta\right)^{3/2}} \quad \text{if} \quad \theta \in [0; \pi] \tag{5.2}$$

where $g \in [-1; 1]$ is an anisotropy factor. This ensures that for isotropic scattering ($g = 0$), the number of photons scattered per solid angle remains constant.

The Henyey–Greenstein function is heuristic and its parameter g, called the *anisotropy factor*, is equal to the mean cosine of the scattering angle

$$g = \int_0^{4\pi} f_\Theta(\theta) \cos\theta \, d\varpi \tag{5.3}$$

The second angle φ can be assumed to be random, which means that its probability distribution is uniform. This assumption is rather strong in microvascular networks. The directions of movement of red blood cells are not random and are determined by the geometry of the microvessels. However, considering that the photons are diffusely distributed in the tissue and their travel distances are longer than inverse of scattering coefficient,the assumption that angles between photons and moving particles are uniformly distributed is reasonable.

It can be noted from Eq. (5.1) that the maximum frequency shift related to the Doppler scattering event is

$$\Delta f_{max} = \frac{2nV_{max}}{\lambda} \tag{5.4}$$

and the amplitude of the Doppler shift for a single photon may have values between 0 and Δf_{max}. The probability distribution of Doppler shifts obtained for a large set of photons depends only on angles θ and φ. It should be noted that for a Doppler scattering event occurring with high anisotropy of light scattering, the sine term in Eq. (5.1) is much smaller than one ($\sin(\theta/2) \ll 1$). Such a situation is typical for scattering of light on red blood cells, for which anisotropy factor is estimated to be about 0.98–0.99 [24]. Thus, for such scattering events, the Doppler frequency shift is usually lower than Δf_{max} for interactions with particle moving at speed greater than V_{max}. This effect should be taken into consideration when defining maximum speed of moving particles $V_{max} = \lambda\Delta f_{max}/2n$ (see Eq. (5.4)), which can be observed in the laser Doppler power density spectra.

The dependence of DSPDs on speed V and concentration of moving particles can be assessed with the use of Monte Carlo simulations (see Figure 5.2). It can be clearly noted that Δf_{max} is related to V and that the amplitude of the DSPDs depends on the concentration of particles c. Spectra shown in Figure 5.2b contain photons that undergo only single Doppler scattering event. The other photons undergoing multiple Doppler scattering were omitted. For large concentration of moving particles, the influence of the number of photons that undergo higher-order Doppler scattering events is significant. Thus, it should be noted that in this case, there is no linear relation between the integral of detected spectra and concentration of moving particles.

The shape of the distribution depends on shape of the scattering angle phase function. The phase function for moving particles can be approximated by Henyey–Greenstein phase function [24], Gegenbauer kernel phase function [28], or Mie theory [29]. In Figure 5.3, DSPD shapes are presented for different anisotropy factors. These shapes were calculated for a Henyey–Greenstein phase function given in Eq. (5.2). It can be noted that for high g values, which are typical for a living tissue [24], the DSPDs become very steep, whereas for low g values, the distribution is rather flat. With the assumption that the Henyey–Greenstein phase function

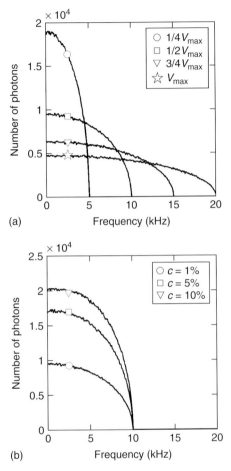

(a)

(b)

Figure 5.2 Dependence of Doppler shift probability distribution on (a) speed and (b) concentration of moving particles in a highly scattering medium with few moving particles, that is, the number of scattering events is much greater than the number of Doppler shift scattering events. Results of Monte Carlo simulations performed for semi-infinite medium, source–detector separation $r = 1$ mm, and laser light wavelength $\lambda = 780$ nm and optical properties of the medium: scattering coefficient $\mu_s = 2$ mm^{-1}, absorption coefficient $\mu_a = 0.01$ mm^{-1}, anisotropy factor $g = 0$, and refractive index $n = 1.4$.

defined in Eq. (5.2) can be applied to the estimation of scattering angle distribution, the DSPDs denoted by h for assumed particle speed V can be calculated analytically [19]. It can be assumed that anisotropy of light scattering on moving particles is high, which leads to small scattering angle θ. As mentioned above, in such cases, the scattering events occurring on particles moving with maximal speed may significantly influence the observed power density spectra. Thus, DSPDs h should be calculated for maximum frequency shift higher than Δf_{max}, and the first part of the h distribution up to Δf_{max} should be taken for further calculations. For

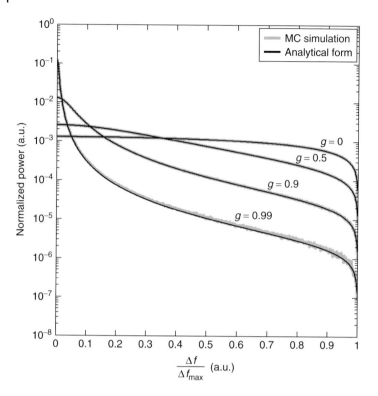

Figure 5.3 Shape of the Doppler shift probability distributions for different values of anisotropy factor *g* of the scattering on moving particles.

example, assuming calculation of *h* for $3\Delta f_{max}$, the DSPD for assumed anisotropy factor of moving particles $g \in [-1, 1]$, moving particles speed $V \in [0, 3V_{max}]$, tissue refractive index *n*, and laser light wavelength λ can be represented as follows:

$$h\left(V, \Delta f\right) = \begin{cases} f_Z\left(\dfrac{\lambda}{2nV}\Delta f\right) & \text{if} \quad \Delta f \in \left[0; \dfrac{2nV}{\lambda}\right] \\ 0 & \text{if} \quad \Delta f \in \left(\dfrac{2nV}{\lambda}; 3\Delta f_{max}\right] \end{cases}$$

$$f_Z\left(x\right) = \frac{4}{\pi} \cdot \frac{\left(1-g\right)\sqrt{1-x^2}}{\left(1-g\right)^2 + 4gx^2} \quad \text{if} \quad x \in [0; 1] \tag{5.5}$$

where $f_Z\left(x\right)$ is a probability distribution function of random variable $x \in [0; 1]$.

Potentially, analytical functions of DSPDs can be calculated for different scattering phase functions. However, the solutions for more complex phase functions become impossible to derive without numerical approaches. It should be noted that the Doppler frequency shift probability distributions can be calculated using numerical methods for any assumed phase function.

As can be observed in Figure 5.2, the DSPDs are scaled along the frequency axis for different speeds of the particles. On the other hand, the DSPDs are scaled along the amplitude axis with concentration of moving particles. Thus, the spectrum of the laser Doppler signal $S(\Delta f)$ can be expressed as a superposition of DSPDs calculated for different speeds $h(V, \Delta f)$. This superposition is schematically illustrated in Figure 5.4 for an assumed distribution of speeds of particles in the medium.

The superposition can be expressed by the following system of linear equations:

$$S(\Delta f_1) = c(V_1) h(V_1, \Delta f_1) + c(V_2) h(V_2, \Delta f_1) + \cdots + c(V_N) h(V_N, \Delta f_1)$$
$$S(\Delta f_2) = c(V_1) h(V_1, \Delta f_2) + c(V_2) h(V_2, \Delta f_2) + \cdots + c(V_N) h(V_N, \Delta f_2),$$
$$\vdots$$
$$S(\Delta f_M) = c(V_1) h(V_1, \Delta f_M) + c(V_2) h(V_2, \Delta f_M) + \cdots + c(V_N) h(V_N, \Delta f_M)$$
$$(5.6)$$

which can be rewritten as matrix equation

$$\mathbf{S}^T = \mathbf{c}^T \mathbf{h} \tag{5.7}$$

where row vector $\mathbf{c}$ contains concentrations $c(V)$ of particles moving with speed V.

The spectrum $\mathbf{S}$ represents the measured data normalized by its integral. The DSPDs, $\mathbf{h}$, can be calculated for assumed g of the scattering anisotropy of the

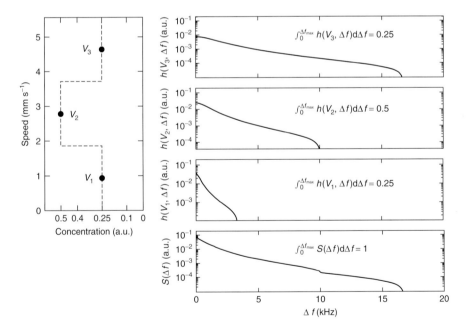

Figure 5.4 Schematic representation of Laser Doppler spectrum $S(\Delta f)$ as a superposition of Doppler shift probability distributions calculated for different speeds $h(V, \Delta f)$.

particles, refractive index n, and light wavelength λ. If the spectrum is sampled at M frequencies, the DSPDs are estimated at $3N$ speeds and sampled at $3M$ frequencies. Furthermore, the unknown moving particles speed distribution $\mathbf{c}$ is sampled at $3N$ speeds. Finally, the laser Doppler spectrum $\mathbf{S}$ corresponds to first M elements of $1 \times 3M$ size row vector $\mathbf{c}^T\mathbf{h}$. This system of equations can be solved for $N \leq M$. However, because of the similarity of the DSPDs, the problem is ill-posed and the solving process is rather difficult.

Moving particles speed distribution $\mathbf{c} = c(V)$ is expressed in arbitrary units. Integral (zeroth moment) of the laser Doppler spectrum is assumed to be proportional to the total concentration of the moving particles [12]. Typically, measured spectrum $\mathbf{S}$ and DSPDs matrix $\mathbf{h}$ are normalized by their integrals. Thus, the integral of the distribution $\mathbf{c}$ is equal 1 when the error of solution of Eq. (5.7) approaches 0. When series of spectra collected during *in vivo* measurement are acquired, the normalization of the spectra can be carried out, considering the integral of selected (or averaged) spectrum from the rest flow period as a reference spectrum. This procedure allows monitoring changes in concentration of moving particles in arbitrary units.

5.2.2
Multiple Scattering

In classical laser Doppler measurements performed on human skin, the combination of optical properties, source–detector separation, and low concentration of moving particles (red blood cells) assure that most of Doppler-shifted photons reaching the detector undergo only a single Doppler scattering event. Higher-order

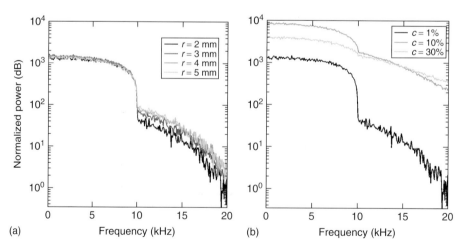

Figure 5.5 Laser Doppler spectra obtained for different source–detector separations (a) and for different concentrations of moving particles (b) with the assumption that the single speed of moving particles corresponds to $\Delta f_{max}/2$.

Doppler scattering events lead to appearance of higher frequencies in measured spectra and cause the spectra to become more flat. This effect is shown in Figure 5.5, where spectra for different concentrations of moving particles and different source–detector separations were presented. The theory of laser Doppler spectrum decomposition for multiple Doppler scattering regimes was proposed to utilize the decomposition method in more general cases.

The theory of multiple Doppler scattering events represents an extension of the method described above. The DSPDs characterizing double-scattering $h_2(V, \Delta f)$ can be expressed as convolutions of single-scattering DSPDs $h_1(V, \Delta f)$ according to the following formula

$$h_2\left(V, \Delta f\right) = h_1\left(V, \Delta f\right) * h_1\left(V, \Delta f\right) \tag{5.8}$$

The results of convolution of DSPDs expressed by Eq. (5.8) for two assumed different speeds of moving particles (V_1 and V_2) yields the results presented in Figure 5.6.

Consequently, the DSPDs for Doppler scattering of order s can be calculated with the use of iterative approach

$$h_s\left(V, \Delta f\right) = h_{s-1}\left(V, \Delta f\right) * h_1\left(V, \Delta f\right) \tag{5.9}$$

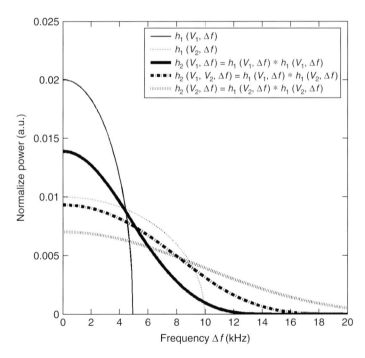

Figure 5.6 DSPDs obtained for a double-Doppler scattering regime by convolutions calculated according to the Eq. (5.8) for two assumed speeds of moving particles V_1 and V_2, which correspond to $\Delta f_{max}/4 = 5\,\text{kHz}$ and $\Delta f_{max}/2 = 10\,\text{kHz}$, respectively.

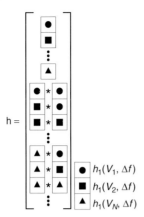

$h_1(V_1, \Delta f)$
$h_1(V_2, \Delta f)$
$h_1(V_N, \Delta f)$

Figure 5.7 Illustration of the calculation of Doppler shift probability distributions matrix for the multiple scattering regime.

Unfortunately, when more than one scattering event is considered, the number of DSPDs that must be included in the analysis grows very quickly. In this way also the number of unknowns in the system of equations increases. All possible variations of convolutions of DSPDs obtained for different speeds must be included. The number of all variations is equal to N^s. However, commutativity of convolution allows one to reduce this number. The convolution procedure is illustrated in Figure 5.7. For two scattering events, the number of derived DSPDs that must be included in the system of equations is given by $Q = N(N + 3)/2$ (where N is the number of speeds considered). More generally, in case of s scattering events, the system of linear equations should cover all possible combinations, with repetitions (multicombinations) from a set of particles moving with N different speeds summed up for the considered number of scattering events from 1 to s. Thus, the number of DSPDs Q, which should be included in the system of equations, is given by

$$Q = \sum_{k=1}^{s} \binom{N + k - 1}{k} \tag{5.10}$$

Table 5.1 Number of unknowns for different number of speeds and Doppler scattering events taken into consideration during decomposition process.

Number of doppler scattering events, s	Number of speeds, N	Number of unknowns, Q
1	10	10
1	20	20
2	10	65
2	20	230
3	10	285
3	20	1770

Some examples of the number of unknowns for different combinations of number of speeds and scattering events are presented in Table 5.1.

It has been shown that for noise-free spectra analyzed for $N = 20$ and $s = 2$, the speed distributions can be estimated. However, for higher numbers of speeds and/or scattering events, the system of equations is ill-posed and hard to solve.

In case of multiple Doppler scattering, Eq. (5.7) can be rewritten as follows:

$$\mathbf{S}^{\mathrm{T}} = \mathbf{a}^{\mathrm{T}}\mathbf{h} \tag{5.11}$$

where row vector $\mathbf{S}$ represents the Doppler spectrum sampled at M frequencies and normalized by its integral and $\mathbf{h}$ is the matrix of convoluted DSPDs normalized by their integrals calculated as shown in Figure 5.7. Row vector $\mathbf{a}$ corresponds to the product of unknown speed distribution $\mathbf{c}$ and a matrix of coefficients $\mathbf{C}$, which describes weights of the different speeds in all convolutions of DSPDs. The repeated variations of convolutions can be omitted, and representation of defined speed in each convoluted DSPD can be considered. Speed distribution $\mathbf{c}$ can be derived utilizing the vector $\mathbf{a}$, which can be obtained by solving Eq. (5.11) and matrix $\mathbf{C}$

$$\mathbf{a}^{\mathrm{T}} = \mathbf{c}^{\mathrm{T}}\mathbf{C}^{\mathrm{T}} \tag{5.12}$$

Solution of the ill-posed problem of decomposition can be found using a constraint-based approach. Methods based on pseudoinverison or minimization of solution error allow the $\mathbf{c}$ row vector in $\mathbf{R}^N$ Euclidean space to be obtained. However, the speed distribution values should be located in $\mathbf{R}^N_+$ subspace, considering that the concentrations of moving particles cannot be negative. This observation applied to the decomposition problem transforms solving of the set of linear equations to a convex minimization problem with constraints. The Eqs. (5.11) and (5.12) can be rewritten as

$$\begin{array}{ll} \text{minimize} & f_1(\mathbf{a}) = \left(\mathbf{S}^{\mathrm{T}} - \mathbf{a}^{\mathrm{T}}\mathbf{h}\right) \cdot \left(\mathbf{S}^{\mathrm{T}} - \mathbf{a}^{\mathrm{T}}\mathbf{h}\right)^{\mathrm{T}} \\ \text{subject to} & \mathbf{a} \geq 0 \\ \text{minimize} & f_2(\mathbf{c}) = \left(\mathbf{a}^{\mathrm{T}} - \mathbf{c}^{\mathrm{T}}\mathbf{C}^{\mathrm{T}}\right) \cdot \left(\mathbf{a}^{\mathrm{T}} - \mathbf{c}^{\mathrm{T}}\mathbf{C}^{\mathrm{T}}\right)^{\mathrm{T}} \\ \text{subject to} & \mathbf{c} \geq 0 \end{array} \tag{5.13}$$

For typical *in vivo* laser Doppler measurements, the influence of higher-order Doppler scattering events may be insignificant for the short source–detector separations used. However, speed distributions for single and higher-order Doppler scattering events can provide depth-resolved information about perfusion of the tissue.

An example of speed distribution decomposition for a medium in which multiple scattering is present is shown in Figure 5.8. Speed distributions were derived for laser Doppler spectra simulated with Monte Carlo code assuming that number of Doppler scattering events was limited to $s = 1, 2,$ and 3. The laser Doppler spectra are shown in Figure 5.8a. Speed distributions derived by decomposition of the laser Doppler spectra are shown in Figure 5.8b. These distributions were obtained from the laser Doppler spectra with the use of only single Doppler scattering DSPDs, while decomposed spectra are affected by multiple Doppler scattering.

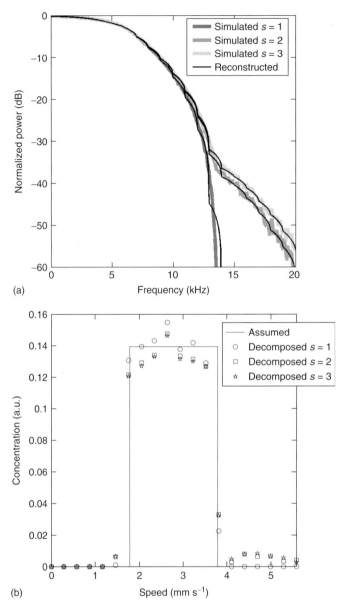

(a)

(b)

Figure 5.8 Laser Doppler spectrum obtained for semi-infinite medium, source–detector separation $r = 1$ mm, laser light wavelength $\lambda = 780$ nm, concentration of moving particles $c = 1\%$, scattering coefficient $\mu_s = 2$ mm^{-1}, absorption coefficient $\mu_a = 0.01$ mm^{-1}, anisotropy factor $g = 0$, and refractive index $n = 1.4$. Components of the spectrum related to the different orders of Doppler scattering events s are presented in (a). Speed distributions derived from laser Doppler spectra shown in (a) were obtained with assumed single Doppler scattering decomposition regime and presented in (b).

Thus, the comparison of obtained speed distributions shows influence of the presence of higher-order Doppler scattering on the results of the decomposition when only single Doppler scattering DSPDs are used. It can be noted that the decomposed distributions contain high-speed components resulting from the simplified procedure utilized.

5.3
Validation of the Spectrum Decomposition Method

5.3.1
Laser Doppler Spectra Generated by Monte Carlo Simulations

The method of laser Doppler spectrum decomposition was validated by the analysis of spectra obtained in Monte Carlo simulations. The spectra were simulated for different assumed speed distributions and concentrations of moving particles. The optical properties of the medium were selected according to the published characteristics data of living tissues [30, 31]. Results of spectra decompositions for assumed uniform and Gaussian speed distributions are presented in Figure 5.9. The decomposition was carried out for the single Doppler scattering regime, and it can be noted that the method allows for successful estimation of speed distributions for nonnoisy spectra obtained by Monte Carlo simulations.

Laser Doppler spectrum decomposition for multiple Doppler scattering regimes requires spectra with high signal-to-noise ratio [18]. For *in vivo* measured laser Doppler spectra, the signal-to-noise ratio is lower than the required value and the decomposition for multiple Doppler scattering regime is not possible. However, for spectra simulated with the Monte Carlo method, the decomposition is possible. An example of such decomposition is presented in Figure 5.10 for two Doppler scattering events. The spectra were generated for two different speed distributions and two source–detector separations r. It should be noted that the relation between speed distributions integrals for first ($s = 1$) and second ($s = 2$) Doppler scattering events corresponds to the relation between the total power of detected photons that undergo only one and those that undergo only two Doppler scattering events.

Furthermore, the system of linear equations (Eq. (5.7)) can be utilized for simulations of laser Doppler power density spectra when the following parameters are assumed:

- moving particles speed distribution;
- scattering anisotropy;
- medium refractive index;
- laser light wavelength;
- sampling frequency of laser Doppler signal;
- cut-off frequencies of the filters implemented in the laser Doppler instrument;
- noise in the measured power density spectra.

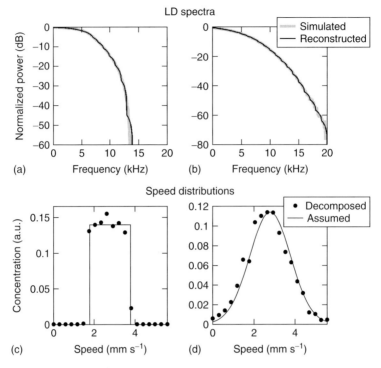

Figure 5.9 Results of decompositions of laser Doppler spectra obtained by Monte Carlo simulations for assumed uniform (a,c) and Gaussian (b,d) speed distributions.

Moreover, time domain signals could be obtained from the spectrum, assuming random phase shift of harmonics [32]. The spectrum could be also used for calculation of perfusion index and simulation of perfusion signals. In other words, the simulation method can be utilized as a tool in development of the signal processing algorithms in LD instrumentation [33].

Assuming a homogeneous medium, where the single Doppler scattering regime dominates, results from Monte Carlo simulations and those obtained from Eq. (5.7) are similar and the difference tends to zero for an infinite number of simulated photons. Thus, Eq. (5.7) represents an analytical form of the time-consuming Monte Carlo algorithm of laser Doppler power density spectra simulation. Comparison of spectra simulated by the Monte Carlo algorithm and analytically calculated laser Doppler spectra for single Doppler scattering regime are shown in Figure 5.11.

5.3.2
Laser Doppler Spectra Measured on the Phantom

The decomposition method described was validated in a series of experiments carried out on a phantom, based on a glass tube (1 mm inner diameter) filled

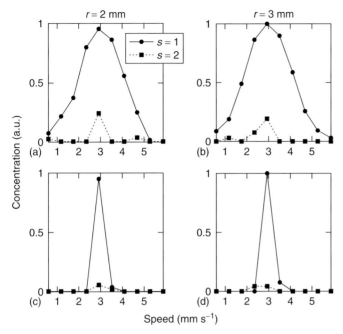

Figure 5.10 (a–d) Results of speed distributions calculation for spectra simulated by Monte Carlo method, obtained by decomposition for two Doppler scattering events ($s = $ 1 and 2) and emitter–detector separations $r = $ 2 and 3 mm. (a,b) results obtained for assumed Gaussian speed distribution with center speed corresponding to $\Delta f_{max}/2$ and standard deviation 1 mm s^{-1}. For (c,d), the single speed of moving particles corresponding to $\Delta f_{max}/2$ was assumed.

with a suspension containing moving particles (intralipid). The tube was mounted in an optically turbid medium (silicone rubber), and the laser Doppler probe was positioned above the tube, covered by 1 mm thick silicon rubber layer, with source and detection fibers (200 μm core multimode fibers, 250 μm separation) fixed perpendicularly to the axis of the tube. The solution was pumped at different speeds achieved by gravitation in order to simulate various perfusion conditions. Actual mean solution speed was assessed measuring volume flowing by the tube in time, with knowledge of the tube diameter. Measurements were performed by using a self-constructed laser Doppler instrument with laser wavelength of 780 nm. The AC components of the signal from photodetector were recorded with a sampling frequency of 40 kHz.

The spectra of laser Doppler signal and derived distributions of speed of moving particles obtained for different speeds of the suspension in the phantom are presented in Figure 5.12. It can be observed that the estimated speed (at which the concentration reaches its maximum) increases gradually with the speed of the suspension pumped through the phantom.

The mean speed of moving particles can be estimated from the speed distribution by calculation of its first moment. First moments of speed distribution related to

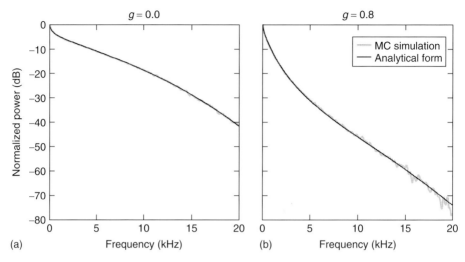

Figure 5.11 Comparison of spectra simulated by the Monte Carlo algorithm and analytically calculated laser Doppler spectra for the single Doppler scattering regime. Results obtained after simulation of 30×10^8 photons for two different anisotropy factors $g = 0.0$ (a) and $g = 0.8$ (b). Analytically obtained spectra were normalized by integrals of Monte-Carlo-simulated spectra.

the mean intralipid flow speed are presented in Figure 5.13. It can be noted that the relationship is linear (correlation $r = 0.96$) with slight saturation observed for high speeds. However, the absolute values of speed derived by proposed method are underestimated in comparison to the actual speed of the suspension in the tube of the phantom.

Gradual increase of speed connected with the maximum concentration in the distribution was reported in the studies carried out by the Linköping group [20, 34] for a suspension with polystyrene particles.

5.4
In Vivo Measurements of Speed Distribution of Red Blood Cells in the Microvascular Network

The technique of laser Doppler spectrum decomposition facilitated recording speed distributions of red blood cells in the microvascular network during stimulation tests. The tests were carried out on healthy volunteers examined in sitting position at room temperature (22 °C). Measurements were performed with a self-constructed laser Doppler instrument operating at laser wavelength of 780 nm and with sampling frequency of 40 kHz. The probe (200 μm core multimode fibers, 250 μm source–detector separation) was fixed on the tip of the middle finger of the left hand using self-adhesive tape. A pressure cuff fixed on the forearm was used to block the blood flow. Results of arterial and venous occlusions are presented in Figures 5.14 and 5.15, respectively. During artery occlusion, the cuff was manually pumped to

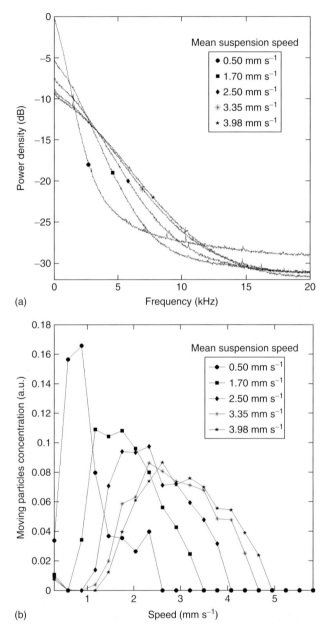

Figure 5.12 Laser Doppler spectra (a) and decomposed speed distributions (b) for various speeds of suspension pumped through the phantom tube. Phantom was based on a glass tube (1 mm inner diameter) filled with a suspension containing moving particles (intralipid) and mounted in an optically turbid medium (silicone rubber). The laser Doppler probe positioned above the tube, covered by 1 mm thick silicon rubber layer, with source and detection fibers (200 μm core multimode fibers) fixed perpendicularly to the axis of the tube at 250 μm separation.

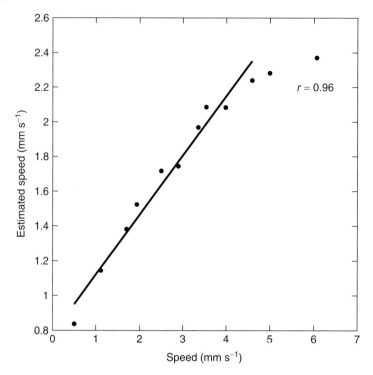

Figure 5.13 Speeds of intralipid estimated from first moments of decomposed speed distributions related to the actual intralipid speed in phantom.

pressure of 200 mmHg. The occlusion was maintained for 2 min. Venous occlusion test started with pressure of 40 mmHg in the cuff, and then the pressure was gradually increased up to 200 mmHg in steps of 20 mmHg. Each step was 15 s long. Resting flow and reperfusion measurements periods took 2.5 and 3.5 min, respectively.

It can be observed that the postocclusive reaction represents a complicated pattern of changes in speed and concentration of red blood cells. It can also be noted that in the venous occlusion phase the velocity drops down, whereas the concentration of red blood cells increases. This effect is connected with filling up the volume of the venous microvascular bed with blood when the outflow is closed.

For thermal stimulation, a thermal chamber was used to provide stable air temperature surrounding the hand. Signals were recorded as follows: first 2 min at 23 °C, next 10 min at 40 °C, then 10 min at 5 °C, and the final 2 min at 23 °C. Considering the time needed to achieve stable thermal conditions, the whole experiment took about 45 min. An example of results of a thermal test is presented in Figure 5.16.

During the thermal stimulation test, an increase of blood concentration combined with a drop of speed can be observed during tissue heating. Cooling down the

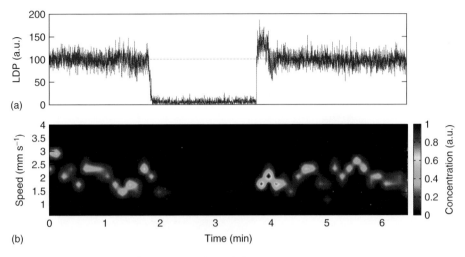

Figure 5.14 Perfusion signal (LDP) (a) and speed distributions (b) obtained during *in vivo* experiment with artery occlusion test.

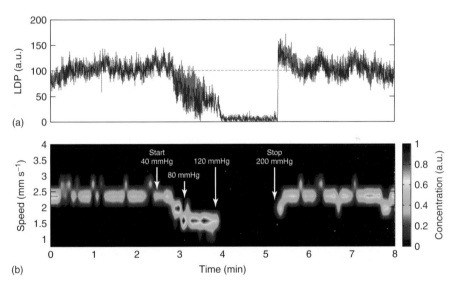

Figure 5.15 Perfusion signal (LDP) (a) and speed distributions (b) obtained during *in vivo* experiment with venous occlusion test.

tissue leads to a fast increase of speed, together with the decrease of concentration of moving red blood cells. These reactions are related to vasodilatation and vasoconstriction effects. Changes of perfusion in three different speed ranges during the thermal challenge test obtained by laser Doppler spectrum decomposition were shown also by Fredriksson [35].

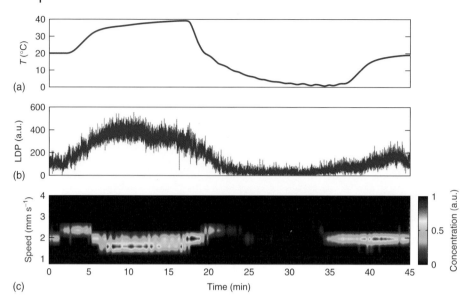

Figure 5.16 Temperature changes in thermal chamber (a), perfusion signal (LDP) (b), and speed distributions (c) during *in vivo* experiment with thermal test.

5.5
Estimation of Anisotropy Factor

The system of equations (Eq. (5.7)) can be solved only for assumed anisotropy factor g. As shown earlier, the g value significantly influences the shape of the DSPDs that form the system of linear equations. The solution of Eq. (5.7) is the least squares fit in which the quality can be assessed. The average difference between the resulting spectra representing superposition of DSPDs can be used for such analysis. The fitting procedure can be carried out for various values of anisotropy factor g used in the derivation of DSPDs. Furthermore, the minimum of mean difference between the fit and measured laser Doppler spectrum can be estimated. This minimum is reached for the anisotropy factor, which is likely the closest to the real anisotropy factor of the scattering of light by the moving particles in the medium under investigation [18]. This procedure of minimum estimation is presented schematically in Figure 5.17.

It should be noted that the theory described here considers only anisotropy of scattering appearing on the moving particles and not on the other (static) inhomogeneities of the medium that influence its optical turbidity. The laser Doppler spectrum does not contain information about the nondynamic scattering events, and thus the anisotropy factor calculated here is only related to the scattering by moving particles.

Results of estimation of anisotropy factor g for phantom experiments (see Section 5.3.2) are shown in Figure 5.18. It can be observed that the estimated

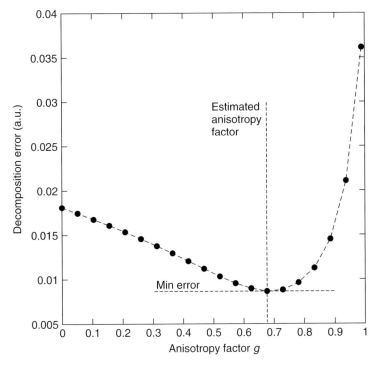

Figure 5.17 An example of estimation of anisotropy factor g from the minimum error of decomposition procedure for *in vivo* experiment during heating (see Section 5.5). Mean difference between the fit and measured laser Doppler spectrum estimated for assumed anisotropy factor of the medium used in calculation of DSPDs. The minimum of the decomposition error is likely the closest to the true anisotropy factor of the dynamic scattering of light in the medium.

g value remains constant for different speeds of suspension in the tube of the phantom phantom.

Estimation of anisotropy factor for *in vivo* measurement during thermal test (see Section 5.4) is presented in Figure 5.19. It can be observed that changes of perfusion caused by the temperature do not have a significant influence of the estimated anisotropy factor value. The estimated anisotropy factor value g = 0.79 ± 0.04 is different from the anisotropy factor of whole blood (≈0.99) reported in review by Cheong *et al.* [30]. This discrepancy can be explained by the fact that the Henyey–Greenstein phase function only approximately describes the scattering angle distribution for red blood cells. The group from Linköping University suggested using another phase function in the decomposition procedure [20, 36]. However, it should be noted that the Henyey–Greenstein phase function allows for analytical derivation of the DSPDs [19] and much faster calculation of nonnoisy components of h matrix.

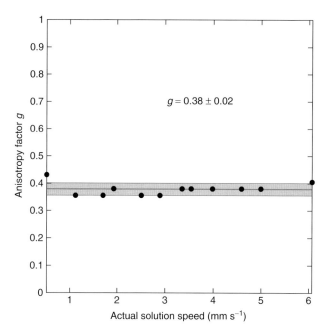

Figure 5.18 Estimated anisotropy factor g from phantom experiments (see Section 5.3.2).

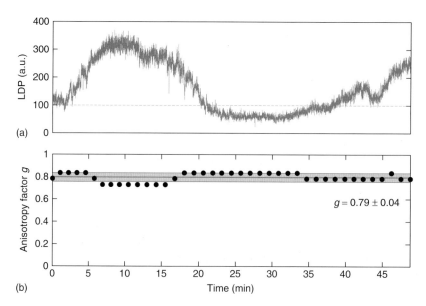

Figure 5.19 Estimation of anisotropy factor for *in vivo* thermal measurements (see Section 5.5): (a) perfusion signal and (b) estimated anisotropy factor.

5.6
Conclusions and Future Developments

The technique presented here is based on the analysis of spectra of the laser Doppler signal. In the classical laser Doppler technique, the first moment of the spectrum is evaluated, and it was shown that this parameter is linearly related to the blood perfusion of the tissue. However, the measured perfusion signals are only relative and the attempts to provide absolute calibration were rather unsuccessful [37, 38]. In the spectrum decomposition technique, the speed distributions can be obtained with the speed expressed in absolute units. However, the concentration of RBCs cannot be calibrated in absolute units because it is related to the number of photons detected, which depends on optical properties of the tissue and many instrumental factors such as photodetector efficiency, numerical aperture of the detection system, and so on. The theory presented here is consistent with the classical laser Doppler flowmetry algorithms – the integral of the decomposed speed distribution is equal to the integral of the laser Doppler spectrum and is a measure of the total concentration of moving particles in the medium.

The presented method may allow for more detailed studies of the human micro-circulation with simultaneous assessment of changes in speed and concentration of red blood cells moving in the volume interrogated by the photons of laser light. The signal processing principle can be applied also in the analysis of data obtained with the use of laser Doppler imaging devices. Potentially, it allows expansion of the information that can be extracted from measurements carried out with these devices. It should be noted that the algorithms based on moments of the laser Doppler spectrum which were used for independent estimation of speed and concentration of red blood cells do not allow for calculation of speed distribution. Because of the limited number of frequencies at which the spectrum is sampled, the calculation of mean speed based on first normalized moment of the spectrum may lead to underestimation of the calculated parameter.

We have shown that the spectrum of the laser Doppler signal depends on the anisotropy of the light scattering on the moving particles. It is worth noting that the spectrum shape does not depend directly on absorption and scattering coefficients of the medium or on anisotropy of scattering of the light on static elements of the structure of the medium. This observation holds true only for the limit of single Doppler scattering, that is, for combinations of optical properties, source–detector separations, and concentrations of moving particles, for which the probability of multiple Doppler scattering for a single photon is very low. Combination of the above-enumerated parameters influences the number of Doppler scattering events that must be considered in decomposition procedure. However, results of Monte Carlo simulations showed that, even in cases in which a small number of detected photons was Doppler scattered more than once, the single Doppler scattering algorithm can be applied and leads to only small deviations between derived and simulated speed distributions.

It was mentioned that the solution of the system of equations, which is a kernel of the decomposition procedure, is rather difficult for noisy spectra. However, this obstacle can be avoided by limiting the number of speeds resolved, which would limit number of unknowns. The method presented here could also be utilized for the estimation of speed distributions of particles in colloidal suspensions. The speed distribution derived may allow for assessment of size of the particles in Brownian motion. The theory presented here also allows for modeling of the laser Doppler spectra for defined speed distributions of particles. This technique in combination with the theory recently presented by Binzoni *et al.* [39] allows simulation of the laser Doppler signals for various perfusion conditions. Such simulations may allow for further analysis of efficiency of different signal processing methods for estimation of blood perfusion in the tissue [33].

5.7
Biography

Dr Adam Liebert is with the Institute of Biocybernetics and Biomedical Engineering of the Polish Academy of Sciences. He is associate professor and head of the Department for Biophysical Measurements and Imaging. He deals with metrological problems connected with the use of optoelectronic techniques in medical diagnosis. His main areas of interest are laser Doppler measurements of tissue perfusion, utilization of near-infrared spectroscopy in brain oxygenation assessment, and evaluation of brain perfusion with the use of optical contrast passage monitored by time-resolved reflectometry.

References

1. Humeau, A. *et al.* (2007) Laser Doppler perfusion monitoring and imaging: novel approaches. *Med. Biol. Eng. Comput.*, **45** (5), 421–435.
2. Rajan, V. *et al.* (2009) Review of methodological developments in laser Doppler flowmetry. *Lasers Med. Sci.*, **24** (2), 269–283.
3. Belcaro, G. *et al.* (1993) *Laser Doppler*, Med-Orion Publishing.
4. Choi, C.M. and Bennett, R.G. (2003) Laser Dopplers to determine cutaneous blood flow. *Dermatol. Surg.*, **29** (3), 272–280.
5. Liebert, A., Leahy, M., and Maniewski, R. (1998) Multichannel laser-Doppler probe for blood perfusion measurements with depth discrimination. *Med. Biol. Eng. Comput.*, **36** (6), 740–747.
6. Varghese, B. *et al.* (2007) Path-length-resolved measurements of multiple scattered photons in static and dynamic turbid media using phase-modulated low-coherence interferometry. *J. Biomed. Opt.*, **12** (2), 024020.
7. Varghese, B. *et al.* (2010) Measurement of particle flux in a static matrix with suppressed influence of optical properties, using low coherence interferometry. *Opt. Express*, **18** (3), 2849–2857.
8. Varghese, B. *et al.* (2007) Path-length-resolved optical Doppler perfusion monitoring. *J. Biomed. Opt.*, **12** (6), 060508.
9. O'Doherty, J. *et al.* (2009) Comparison of instruments for investigation of microcirculatory blood flow and red blood cell concentration. *J. Biomed. Opt.*, **14** (3), 034025.
10. Wardell, K. *et al.* (1994) Spatial heterogeneity in normal skin perfusion recorded with laser Doppler imaging

and flowmetry. *Microvasc. Res.*, **48** (1), 26–38.

11. Wardell, K., Jakobsson, A., and Nilsson, G.E. (1993) Laser Doppler perfusion imaging by dynamic light scattering. *IEEE Trans. Biomed. Eng.*, **40** (4), 309–316.

12. Leahy, M.J. *et al.* (1999) Principles and practice of the laser-Doppler perfusion technique. *Technol. Health Care*, **7** (2–3), 143–162.

13. Binzoni, T. *et al.* (2006) Absorption and scattering coefficient dependence of laser-Doppler flowmetry models for large tissue volumes. *Phys. Med. Biol.*, **51** (2), 311–333.

14. Larsson, M., Nilsson, H., and Stromberg, T. (2003) In vivo determination of local skin optical properties and photon path length by use of spatially resolved diffuse reflectance with applications in laser Doppler flowmetry. *Appl. Opt.*, **42** (1), 124–134.

15. Nilsson, H. *et al.* (2002) Photon pathlength determination based on spatially resolved diffuse reflectance. *J. Biomed. Opt.*, **7** (3), 478–485.

16. Bonner, R.F. *et al.* (1987) Model for photon migration in turbid biological media. *J. Opt. Soc. Am. A*, **4** (3), 423–432.

17. Stern, M.D. (1975) In vivo evaluation of microcirculation by coherent light scattering. *Nature*, **254** (5495), 56–58.

18. Liebert, A., Zolek, N., and Maniewski, R. (2006) Decomposition of a laser-Doppler spectrum for estimation of speed distribution of particles moving in an optically turbid medium: monte carlo validation study. *Phys. Med. Biol.*, **51** (22), 5737–5751.

19. Wojtkiewicz, S. *et al.* (2009) Laser-Doppler spectrum decomposition applied for the estimation of speed distribution of particles moving in a multiple scattering medium. *Phys. Med. Biol.*, **54** (3), 679–697.

20. Larsson, M. and Stromberg, T. (2006) Toward a velocity-resolved microvascular blood flow measure by decomposition of the laser Doppler spectrum. *J. Biomed. Opt.*, **11** (1), 014024.

21. Binzoni, T. *et al.* (2004) Translational and Brownian motion in laser-Doppler flowmetry of large tissue volumes. *Phys. Med. Biol.*, **49** (24), 5445–5458.

22. Dorschel, K. and Muller, G. (1999) Velocity resolved laser Doppler blood flow measurements in skin. *Laser Phys.*, **9** (1), 363–368.

23. Henyey, L.G. and Greenstein, J.L. (1941) Diffuse radiation in the galaxy. *Astrophysics*, **93**, 70–83.

24. Jacques, S., Alter, C., and Prahl, S. (1987) Angular dependence of helium-neon laser light scattering by human dermis. *Lasers Life Sci.*, **4**, 309–333.

25. Zolek, N., Wojtkiewicz, S., and Liebert, A. (2008) Correction of anisotropy coefficient in original Henyey Greenstein phase function for Monte Carlo simulations of light transport in tissue. *Biocybern. Biomed. Eng.*, **28** (4), 59–73.

26. Binzoni, T. *et al.* (2006) Comment on 'the use of the Henyey-Greenstein phase function in Monte Carlo simulations in biomedical optics'. *Phys. Med. Biol.*, **51** (22), L39–L41.

27. Binzoni, T. *et al.* (2006) The use of the Henyey-Greenstein phase function in Monte Carlo simulations in biomedical optics. *Phys. Med. Biol.*, **51** (17), N313–N322.

28. Reynolds, L.O. and McCormick, N.J. (1980) Approximate two-parameter phase function for light scattering. *J. Opt. Soc. Am.*, **70** (10), 6.

29. Hammer, M. *et al.* (1998) Single scattering by red blood cells. *Appl. Opt.*, **37** (31), 7410–7418.

30. Cheong, W., Prahl, S., and Welch, A. (1990) A review of the optical properties of biological tissues. *IEEE J. Quantum Electron.*, **26**, 2166–2185.

31. Niemz, M. (2003) *Laser-Tissue Interactions Fundamentals and Applications*, 3rd enlarged edn, Springer-Verlag, Berlin, Heidelberg.

32. Binzoni, T., Seelamantula, C.S., and Van De Ville, D. (2010) A fast time-domain algorithm for the assessment of tissue blood flow in laser-Doppler flowmetry. *Phys. Med. Biol.*, **55** (13), N383–N394.

33. Wojtkiewicz, S. *et al.* (2011) Evaluation of algorithms for microperfusion assessment by fast simulations of laser Doppler power spectral density. *Phys. Med. Biol.*, **56** (24), 7709–7723.

34. Fredriksson, I., Larsson, M., and Strömberg, T. (2006) Absolute flow velocity components in laser Doppler flowmetry, *Optical Diagnostics and Sensing VI*, SPIE, **6094**, 60940A.

35. Fredriksson, I. (2009) Quantitative laser-Doppler flowmetry, *Department of Biomedical Engineering*, Linkoping University, Linkoping.

36. Lindbergh, T. *et al.* (2009) Spectral determination of a two-parametric phase function for polydispersive scattering liquids. *Opt. Express*, **17** (3), 1610–1621.

37. Steenbergen, W. and de Mul, F.F.M. (1998) A perfusion simulator for testing and calibrating laser Doppler blood flow meters. *J. Vasc. Res.*, **35**, p. 240.

38. Liebert, A., Leahy, M., and Maniewski, R. (1995) A calibration standard for laser-Doppler measurements. *Rev. Sci. Instrum.*, **66**, 5169.

39. Binzoni, T., Leung, T.S., and Van De Ville, D. (2009) The photo-electric current in laser-Doppler flowmetry by Monte Carlo simulations. *Phys. Med. Biol.*, **54** (14), N303–N318.

6
Fast Full-Field Laser Doppler Perfusion Imaging

Wiendelt Steenbergen

6.1
Introduction

As described in Chapter 4, the technology of laser Doppler flowmetry (LDF) was developed in the late 1970s and early 1980s and has been given two different implementations: laser Doppler perfusion monitoring (LDPM) and laser Doppler perfusion imaging (LDPI). In LDPM, mostly fiber-optic probes are attached to the tissue, and the measurement results in a time signal representing the temporal changes of perfusion in a single fixed volume located at the tissue surface. In LDPI, microcirculatory perfusion is evaluated in a larger tissue area, leading to a two-dimensional spatial distribution of perfusion levels. Traditionally, spatial information is gathered by scanning the tissue with a collimated laser beam.

Since the introduction of LDPI in the early 1990s and their commercial introduction in the mid-1990s, the technology of commercial devices has not fundamentally changed. Modifications that were introduced and technological variations between manufacturers mainly concerned specific parts of the technology. Examples are (i) the introduction of semiconductor lasers replacing helium–neon lasers, (ii) the use of lenses to improve the amount of detected light, (iii) the use of optical bandpass filters to reduce disturbances due to ambient light, (iv) stepwise scanning versus continuous scanning of the laser beam, and (v) analog versus digital signal processing. Not only from the clinical point of view but also from the point of view of technology advancement, the evolution of the technology in terms of imaging speed and quality is a logical one. While the quality of perfusion imaging has improved through the above-mentioned modifications, the imaging speed has essentially remained the same. Here, *imaging speed* is defined as the number of perfusion images that can be obtained per unit of time. This imaging speed is essentially limited by the principle of tissue scanning adopted. As for the improvement of imaging speed, new developments have been made possible by the introduction of high-speed optical imaging arrays based on complementary metal oxide semiconductor (CMOS) technology. In this chapter, the reader is introduced to the field of fast full-field LDPI. We discuss the design and algorithms of such

Microcirculation Imaging, First Edition. Edited by Martin J. Leahy.
© 2012 Wiley-VCH Verlag GmbH & Co. KGaA. Published 2012 by Wiley-VCH Verlag GmbH & Co. KGaA.

devices, some practical implementations and results obtained, and the behavior of these devices compared to scanning beam devices.

6.2
Fast Full-Field Laser Doppler Perfusion Imaging: Why and How?

First, it is important to specify what we mean by full-field laser Doppler perfusion imaging (ffLDPI). The term *full field* refers to the property that all information regarding the Doppler content of the detected light is obtained at once, rather than by sequentially addressing all points within a certain tissue area by scanning a laser beam over the tissue surface. Furthermore, we require that the extraction of the perfusion information be based on the optical Doppler effect. This, in general, will mean that the perfusion is estimated from the first-order moment of the power spectrum of the photocurrent fluctuations $M_1 = \int P(\omega)\omega \, d\omega$. This algorithm is based on the theoretical model by Bonner and Nossal [1], which is adopted in all current devices for LDF. Hence, in this chapter, we exclude the full-field methods based on laser speckle contrast imaging [2].

The inherent slowness of scanning beam LDPI devices is related to the fact that the erythrocyte speeds in the microcirculation might lead to Doppler shifts as low as 10–20 Hz. In order to resolve these low Doppler shifts, in each tissue point, intensity fluctuations must be recorded during at least one fluctuation cycle, hence with a duration of 50–100 ms. In stepwise scanning systems, this implies that for an image of 64 × 64 tissue points, a scanning time of 3.5–7 min would be needed. Often, the lower cut-off frequency is taken a little higher (e.g., 50 Hz) to decrease the scanning time. However, for various reasons and in various situations as explained below, a scanning time of several minutes is too large:

1) Scanning times of minutes will not allow studying fast transients in tissue perfusion, such as those caused by the cardiac cycle, breathing, fast temperature changes, and, in particular, occlusion and reperfusion. Even in case of humans, where the fundamental frequency of the cardiac cycle is of the order of 1 Hz, there are components of the dichrotic notch close to 10 Hz. To avoid aliasing, sampling rate must be at least twice this. Thus to be able to visualize even the fastest perfusion variations, a system must render the perfusion at video rate (≈25 fps).
2) Long scanning times may easily lead to movement artifacts because of motions that are likely to occur in a time frame of minutes.
3) This will be more so when carrying out measurements on young children, in particular, those suffering from burn trauma, and on lower limbs of elderly patients, for instance, in the case of ulcers.
4) Long scanning times will make the technology less attractive for clinical use, in terms of planning and logistics.

Compared to the scanning beam imagers, a step ahead in terms of scanning time was realized recently by a line scanning system introduced by Moor Instruments

Ltd (Axminster, Devon, UK). In this system, the tissue is scanned by a planar 780 nm laser beam, creating linear illumination of the tissue. The light is detected by a linear array of photodetectors. This allows a perfusion image of 64 × 64 pixels to be obtained in 4 s. The minimum image acquisition time is dependent on the number of data points per fast Fourier transform (FFT): at maximum resolution (256 × 64 pixels), the best image acquisition time is 13 s for 256 FFTs and 20 s for 1024 FFTs. The best image acquisition time for 64 × 64 pixels is 4 s. The maximum scan area is 20 cm × 15 cm, and the scan distances to the tissue surface (given by the manufacturer) are between 10 and 20 cm. The device is also capable of single-point multichannel acquisition at the sampling rate up to 40 Hz for the entire line of detectors simultaneously [3].

Such imaging times will increase the applicability of LDPI in terms of patient groups and logistics, but will still not allow imaging of the fastest perfusion variations. For this, we need to use two-dimensional image sensors that can be read out with a frame rate twice the maximum Doppler frequency to be measured, following the Nyquist criterion. For typical highest Doppler frequencies of 12.5 kHz, we need frame rates of at least 25 kHz. Nowadays, such frame rates are possible by using CMOS image sensors. CMOS image sensors can achieve such large frame rates since they allow reading out pixels in a selected region within the entire array. Charge-coupled device (CCD) image sensors are not suitable since reading out only a selected number of pixels is not possible.

Let us consider what a complete camera system should be capable of. With a frame rate of 25 kHz, for obtaining Doppler information in the Doppler frequency range of 20 Hz to 12.5 kHz, we need a raw frame rate of 25 kHz and the capability to acquire images at this frame rate for at least 50 ms, leading to 1250 raw frames. For a perfusion image of 128 × 128 pixels, this leads to 30 Mb of raw data, which can be processed into a single perfusion frame of 128 × 128 pixels. Such numbers for camera speed and memory are easy to realize with several of today's commercial high-speed cameras. Hence, as for imaging speed and internal memory, today's high-speed cameras allow taking a single perfusion image with an acquisition time of 50 ms, which is sufficiently short to be regarded as a perfusion snapshot, even in cases of fast perfusion transients. However, the frame rate of a perfusion movie will depend on the speed of raw data transmission and the speed of the algorithm to determine M_1 in all involved pixels (in the above example: 16384 pixels). This issue is addressed in Section 6.4.1. Furthermore, the specifications of the CMOS image array should allow the perfusion-related intensity fluctuations to be measured at sufficient signal-to-noise ratio (SNR). This issue is elaborated in Section 6.3.1.

A full-field method for LDPI using a CMOS array was developed by Atlan et al. [4–7], based on heterodyne holography. In their setup, a frequency-shifted Bragg cell in a reference beam was used to map the spatial occurrence of Doppler shifts in a specific frequency band. By scanning the frequency of the Bragg cell, the entire laser Doppler spectrum could be reconstructed. The holographic approach implies that this is a lensless imaging method. Advantages are the potentially higher SNR, thanks to the use of a reference beam, and the possibility to acquire the Doppler spectrum with only a slow CCD camera. Also, no large amounts of raw image data need to be transferred and analyzed. However, for real-time perfusion imaging, a still higher speed camera is needed. Furthermore, the need of one or more Bragg cells and a reference beam makes the system optically more complicated and expensive than the systems discussed below.

In this chapter, we focus on the systems whose detection apparatus consists of a CMOS imaging array on which the tissue is imaged by a lens system.

6.3
Characteristics of a CMOS-Based Full-Field Laser Doppler Perfusion Imager

In this section we analyze the various parts and characteristics of an ffLDPI system. We describe the aspects that will lead to the choice of a certain camera, the prediction of the SNR based on a model for the generation of photocurrent intensity fluctuations, noise reduction in the perfusion images, and some considerations regarding signal processing.

6.3.1
Choice of a CMOS Camera: General Considerations

When developing a high-speed LDPI device based on a CMOS imaging array, we will have to make various choices that are briefly elaborated below.

6.3.1.1   Commercial Device versus Tailor-Made Device?
Here we assume that we will make use of a commercially available high-speed CMOS camera, rather than building the camera ourselves around a CMOS image sensor, or even developing a specialized CMOS image sensor. It should be emphasized that using a commercially available high-speed camera will lead to a suboptimal design. CMOS image sensors are designed to acquire high-speed images in which the distribution of the DC value will contain the information. In the case of LDPI, however, the perfusion is estimated from the local photocurrent fluctuations per pixel. Each pixel is illuminated by a dynamic speckle pattern. Since each speckle can be regarded as an independent oscillator, the central limit theorem shows that if a pixel is illuminated by N speckles, with $N \gg 1$, the modulation depth M is $M \equiv \langle i_{AC}^2 \rangle / i_{DC}^2 = 1/N$ with i_{AC} and i_{DC} being the photocurrent fluctuations and average photocurrent, respectively. For more information about the relationship between the speckle phenomenon and LDF, the reader is referred to Chapter 7. Since each pixel is illuminated by many speckles, the modulation depth in ffLDPI will be $M \ll 1$. Ideally, the AC and DC signals should be separated electronically and the AC signal amplified so as to completely exploit the dynamic range of the analog-to-digital converter. Such a separate treatment of the AC and DC components, however, is not possible in standard CMOS imaging arrays. Hence the AC part of the signal occupies only a limited number of bits, which might lead to a loss of information. Furthermore, no analog filtering is performed before digitization, potentially leading to aliasing of high-frequency noise into the system's frequency range.

The University of Nottingham [8, 9] developed CMOS arrays that are optimized for LDPI. Their most recent CMOS array comprises 16 × 1 pixels. In each pixel, the AC and DC components are separated and individually amplified and filtered. Furthermore, the AC component is digitized and ω-weighted and averaged to yield the first-order moment of the power spectrum. In the remainder of this chapter, we restrict ourselves to CMOS imaging arrays in which digitization is performed on the complete photocurrent, without prior signal conditioning.

6.3.1.2 Color Sensor versus Monochrome Sensor?
The advantage of using a CMOS image sensor for ffLDPI, apart from its speed, is the possibility to combine perfusion sensing with photography on the same sensor. This will solve the problem of image merging (coregistration) that is needed when two different devices are used for these purposes. From that point of view, using a color sensor would be advantageous. However, since for the speckle sensing only one of the pixels of the RGB chip will be used, this will strongly reduce the effective area of light collection. Therefore, for the current technology, it seems better to use monochrome image sensors.

6.3.1.3 Rolling Shutter versus Global Shutter?
CMOS cameras can be split into devices having a rolling shutter or a global shutter. A rolling shutter means that the pixel lines in the array will be addressed sequentially rather than simultaneously, as is the case for the global shutter. In motion capturing, this will lead to distortion of the image, whereas for ffLDPI, the consequence will not be large, since the method analyzes temporal signals for all pixels simultaneously. Using a global shutter will create a temporal spread in a perfusion movie equal to the acquisition time of a single raw frame, which will typically be in the order of 0.05 ms. This timescale is much smaller than that of perfusion variations.

6.3.1.4 Logarithmic versus Linear Response?
Cameras with logarithmic sensitivity will be useful for recording scenes with a large intensity variation, such as those caused by directly visible concentrated light sources. In LDPI, however, a much more uniform intensity distribution can be expected. Hence, for ffLDPI, devices with a linear response seem the most obvious choice.

6.3.1.5 What Frame Rate and Frame Size is Required?
As mentioned earlier, for ffLDPI, acquisition rates of the raw frames should be sufficiently high to resolve the highest possible Doppler shifts. Based on general experience, a maximum measurable Doppler shift of 12.5 kHz is sufficient. Using the Nyquist theorem, this leads to a frame capture rate of 25 000 fps. In CMOS cameras, this high-frame rate is achieved by acquiring data in selected pixels only. For perfusion imaging, acquiring high-speed images in a square region of interest consisting of 128 × 128 pixels can be considered sufficient.

6.3.2
Model-Based Prediction of CMOS Performance

There are many cameras that are able to capture images at the above-mentioned frame rate within a specific region of interest. It is important that the selection of the camera be based on a prediction of the SNR, using a model that uses the camera specifications as input parameters. In this section, we briefly present such a model. Details are given by Draijer *et al.* [10].

The distinction between noise and signal can be easily made from a power spectrum of the photocurrent fluctuations. Such a power spectrum is shown schematically in Figure 6.1 and is composed of a noise part whose spectrum is assumed to be flat and a more or less exponential signal part. Here we define the SNR as the ratio of the variances of the interferometric photocurrent fluctuations and the noise variance. Hence, $\text{SNR} \equiv \langle i_{\text{signal}}^2 \rangle \big/ \langle i_{\text{noise}}^2 \rangle$. The numerator and denominator are the zero-order moments of the power spectra for the signal and the noise, as indicated in Figure 6.1.

We now treat the signal and the noise separately. The variance of the Doppler-related photocurrent fluctuations is

$$\langle i_{\text{signal}}^2 \rangle = f(2-f)\frac{i_{\text{DC}}^2}{2N} = f(2-f)\frac{i_{\text{DC}}^2 A_{\text{sp}}}{2A_{\text{p}}} \tag{6.1}$$

where f is the fraction of Doppler-shifted light, N the number of speckles per pixel, A_{sp} the area of one speckle, A_{p} the pixel area, and i_{DC} the average photocurrent per pixel. The factor $1/2$ accounts for the assumed depolarization of the initially linearly polarized light by multiple scattering in the tissue. Without the use of a linear polarizer in front of the image sensor, the effect of depolarization is that actually two independent speckle patterns are created, leading to less efficient interference.

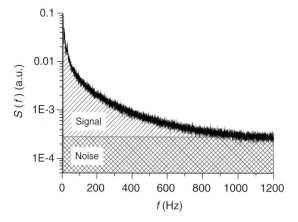

Figure 6.1 Power spectrum of photocurrent fluctuations, composed of a noise part (assumed flat) and an interferometric part containing perfusion information.

The average photocurrent per pixel i_{DC} will depend on the laser power, the diffuse backscattering by the tissue, and the collection efficiency of the camera lens. We find

$$i_{DC}^2 = \frac{R_d P_{laser}}{N_p} \frac{\pi r^2}{4Z^2} \frac{\lambda}{hc} \eta Q q_e \tag{6.2}$$

with R_d the relative diffuse backscattering, P_{laser} the total laser power, N_p the number of pixels involved in the image, r the radius of the lens, Z the distance between lens and tissue, λ the wavelength, h Planck's constant, c the speed of light, η the so-called fill factor of the CMOS chip (the relative effective area of one pixel), Q the quantum efficiency of the CMOS chip, and q_e the charge of an electron. In this expression, we have assumed that the tissue area illuminated by the laser beam is exactly imaged onto the region of interest on the CMOS chip. Furthermore, we have assumed isotropic diffuse backscattering from the tissue. The speckle area A_{sp} in Eq. (6.1) can be written (see Chapter 7) as

$$A_{speckle} = \frac{\lambda^2}{\Omega} = \frac{R^2 \lambda^2}{\pi r^2} \tag{6.3}$$

with Ω being the solid angle of the light incident on the CMOS chip and R the distance between the lens and the chip. Finally, the noise is composed of shot noise, dark noise, and quantization noise. For the light levels considered in LDPI, the dominant noise source will be shot noise, leading to

$$i_{noise}^2 = 2 q_e i_{DC} B \tag{6.4}$$

where B is the detection bandwidth. Equations (6.1–6.4) allow for predicting the SNR based on the specifications of the CMOS imaging array and the optical imaging system and the assumptions regarding the medium. For the medium, we can typically assume for the Doppler fraction of the remitted light that $f = 0.2$, since in most tissues a lower Doppler fraction will hardly be feasible. Furthermore, we can assume the relative diffuse reflection to be typically $R_d = 0.5$. The suitability of the model presented has been verified experimentally [10].

When comparing various cameras, the imaged tissue area, the number of pixels N_p in the perfusion image, and the radius r of the imaging lens should be kept at a fixed value. Furthermore, it is convenient to also use a fixed value for the distance R between the lens and the chip, since in most cases, this distance is given by the type of camera mount (e.g., a C-mount). The set of values chosen will make the distance Z between the lens and the tissue dependent on the size of the pixels, since a fixed amount (say 128×128) of pixels of different size will lead to different values for the required magnification.

The results for three cameras are given in Figure 6.2 (see Ref. [10] for more information). It can be observed that when the amount of injected power exceeds a certain level, the SNR is truncated: at this level, the number of electrons in the pixel reaches the so-called full well capacity, which is different for each CMOS chip. The light intensity for which this full well capacity is reached will also depend on the quantum efficiency, Q, which was highest for camera A. This also leads to the

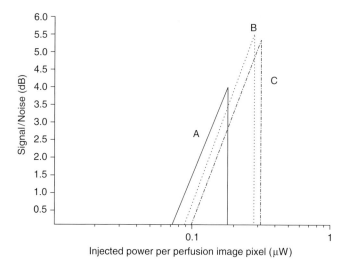

Figure 6.2 Predicted signal-to-noise ratios for three CMOS cameras as a function of the amount of injected power per perfusion image pixel.

largest SNR for camera B. However, due to the saturation at a lower laser power per pixel, this camera is not preferred.

The results in Figure 6.2 were obtained when the camera diaphragm was completely opened. In practice, a diaphragm will be used to decrease the effective lens radius r. However, this will lead to a larger modulation depth of the photocurrent fluctuations to a smaller absolute value of these fluctuations. This signal loss can be restored by further increasing the laser power until saturation is almost reached. The overall result is a higher SNR. In this case, the limiting factor will either be the optical exposure limit of the tissue or the saturation of the camera. For a continuous wave laser in the visible range, the IEC 60825-1 safety limit is a power of $2000\,W\,m^{-2}$. For a typical illuminated area of $0.1 \times 0.1\,m^2$, this would lead to a maximum allowable skin exposure of $20\,W$. The use of such a high-power laser source is unrealistic. In practice, the laser power will be a fixed quantity. If with a completely opened diaphragm the camera will be saturated, the maximum SNR will be reached when the diaphragm is gradually closed until the camera leaves the state of saturation.

6.3.3
Noise Correction in CMOS Based ffLDPI Systems

For any ffLDPI to obtain reliable results, it is essential that the effect of noise in the raw signals be accounted for. As can be expected from the spectrum in Figure 6.1, signal noise will lead to an offset in the perfusion images. In view of Eq. (6.4), it is expected that this offset will increase with the DC level of the photocurrent and therefore with light intensity. In view of the SNR values to be expected, this offset can be significant. In scanning beam LDPI devices, this calibration can be performed by exposing the single detection channel to a range of light levels, leading to an empirical relation between the DC signal and the offset in the perfusion estimations. In our ffLDPI device, a similar procedure can be followed; however, this empirical relation must be established for each individual pixel. This is necessary since in CMOS arrays (in contrast to CCDarrays) each pixel has its own analog circuitry, leading to significant pixel-to-pixel variations of the noise characteristics.

To establish the empirical relationship between the DC level and the perfusion offset, the CMOS array is exposed to light, which is diffusely backscattered from a white Delrin block illuminated by the incoherent light of an LED. The result at a single pixel is given in Figure 6.3. The measurement has been performed on two different days, leading to different results. The relationship between the offset and the DC level cannot be completely understood from the model presented before: deviations are observed for low light levels, but in particular, for light levels exceeding ~60% of the saturation value where the offset decreases with the DC level. We assumed that the spectral shape of the noise would be independent of the DC level. However, it is likely that the electronic characteristics are affected by the local light level, leading to a nonlinear noise behavior. The offset results for different days have been approximated by a third-order polynomial. Since each pixel will behave differently, this is done on a pixel-by-pixel basis, leading to a correction curve for each individual pixel.

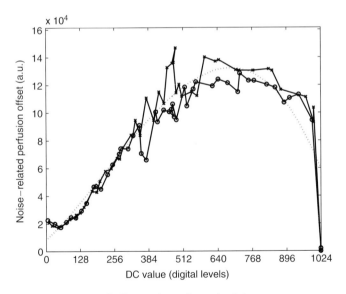

Figure 6.3 Measured offset in the perfusion level due to the pixel noise, generated by one pixel on two different days (symbols), and best fitting third-order polynomial (line).

The above-mentioned procedure for correcting the perfusion images for the effect of signal noise will remove a large part of the noise offset. Complete correction is impossible since the polynomial does not provide a perfect fit and because the offset as a function of DC level changes over time.

6.3.4
Signal Processing Aspects

CMOS-based ffLDPI gives a direct outlook on "online real-time" perfusion imaging. This term means that even the fastest perfusion variations can be visualized and rendered immediately, with minimum time delay. This obviously is an attractive feature in itself, but is particularly useful in those contexts in which instantaneous perfusion variations require immediate actions, such as in surgery. As is shown later in this chapter, at present, only "off-line real-time" perfusion imaging is possible. A single perfusion frame of 128 × 128 pixels, based on 1024 raw frames, currently takes some 0.5 s processing time, excluding the transfer time from camera to computer. This number holds for a straightforward FFT-based algorithm. The data transfer step can be circumvented by processing the raw frames within the camera. While it is to be expected that progress will be made in the coming years in terms of computational speed, it nevertheless will be important and challenging to increase the computational efficiency. The current procedure in which 1024 signal samples are reduced to a single perfusion number, with a power spectrum as intermediate stage, might be called a waste of data. An effort to reduce the data intensity of LDPI was made by Draijer *et al.* [11] who developed a time domain (TD) algorithm for determining the first-order moment M_1 of the power spectrum. *"Time domain"* refers to the property that M is directly estimated from the photocurrent time series $f(t)$, rather than via the power spectrum. The estimator presented has the form:

$$M_1 \approx 2\pi \left\langle \left| f(t) \frac{df}{dt} \right| \right\rangle \approx \frac{2\pi \nu_s}{N} \sum_{i=0}^{N-1} \left| f_i \left(f_{i+1} - f_i \right) \right| \tag{6.5}$$

with ν_s the sample frequency and N the number of samples in the time series. The use of $\approx$ denotes the fact that this estimation is an approximation, partly based on a crude simplification explained in [11], while the second step is a discretization of the first step. In Figure 6.4, the result of this TD algorithm is compared with the traditional FFT-based estimation. This signal is measured on the wrist during reperfusion after arm occlusion and is the perfusion averaged in a window of 128 × 32 pixels. In these results, no noise correction has been applied, which explains the rather large perfusion value during the occlusion. Furthermore, we notice an offset between the algorithms, which is larger during the occlusion than during the reperfusion episode. Both the TD and FFT results show the heartbeat, however, the TD time trace, in general, is a little less smooth. The explanation is that the current simple version of Eq. (6.5) gives an estimation of the first-order moment of the power spectrum starting at 0 Hz, while the high-pass frequency in the FFT algorithm is 50 Hz. Hence, motion artifacts that give rise to low-frequency components are currently not corrected for in the TD algorithm. Our main finding is that

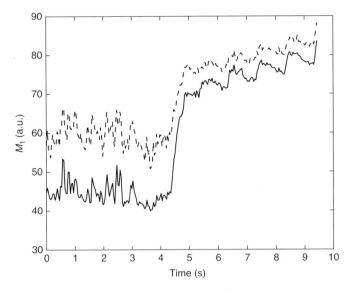

Figure 6.4 Perfusion estimated with the time domain (dashed line) and FFT algorithm (solid line), measured on the wrist during reperfusion after an upper arm occlusion.

the two algorithms give perfusion estimations with a systematic difference within 15%. In practice, the clinical decisions taken on the basis of images obtained with both algorithms will be the same. As for the calculation time, when implemented in LabView (version 7.1), the TD algorithm is twice as fast as the FFT algorithm.

An advantage of the TD algorithm is that it gives the option of a moving average estimation of the perfusion: in this manner, the estimation of perfusion at time t can be updated on the basis of two new raw frames, taken at $t + \Delta t$ and $t + 2\Delta t$. This will greatly reduce the amount of data to be stored and transported. Furthermore, slightly more sophisticated versions of the TD algorithm might allow for high-pass filtering, leading to a reduction of motion artifacts.

6.4
Overview of ffLDPI Systems and Obtained Results

This section deals with the CMOS-camera-based ffLDPI systems that have been described in the literature and gives an impression of the current performance. It must be emphasized that since then, probably progress has been made in terms of image noise and the potential of the method to provide real-time perfusion images. In this chapter we focus on the systems developed by the Ecole Polytechnique Fédérale de Lausanne (EPFL) [12, 13] and the University of Twente (UT) [10]. A concise overview of these systems is given in Table 6.1. A common feature in these systems is the wavelength of 671 nm, produced by a DPSS laser. This is

Table 6.1 Overview of specifications of published ffLDPI systems.

	EPFL [13]	EPFL [12]	UTwente [10]
Wavelength (nm)	671	671	671
Laser power (mW)	50	250	400
Imaged tissue area demonstrated	Ø40 mm	$5.5 \times 5.5\,cm^2$	$7 \times 7\,cm^2$
High-speed camera	iMVS 155, Fastcom Ttechnologies	Home-built	Fastcam 1024PCI, Photron
CMOS array	Fuga1000, FillFactory (logarithmic sensor)	VCA1281, Symagery (integrating sensor)	Not specified
Raw frame rate in ROI	16 800 fps in 64×8 pixels	12 000 fps in unknown subwindow inside 256×256 pixels window	27 000 fps in 128×128 pixels
Perfusion frame rate, or refresh time	90 s, for 256×256 pixels	3.5–10 s, for 128 and 512 raw frames, respectively, of 256×256 pixels	5 s, for 1024 raw frames of 128×128 pixels
Remark	Real-time monitoring at single pixel possible	–	Video rate perfusion movies (26 fps) possible with offline processing

currently the only laser that is able to produce visible light of a suitable wavelength at a sufficient power and coherence length. A potential disadvantage of 671 nm is the sensitivity of optical absorption at this wavelength to the oxygenation of hemoglobin in blood. This might make the response of the system dependent on the oxygenation level. For instance, the path length of the photons through the tissue and the penetration depth of the light into the blood vessels might be reduced with decreasing oxygenation. However, at 671 nm, the absorption level at any physiological oxygenation level is sufficiently low to consider this effect negligible. In general, because of eye safety for ffLDPI, the use of visible light is preferred over the potentially better wavelength of 795 nm, at which light absorption is independent of oxygenation (a so-called isosbestic wavelength). If 795 nm is used, a visible guiding beam should be used to delineate the location of the invisible near-infrared laser beam.

6.4.1
Systems Developed by EPFL Lausanne

EPFL Lausanne developed two different ffLDPI systems [12, 13] based on high-speed CMOS camera. In both systems, a CMOS camera that can only achieve a reasonable frame rate in terms of resolvable Doppler frequencies, in a small region of interest, such as 64×8 pixels, is used. Hence, a total perfusion image of, for instance, 256×256 pixels is built up by merging images obtained in smaller subwindows. Their first system [13] was able to perform a scan of 256×256 pixels and produce a perfusion image in 90 s. A tissue domain with a diameter of $\sim$40 mm could be imaged. Furthermore, real-time perfusion monitoring was possible by reading out a single pixel. The performance of the system was limited by the 8-bit resolution of the Analog-to-Digital converter (ADC) and the logarithmic response of the camera. It is not clear how the noise level is established and how the noise-associated perfusion offset is accounted for.

Their second system [12] showed an increased performance both in speed and imaged tissue area; see Table 6.1. The time to perform and present a complete perfusion scan in 256×256 pixels was decreased to 3.5–10 s, depending on the number of raw images on which a single perfusion frame was based. A fundamental difference between the two systems is that for the second system an integrating sensor is used, which accumulates charges depending on the number of photons hitting each pixel during a certain integration time. This will lead to a higher SNR: for an integration time increasing from 40 to 100 μs, the SNR increased by a factor of 3. Apart from this aspect, integrating CMOS sensors have better characteristics in terms of thermal noise and readout noise and the bandwidth is independent of the signal level. Furthermore, integration provides a means of antialiasing filtering, which nonintegrating sensors lack. The system was applied [14] for intraoperative function brain imaging on a human patient. The perfusion in an area of $3.5 \times 4 \, cm^2$ was imaged in 140×120 pixels at 1.5 fps. A diode laser at 808 nm was used, which is the isosbestic wavelength. Perfusion images were taken while the patient performed a finger-tapping provocation. Significant perfusion variations of 10–20% relative to the baseline value were observed, also correlating with preoperational functional MRI.

One of the Lausanne systems has been commercialized under the name Flux-EXPLORER. Schlosser *et al.* [15] have used this device to study the feasibility of planning flap surgery and monitoring its result. Their finding was that the method is unsuitable for identifying the main blood vessel supplying a tissue flap; however, tissue ischemia could be detected. The FluxEXPLORER systems feature raw frame acquisition rates that are on the low side compared to the usual bandwidths in laser Doppler systems. This in particular is true for the integrating sensor [12] with a frame rate of 12 000 fps, leading to a Doppler bandwidth of 6 kHz only. Usually, scanning beam laser Doppler perfusion imagers and fiber-optic laser Doppler perfusion monitors have bandwidths of at least 12.5 kHz for red laser sources.

More recently, a fast LDPI system based on the technology developed by EPFL Lausanne has been commercialized by a new spin-off company called *Aïmago*. A frame rate of 16 fps is specified, and it images a region of 7×7 cm.

6.4.2
Systems Developed by the University of Twente

The first ffLDPI system was realized by Serov *et al.* [16]. It was based on a Fuga15d camera, sampling a region of interest of 64 × 64 pixels with a frame acquisition rate of 9000 fps. Actually, this system rendered images of the zero-order moment of the power spectrum only, providing information on the concentration of moving red blood cells. An image was acquired and processed in 7 s. The capabilities of the method were shown both *in vitro*, using Intralipid inside a cavity made in a static Delrin environment, and *in vivo*, on an occluded and reperfused finger.

Draijer *et al.* realized the Twente Optical Perfusion Camera (TOPCam) [10]. The main features of this system are given in Table 6.1.The TOPCam is based on the Photron 1024 Fastcam high-speed camera. This camera is able to acquire images at a frame rate of 27 000 fps in a region of interest of 128 × 128 pixels. This gives a detection bandwidth of 13.5 kHz, which is considered sufficient for recording even the highest Doppler shifts produced by microcirculatory blood flow. For creating a desired illumination pattern, the so-called engineered diffusers are used. These are compact beam-shaping elements made of polymer, which diverge a narrow collimated beam to realize an illumination pattern by the diffractive action of the micropattern on the element's surface. In the TOPCam, square beams are produced with linear sizes up to 15 cm. Such beam patterns can be obtained using commercially available diffractive optical elements. The intensity distribution is uniform within ±10%. Another option for creating a homogeneous beam is to couple the light into a multimode fiber to produce a magnified image of the fiber core on the tissue. This method was applied by Serov and Lasser [12] and may produce a better homogeneity than diffractive optics. However, using a circular illumination pattern is less efficient in combination with the usually rectangular regions of interest on the CMOS arrays.

The TOPCam can produce a perfusion frame in 5 s. This time is dominated by the transfer speed between the camera and the computer, since data acquisition by the camera and processing by the computer only take 380 ms and 1 s, respectively. However, since the entire region of 128 × 128 pixels can be read out at once, video rate perfusion images at a frame speed of 26 fps can be produced by acquiring data until the camera memory is full. For perfusion images of 128 × 128 pixels, with a maximum internal camera memory of 24 Gb, a perfusion movie of 45 s duration can be recorded.

The ability of the TOPCam system to image skin perfusion has been demonstrated in various ways. An example of perfusion data obtained at video rate was already shown in Figure 6.4. The slow increase of skin perfusion in response to topical application of a capsicum cream was measured in a region of 5 × 5 cm on the back of the hand of a healthy volunteer [10]. The perfusion image after 14 min 29 s is shown in Figure 6.5. This figure visualizes the first-order moment for each pixel normalized with the DC value of the photocurrent. DC normalization (rather than DC^2 normalization) has become common practice in commercial devices for LDPI. While DC^2 normalization is suitable for correction variations

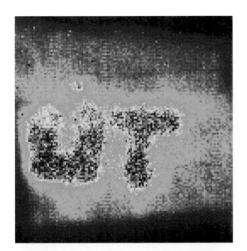

Figure 6.5 Skin perfusion image (M_1/DC) of the back of the hand in response to topically applied capsicum cream. The image is recorded 14 min after cream application. "UT" denotes "University of Twente."

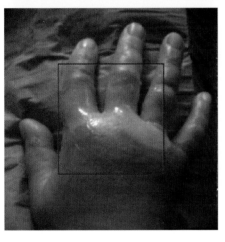

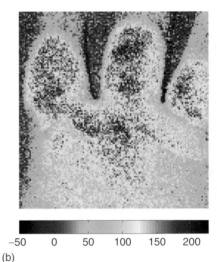

-50   0   50   100   150   200

(a)   (b)

Figure 6.6 Perfusion of a second-degree burn at two days postburn [17]. (a) Image of DC values, and indication of the 128 × 128 pixel region of interest (ROI) for perfusion imaging. (b) Perfusion within ROI, expressed by M_1/DC. (Reprinted with permission of Elsevier.)

in laser power, normalization by DC may enable a better correction for inhomogeneities in the tissue surface condition. Such inhomogeneities may become dominant if no cross-polarizers are used to suppress the reflection from the tissue surface.

The suitability of the TOPCam to image burn perfusion has been tested in a pilot study [17]. The result of imaging a second-degree burn of the hand is shown in Figure 6.6, where panel (a) shows the raw image taken with the entire CMOS array and panel (b), the perfusion as measured within the indicated region of interest. These images show both an advantage and a disadvantage of using CMOS imaging arrays for perfusion imaging. An advantageous feature is that the wound topography and the perfusion information can be obtained with the same sensor, which facilitates fusing both types of information. This is important, since burn diagnosis will be based on both the wound appearance and the perfusion image. A disadvantage is the absence of color and the moderate quality of the photograph taken with the CMOS image. However, taking high-quality color images with a monochrome imaging array is feasible and is a matter of further sophistication of the entire system. The general finding in the burn center setting was that the imaging speed of the system is a big advantage, which balances against the slightly lower imaging quality in terms of SNR. In general, the sensitivity and resolution of the method are sufficient. Furthermore, practical issues, such as the presence of crusts, creams and blisters, and tissue curvature, have a similar impact as identified by Droog *et al.* [18] for scanning beam systems.

6.5
Comparative Behavior of CMOS-Based Systems: How Good Are They to Measure Perfusion?

6.5.1
General Considerations

The generic methodology of LDF is able to quantitatively measure microcirculatory perfusion in a relative manner, provided that the fraction of Doppler-shifted photons involved in signal generation is much smaller than one. This is known from the early work on LDF, both from the theory by Bonner and Nossal [1] and the experiments by Nilsson *et al.* [19, 20]. Usually, this condition is met in moderately perfused tissues, using fiber-optic probes with a small distance between the fibers for illumination and detection. For scanning beam laser Doppler perfusion imagers, this aspect has not been studied in great detail.

The question may arise to what extent ffLDPI based on CMOS arrays is able to measure perfusion, and how it compares against other methods providing similar information. Binzoni and Van de Ville [21] used Monte Carlo simulations to study the performance of ffLDPI systems. They concluded that the first-order moment M_1 could properly describe perfusion, whereas the zero-order moment M_0 was hardly sensitive to blood volume when the probability of interaction of light with moving red blood cells exceeded a value of 0.05. They attribute this to the strong forward scattering of light in tissues. This is only one of the various conditions that leads to an excessive fraction of Doppler-shifted light, along with too large a distance between the points of injection and detection of photons. Unlike fiber-optic probes, in ffLDPI systems, the use of a broad laser beam may lead to relatively large photon trajectories, and hence to a relatively large probability of interaction of photons with moving red blood cells.

6.5.2
Comparison with Scanning Beam Systems

While most experience in the use of LDPI is built on the use of scanning beam systems, it is to be expected that eventually, these systems will be discarded in favor of either CMOS-based ffLDPI devices or laser speckle contrast perfusion imaging (referred to as *LCSPI*). In this and the next subsection, we briefly compare ffLDPI with scanning beam LDPI and LSCPI methods, respectively.

In a few yet unpublished studies performed in our group, when comparing ffLDPI and scanning beam LDPI images on similar objects, the following features immediately attracted attention:

- Perfusion images formed by ffLDPI suffer from structured noise (so-called fixed pattern noise) and a higher random noise than scanning beam LDPI images. The fixed pattern noise is a well-known feature of CMOS arrays, which can be partly suppressed by calibration. The higher random noise is the consequence of the much smaller detector size in ffLDPI systems. We can regard an ffLDPI device as having $p \times q$ individual detection channels, with p and q denoting the perfusion image size, compared with a single detection channel in scanning beam systems.
- Boundaries between dynamic media (e.g., Intralipid) and static media (e.g., Delrin) are rendered at a higher resolution with scanning beam systems than with ffLDPI systems. In tissues, this difference is less pronounced in the absence of sharp transitions. While for many diagnostic decisions the potentially worse resolution of ffLDPI systems is not important, it is an interesting feature that will be elaborated below.

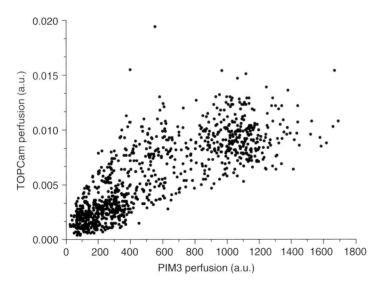

Figure 6.7 Pixel-by-pixel comparison of perfusion values obtained with PIM3 (Perimed AB) versus' TOPCam, imaging skin tissue with topically applied capsicum cream.

- Scanning beam systems appear to be more sensitive to variations in tissue optical properties than ffLDPI systems. An example is shown in Figure 6.7, which reveals that the skin perfusion increase generated by capsicum cream as recorded with scanning beam device PIM3 (Perimed AB) is larger than that recorded with the TOPCam.

It is tempting to state that scanning beam devices should have a better resolution than ffLDPI devices, because the latter uses a much broader beam. However, a closer look reveals that the difference in beam sizes as such cannot lead to a different imaging resolution. This is illustrated in Figure 6.8. In a scanning beam device, light is injected into a point and follows shallow or deep trajectories back to the surface at positions remote from or nearby the injection point. Part of this light is imaged on a large photodetector. In a full-field device, light is injected in a broad beam, which we can regard as a large number of collimated beams. A certain pixel, imaged on the tissue surface, is illuminated by light that followed shallow or deep trajectories, coming from remote or nearby collimated beams. Hence, from the point of view of photon migration, there is no fundamental difference between the two modalities. In other words, the better resolution of scanning beam devices is not obvious from the fact that they use a narrower beam.

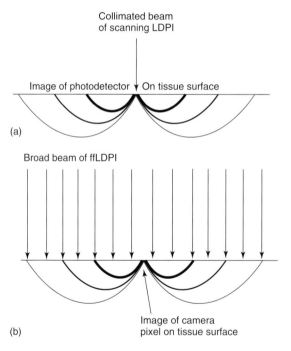

(a)

(b)

Figure 6.8 Comparison of beam configurations and light trajectories. (a) Scanning beam LDPI with a collimated beam and light trajectories ending on a large photodetector projected on the tissue; (b) ffLDPI with a broad beam and light trajectories ending on one camera pixel. The relative trajectory thicknesses indicate the decay of intensity with penetration depth.

A more probable explanation can be found in the physics behind Eqs. (6.1) and (6.3) and, in particular, in the role of the number of speckles N on the photodetector. This is defined as $N = A_{\text{det}}/A_{\text{sp}}$, with A_{sp} being the average speckle area and A_{det} the effective detection area. According to Eq. (6.3), the speckle area A_{sp} is governed by the solid angle Ω of the light hitting the detector and therefore only dependent on the detection geometry. However, while the effective detection area A_{det} is equal to the pixel size A_{p} in ffLDPI (see Eq. (6.1)), in scanning beam systems, A_{det} will be related to the size of the light-emitting spot on the tissue surface. This size will depend on the tissue optical properties. This gives scanning beam LDPI an independent source of cross talk between perfusion readings and optical properties. This issue is treated in much more detail in Chapter 7 and in its references.

To study the relationship between perfusion readings with ffLDPI and scanning beam LDPI, perfusion measurements have been performed in Intralipid samples at various levels of the reduced scattering coefficient. The results are shown in Figure 6.9. Panel (a) shows a nonlinear relationship between the perfusion values of the PIM3 and the TOPCam, in a manner that has some qualitative similarity to the *in vivo* result in Figure 6.7. Since these samples, unlike perfused tissue, are

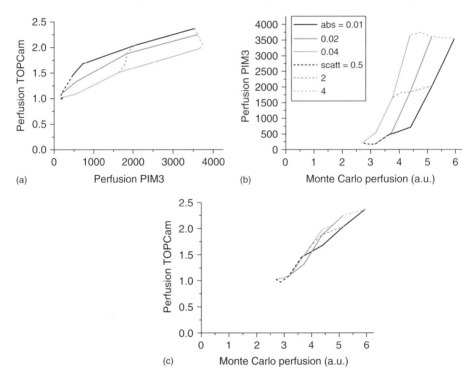

(a)

(b)

(c)

Figure 6.9 Comparison of perfusion values measured with the PIM3 (Perimed AB) and the TOPCam in Intralipid samples with various scattering and absorption levels. (a) TOPCam versus PIM3. (b) PIM3 versus Monte Carlo simulation results. (c) TOPCam versus Monte Carlo. Values in the legend are the absorption and reduced scattering coefficients in mm^{-1}.

completely dynamic, it is difficult to define their "perfusion level." However, it is possible to predict the ideal laser Doppler perfusion reading in terms of the first moment of the power spectrum by performing Monte Carlo simulations. We can regard the Monte Carlo predictions as a reference method, in that they show how the Doppler statistics of the detected photons are related to and affected by the tissue optical properties. The result is shown for the PIM3 and the TOPCam in panels (b,c), respectively. These figures reveal that the PIM3 perfusion readings are highly nonlinear with the Monte Carlo values. For varying scattering, the TOPCam-measured perfusion value hardly changes, while the scanning beam device shows an extreme sensitivity to varying scattering levels. This opposite response is related to the effect that the optical properties have on A_{det} in the case of the scanning beam device. The TOPCam perfusion readings, however, are quite proportional to the predicted values. We emphasize that these "perfusion readings" in these entirely liquid samples do not estimate the flux of particles, but the Doppler statistics of the detected light. However, we must conclude that scanning beam devices are less able than ffLDPI devices to give a one-to-one relation with the Doppler statistics of the detected light. The difference between these two modalities must be attributed to the speckle phenomenon that affects ffLDPI and scanning beam LDPI measurements in a fundamentally different way.

This difference also forms the explanation for the better spatial resolution of scanning beam devices. As described in Chapter 7 (see, in particular, Figure 7.6), the speckle effect reduces the effective probed depth by ~50% with, as a side effect, an improved spatial resolution.

6.6
Concluding Remarks

The early results of ffLDPI devices illustrate their potential and their relative advantages over scanning beam devices. In particular, in view of their improved imaging speed, it seems inevitable that in the long term, the scanning beam approach will be replaced by the full-field approach. In addition to a faster speed, it was also illustrated in this chapter that ffLDPI systems seem to have a better ability to render the Doppler information contained by the detected light, which may be regarded as an advantage.

The future of ffLDPI cannot be viewed independently from that of laser speckle contrast perfusion imaging (LSCPI) [2], which must be regarded as its main competitor. LSCPI has the advantage of being relatively simple and cheap, since it does not need a high-speed imaging array. On the other hand, LSCPI is less quantitative in that the relation between speckle contrast and perfusion is not described by a physical model, unlike laser Doppler methods, which are supported by the model of Bonner and Nossal [1].

A theory by Draijer et al. [22] suggests that LSCPI is more sensitive to concentration variations of moving red blood cells than to variations of red blood cell velocity.

Furthermore, Thompson and Andrews [23] showed that combining speckle contrast values measured at various exposure times may lead to the prediction of laser Doppler spectra. This would make multiple-exposure LSCPI equivalent to LDPI, although at the expense of acquisition speed.

Probably there will be a future for both modalities, where the choice for a specific technology will depend on the need for quantitative imaging. Since almost all experience in LDPI has been gained with the use of scanning beam LDPI, the introduction of both ffLDPI and LSCPI will make it necessary to reconsider existing practices, protocols, and procedures.

References

1. Bonner, R. and Nossal, R. (1981) Model for laser Doppler measurements of blood-flow in tissue. *Appl. Opt.*, **20** (12), 2097–2107.

2. Draijer, M., Hondebrink, E., van Leeuwen, T., and Steenbergen, W. (2009) Review of laser speckle contrast techniques for visualizing tissue perfusion. *Lasers Med. Sci.*, **24** (4), 639–651.

3. Leahy, M.J. (2009) Microvascular blood flow: microcirculation imaging, in *Handbook of Biophotonics*, vol. 2, Chapter 26, (eds J. Popp and V.V. Tuchin), Wiley-VCH Verlag GmbH, pp. 403–444.

4. Atlan, M. and Gross, M. (2006) Laser Doppler imaging, revisited. *Rev. Sci. Instrum.*, **77** (11), 116103.

5. Atlan, M. and Gross, M. (2007) Wide-field fourier transform spectral imaging. *Appl. Phys. Lett.*, **91**, 113510.

6. Atlan, M., Gross, M., Forget, B.C., Vitalis, T., Rancillac, A., and Dunn, A.K. (2006) Frequency-domain wide-field laser Doppler in vivo imaging. *Opt. Lett.*, **31** (18), 2762–2764.

7. Atlan, M., Gross, M., Vitalis, T., Rancillac, A., Rossier, J., and Boccara, A.C. (2008) High-speed wave-mixing laser Doppler imaging in vivo. *Opt. Lett.*, **33** (8), 842–844.

8. Gu, Q., Hayes-Gill, B.R., and Morgan, S.P. (2008) Laser Doppler blood flow complementary metal oxide semiconductor imaging sensor with analog on-chip processing. *Appl. Opt.*, **47** (12), 2061–2069.

9. Kongsavatsak, C., He, D.W., Hayes-Gill, B.R., Crowe, J.A., and Morgan, S.P. (2008) Complementary metal-oxide-semiconductor imaging array with laser Doppler blood flow processing. *Opt. Eng.*, **47** (10), 14.

10. Draijer, M., Hondebrink, E., van Leeuwen, T., and Steenbergen, W. (2009) Twente optical perfusion camera: system overview and performance for video rate laser Doppler perfusion imaging. *Opt. Express*, **17** (5), 3211–3225.

11. Draijer, M., Hondebrink, E., van Leeuwen, T., and Steenbergen, W. (2009) Time domain algorithm for accelerated determination of the first order moment of photo current fluctuations in high speed laser Doppler perfusion imaging. *Med. Biol. Eng. Comput.*, **47** (10), 1103–1109.

12. Serov, A. and Lasser, T. (2005) High-speed laser Doppler perfusion imaging using an integrating CMOS image sensor. *Opt. Express*, **13** (17), 6416–6428.

13. Serov, A., Steinacher, B., and Lasser, T. (2005) Full-field laser Doppler perfusion imaging and monitoring with an intelligent CMOS camera. *Opt. Express*, **13** (10), 3681–3689.

14. Raabe, A., De Ville, D.V., Leutenegger, M., Szelenyi, A., Hattingen, E., Gerlach, R., Seifert, V., Hauger, C., Lopez, A., Leitgeb, R., Unser, M., Martin-Williams, E.J., and Lasser, T. (2009) Laser Doppler imaging for intraoperative human brain mapping. *Neuroimage*, **44** (4), 1284–1289.

15. Schlosser, S., Wirth, R., Plock, J.A., Serov, A., Banic, A., and Erni, D. (2010)

Application of a new laser Doppler imaging system in planning and monitoring of surgical flaps. *J. Biomed. Opt.*, **15** (3), 036023–036026.

16. Serov, A., Steenbergen, W., and de Mul, F. (2002) Laser Doppler perfusion imaging with a complimentary metal oxide semiconductor image sensor. *Opt. Lett.*, **27** (5), 300–302.

17. van Herpt, H., Draijer, M., Hondebrink, E., Nieuwenhuis, M., Beerthuizen, G., van Leeuwen, T., and Steenbergen, W. (2010) Burn imaging with a whole field laser Doppler perfusion imager based on a CMOS imaging array. *Burns*, **36** (3), 389–396.

18. Droog, E.J., Steenbergen, W., and Sjoberg, F. (2001) Measurement of depth of burns by laser Doppler perfusion imaging. *Burns*, **27** (6), 561–568.

19. Nilsson, G.E., Tenland, T., and Oberg, P.A. (1980) New instrument for continuous measurement of tissue blood-flow by light beating spectroscopy. *IEEE Trans. Biomed. Eng.*, **27** (1), 12–19.

20. Nilsson, G.E., Tenland, T., and Oberg, P.A. (1980) Evaluation of a laser Doppler flowmeter for measurement of tissue blood-flow. *IEEE Trans. Biomed. Eng.*, **27** (10), 597–604.

21. Binzoni, T. and Van De Ville, D. (2008) Full-field laser-Doppler imaging and its physiological significance for tissue blood perfusion. *Phys. Med. Biol.*, **53** (23), 6673–6694.

22. Draijer, M.J., Hondebrink, E., Larsson, M., van Leeuwen, T.G., and Steenbergen, W. (2010) Relation between the contrast in time integrated dynamic speckle patterns an the power spectral density of their temporal intensity fluctuations. *Opt. Express*, **18** (21), 21883–21891.

23. Thompson, O.B. and Andrews, M.K. (2010) Tissue perfusion measurements: multiple-exposure laser speckle analysis generates laser Doppler-like spectra. *J. Biomed. Opt.*, **15** (2), 027015.

7
Speckle Effects in Laser Doppler Perfusion Imaging

Wiendelt Steenbergen

7.1
Introduction

For those observing laser light, speckles are an inevitable phenomenon. Images of static objects illuminated by laser light with a sufficient coherence length are characterized by a grainy or speckled structure, or in other words, they are composed of speckles. Speckles on the retina are always "in focus," even when the object plane is not imaged on the retina.

When laser light is scattered off a partially dynamic object, for instance, a scattering medium with slow internal motion of scattering centers, such as many biological samples, the speckle pattern exhibits slow changes in time. Faster motion of scatterers will generate more rapid speckle motion and, above a certain typical speed of scatterers, the speckle motion is too fast to be observed by the naked eye. However, a photodetector that is sufficiently fast will still be able to record the associated intensity fluctuations.

The dynamic speckle pattern, which is the result of the interaction of coherent light with red blood cells moving within a static tissue matrix, and the associated fluctuations of the light intensity of the detector are an essential aspect of laser Doppler perfusion monitoring (LDPM) and laser Doppler perfusion imaging (LDPI). In the past, some confusion has been caused by the parallel use of "speckle flowmetry" [1–4] and "laser Doppler flowmetry" [5, 6] for the same method in which the intensity fluctuation signal is recorded and a perfusion signal is derived from its power spectrum. Although not all speckle motion is caused by the Doppler effect, intensity fluctuations in laser Doppler methods are essentially caused by speckle motion. The distinction between "Doppler" and "speckle" may be described as follows: dynamic speckle is the *phenomenon* that is being recorded, while Doppler effect provides the framework for the *interpretation* of intensity fluctuations in terms of perfusion.

Microcirculation Imaging, First Edition. Edited by Martin J. Leahy.
© 2012 Wiley-VCH Verlag GmbH & Co. KGaA. Published 2012 by Wiley-VCH Verlag GmbH & Co. KGaA.

7.2
What Are Speckles? Basic Properties

Speckles are the result of the interference of a very large number of light waves. A condition for obtaining observable speckles is that the phases of these waves remain fairly constant within a certain time scale, or in other words, the waves should be sufficiently coherent. Without such correlation, no interference can be observed by the eye or with a normal photodetector or imaging array. A second condition is that these multiple waves have a certain angular spread. The situation is illustrated in Figure 7.1a for spherical waves emitted from a plane such as an optically rough reflector illuminated by coherent light. Here, optically rough means a roughness on the scale of the wavelength of light used. Because of the roughness of the screen, a perfectly smooth wave front hitting the screen will lead to a spatial randomization of the phases of the reflected wave. We can also regard this as a collection of spherical waves, with mutually random phases. Since the light is coherent, the waves, although they have a random distribution of phases, are coherent too and are therefore able to interfere. If a screen is placed at a certain distance from the rough surface, the waves arrive as planar waves. The phase of each wave varies with the position on the screen, and the phase difference between two points on the screen will be larger for skew waves than for waves that are almost perpendicular. Therefore, at each location on the screen, the local electric field and the intensity are the result of the addition of many electric fields with mutual phase differences that vary with screen position. The result is the speckle pattern as shown in Figure 7.1b, which was generated by observing light emitted by a paper that was illuminated by a He–Ne laser. Actually, two interference patterns are formed, each associated with two perpendicular polarizations of the incident

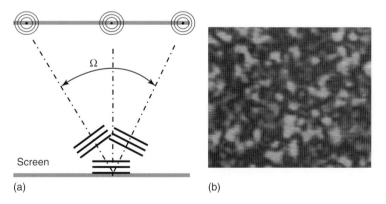

(a)   (b)

Figure 7.1 (a) Waves emitted by an optically rough surface and hitting a distant screen at an angular spread given by solid angle Ω. The phases of the waves vary with the position on the screen. (b) The resulting interference pattern on screen.

light. The speckle pattern shown here is one of the two, selected by placing a linear polarizer between the paper and the screen. This is called *polarized speckle*. It is important to realize that the above principle also holds for coherent waves backscattered from turbid media, such as tissue, as long as the difference in the diffuse path lengths of the interfering photons is less than the coherence length of the light. The visibility of the interference pattern decays exponentially with increasing optical path difference.

The basic properties of speckle patterns have been investigated by Goodman [7, 8]. The most relevant for the topic of this chapter are briefly mentioned here. We restrict ourselves to the case of a single polarized speckle pattern.

7.2.1
Distributions of Field Amplitude and Intensity

Since speckle is formed by the amplitude addition of many coherent waves whose phases are randomized, the local field complex amplitude can be described by a phasor that results from the addition of many phasors, as shown in Figure 7.2. Because speckle is the result of the addition of a large number of randomly oriented phasors, the resulting amplitude has a circular Gaussian distribution in the complex plane. That the resulting distribution is Gaussian follows from the central limit theorem, which is applicable to this situation. As a consequence of the Gaussian distribution of the complex field amplitude, the intensity distribution has an exponential (or Poisson) distribution.

7.2.2
Speckle Contrast

The speckle contrast quantifies the visibility of the speckles, or the modulation depth of the speckle pattern. For a statistically homogeneous static speckle pattern, the contrast is defined as

$$K \equiv \frac{\sigma_I}{\langle I \rangle} \tag{7.1}$$

where σ_I is the standard deviation of the intensity I and $\langle \rangle$ denotes spatial averaging.

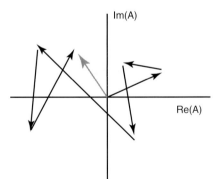

Figure 7.2 Complex amplitude (gray phasor) of the local field as a result of the addition of multiple phasors.

For a single linearly polarized speckle pattern, caused by a static object, the Poisson intensity distribution leads to a value $K = 1$, which means that the standard deviation of the intensity fluctuations is equal to the average intensity. This fact is important later in this chapter.

7.2.3
Speckle Size

Owing to the stochastic nature of laser speckle patterns, speckle size can only be expressed in terms of an average size, to be derived from a function that describes the distribution of the width or diameter of the speckles. For laser Doppler flowmetry, the speckle area, or coherence area, appears to be the quantity of relevance. It is not exactly defined which feature in a speckle pattern such as in Figure 7.1 can be called "a *speckle*." Therefore, we analyze the complete speckle pattern in terms of the spatial correlation function $R_I(\Delta x) \equiv \langle I(x)I(x + \Delta x)\rangle / \langle I\rangle^2$ of the intensity distribution $I(x)$. Here we have assumed that the speckle pattern is statistically homogeneous and isotropic. While $R_I(\Delta x)$ can be analyzed in terms of speckle width or speckle area in various ways, the expression for the area of one speckle that is most relevant for laser Doppler flowmetry can be shown [9] to be

$$A_{\text{speckle}} = 2\pi \int_0^\infty R_I(\Delta x)\Delta x d\Delta x \qquad (7.2)$$

A_{speckle} can be regarded as an "effective speckle area" because a dynamic speckle pattern that would consist of areas of uniform intensity with an area of exactly A_{speckle} will generate the same photocurrent fluctuations as the real dynamic speckle pattern.

The spatial correlation function $R_I(\Delta x)$ is related to the angular intensity distribution of the incoming light and therefore to the intensity distribution $I(x', y')$ in the light-emitting plane. The wider this distribution function, for instance expressed by the solid angle Ω in Figure 7.1, the smaller the speckles will be. This relation is obtained in two steps. First, for light that has a Gaussian amplitude distribution, the spatial correlations of the intensity $R_I(\Delta x)$ and the field amplitude $R_E(\Delta x)$ are related by

$$R_I(\Delta x) = \langle I\rangle^2 + \left|R_E(\Delta x)\right|^2 \qquad (7.3)$$

which is called *Siegert's relation*. The observation plane and the source plane, as shown schematically in Figure 7.3, are related by the Zernike–Van Cittert theorem [10]. This theorem states that $R_E(\Delta x)$ and $I(x', y')$ are related in the same manner as the electric field amplitude distribution $E(x,y)$ in the xy-plane would be related to the electric field amplitude distribution $E(x', y')$ in the x'y'-plane, with amplitude distribution $E(x', y')$ mathematically equal to the intensity distribution $I(x', y')$. This fact mathematically links the problem of coherence of randomly phased waves emitted by a plane to the phenomenon of diffraction. Hence, $R_E(\Delta x)$, or the more

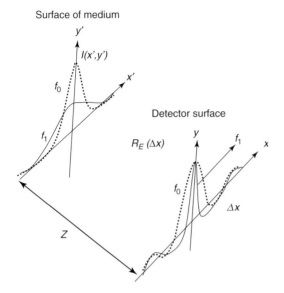

Figure 7.3 Definition of coordinates on the surface of the medium and on the detector surface. f_1 and f_0 refer to two different fractions in which the light can be divided, such as Doppler shifted and non-Doppler shifted light.

general form $R_E(\Delta x, \Delta y)$ and $I(x', y')$ are related by

$$R_E(\Delta X, \Delta Y) = \frac{\int \int_{\text{source}} I(x', y') \exp\left[-i\frac{2\pi}{\lambda Z}(x'\Delta x + y'\Delta y)\right] dx'dy'}{\int \int_{\text{source}} I(x', y')dx'dy'} \tag{7.4}$$

Now, if we know the intensity distribution $I(x', y')$ of the light emitted at the source plane, we can calculate $R_E(\Delta x)$ with Eq. (7.4), $R_I(\Delta x)$ with Eq. (7.3), and eventually A_{speckle} using Eq. (7.2). Remember that this "source" can be a tissue that diffusely and specularly reflects some of the light that it is illuminated with.

For the simple case of a circular homogeneous source, we find that

$$A_{\text{speckle}} = \frac{\lambda^2}{\Omega} \tag{7.5}$$

with angle Ω being the solid angle of the incoming light. Equation (7.5) is a rule of thumb often used for estimating the speckle size when Ω is approximately known.

7.3
Significance of Speckles in LDPI

In the previous section, we only took into account the properties of static speckle patterns. In LDPI, we deal with dynamic speckle patterns, with sometimes a certain static component. The presence of a static component in the speckle pattern will

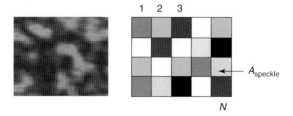

Figure 7.4 Instantaneous speckle pattern with speckle area A_{spec} and an equivalent instantaneous "speckle pattern" consisting of N speckles with equal area $A_{speckle}$ and uniform intensity within each speckle.

depend on the nature of the medium in which the light is scattered. If the medium contains moving particles at a sufficient concentration, all light will be Doppler shifted, leading to a completely dynamic speckle pattern. If a part of the light, which is diffusely scattered by the medium, has not undergone a Doppler shift, a part of the speckle pattern will be static. Here, we first assume a completely dynamic speckle pattern, generated only by Doppler-shifted light. We now analyze the consequence of the speckled nature of the intensity distribution on the photodetector. Instead of a natural speckle pattern as shown in Figure 7.4, we now assume an equivalent pattern such as the one shown in Figure 7.4, consisting of N speckles with equal area $A_{speckle}$ and uniform intensity. "Equivalent" here means that both speckle patterns will generate the same photocurrent fluctuations.

We assume that all speckles are statistically identical, having the same average intensity $\langle i_{sp} \rangle$ and distribution of intensity fluctuations $\delta i_{sp}(t)$. The photocurrent generated by any speckle can then be written as $i_{sp}(t) = \langle i_{sp} \rangle + \delta i_{sp}(t)$. The current $i_{tot}(t)$ generated by the total speckle pattern is the sum of the currents of the individual speckles. For the variance of the total photocurrent we find

$$\langle i_{tot}^2 \rangle = \left\langle \sum_{j=1}^{N} \sum_{k=1}^{N} i_j(t)\, i_k(t) \right\rangle = N^2 \langle i_{sp} \rangle^2 + N \langle \delta i_{sp}^2 \rangle = N^2 \langle i_{sp} \rangle^2 + N \langle i_{sp} \rangle^2 \quad (7.6)$$

This result is obtained if we assume that the intensity fluctuations of all speckles are mutually uncorrelated. In fact, this could be called the definition of the speckle concept within the framework of laser Doppler flowmetry. The second step in Eq. (7.6) can be made, thanks to the Poisson intensity distribution of speckle patterns. We earlier invoked this property to conclude that for polarized speckle the contrast $K = 1$. While this was stated for the spatial variations in a static speckle pattern, it also holds for the temporal fluctuations at one position within a dynamic speckle pattern, that is, there is a Poisson intensity distribution in space and time. The first term of the right-hand side of Eq. (7.6) is related to the DC part of the photocurrent, while the second term is caused by the photocurrent fluctuations. From Eq. (7.6), it follows that the modulation depth of the total photodetector current is

$$M \equiv \frac{\langle i_{AC}^2 \rangle}{\langle i_{DC} \rangle^2} = \frac{1}{N} \quad (7.7)$$

For a mixed static–dynamic speckle pattern, generated by light of which a fraction f has been Doppler shifted, it can be shown [9] that

$$M = \frac{1}{N} f(2 - f) \tag{7.8}$$

For simplicity, we have assumed that the spatial intensity distributions on the tissue surface of Doppler-shifted light and nonshifted light are identical. In general, this will not be the case because Doppler-shifted photons will, on average, have a wider path length distribution and a wider intensity distribution at the tissue surface. The problem is treated in its full complexity by Steenbergen and coworkers [9]. This reference provide a theory for the general case that all photons can be divided into fractions according to relevant criteria, for instance, Doppler shifted versus nonshifted and photons with large penetration depth versus photons with small penetration depth.

Suppose that we can divide the detected light in a static fraction f_0 and Doppler-shifted fractions $f_1, f_2, \ldots, f_N$ whose sum, by definition, is $1 - f_0$. The situation for two fractions is indicated in Figure 7.3. Now, for the modulation depth of the photodetector signal we find

$$M = 2 \sum_i^M f_0 f_i \frac{A^{0i}_{\text{speckle}}}{A_{\text{det}}} + \sum_{i=1}^M \sum_{j=1}^M f_i f_j \frac{A^{ij}_{\text{speckle}}}{A_{\text{det}}} \tag{7.9}$$

Here, A^{ij}_{speckle} is the so-called fractional speckle area, which can be calculated from the field correlation functions $R^i_E(\Delta x)$ and $R^j_E(\Delta x)$ of each fraction f_i and f_j as

$$A^{ij}_{\text{coh}} = 2\pi \int_0^\infty R^i_E(\Delta x) R^{*j}_E(\Delta x) \Delta x \, \mathrm{d}\Delta x \tag{7.10}$$

For each fraction i, the field correlation function $R^i_E(\Delta x)$ can be obtained from the intensity distribution $I^i(x', y')$ of that fraction, by using Eq. (7.4). This theory will allow us to predict signal levels generated by light composed of the arbitrary fraction of Doppler-shifted light and to calculate the relative contribution of each fraction to the total photodetector current.

7.4
Further Analysis of the Consequence of Speckle in LDPI

From Eqs. (7.5) and (7.6), it can be concluded that the number of speckles N involved in signal generation, and therefore the speckle size, determines the overall response of the system. How can the number of speckles N involved in speckle generation vary? The LDPI geometry that we will consider here is that of a scanning laser beam and a lens that images the tissue onto a photodetector. The situation is depicted in Figure 7.5. For a given optical system, the solid angle Ω is constant. However, the effective detector size A_{det} will vary with the tissue optical properties as indicated in the figure, and therefore N will vary. For a given detector area and a given average light intensity, small speckles (large N) generate small

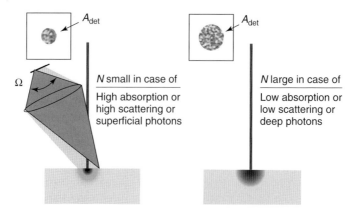

Figure 7.5 Essentials of a laser Doppler perfusion imager. Two effective detector sizes A_{det} are indicated, associated with high or low levels of scattering and/or absorption and with photons with a large or small penetration depth.

photocurrent fluctuations and large speckles (small N) generate large fluctuations of the photocurrent. Furthermore, from our theory [9], it can be concluded that if a certain category of photons generates by itself speckles smaller than the average size, its contribution to the total photocurrent fluctuations will be relatively suppressed. Such a category could be the photons that reached at least a certain depth. This category will occupy a larger detector area than the superficial photons, and the associated value of N will be relatively large.

For scanning beam LDPI devices without a lens, the solid angle Ω will vary with tissue optical properties or photon penetration depth, and in this case, A_{det} is determined by the physical size of the photodetector. It has been shown [11] that the conclusions drawn in this chapter also hold for this configuration.

Hence, we restrict ourselves to the category of scanning beam perfusion imagers [12, 13]. The conclusions will *not* hold for the recent wide-field LDPI devices with high-speed cameras [14–18]. In these, the number of speckles N will only depend on the properties of the imaging system.

The above concept is now elaborated for the following properties of scanning beam LDPI devices:

- The overall sensitivity of a laser Doppler system in relation to the beam size and the tissue optical properties.
- The depth sensitivity of LDPI.
- The width of the power spectrum of photocurrent fluctuations.

7.4.1
Overall Sensitivity

As a measure of sensitivity, we take the modulation depth of the photodetector signal, as defined in Eq. (7.7). The overall sensitivity of an LDPI system for a range of absorption and scattering coefficients was studied by Monte Carlo simulations. We simulated [19] the situation of a system with a Gaussian beam with $1/e^2$ diameter of 1 mm. The simulated tissue configuration was a static matrix with thin dynamic layers at a mutual spacing of 0.25 mm. We recorded both the detection positions on the tissue surface and the Doppler shift of all detected photons. From these, the fractions of Doppler-shifted photons f_1 and unshifted photons f_0, and the intensity distributions of Doppler-shifted and unshifted light, can be calculated for use in Eqs. (7.9) and (7.10). While the properties of the dynamic layers were kept constant, the levels of absorption and scattering were varied. The results are shown in Figure 7.6a for only the photon statistics and in Figure 7.6b for both

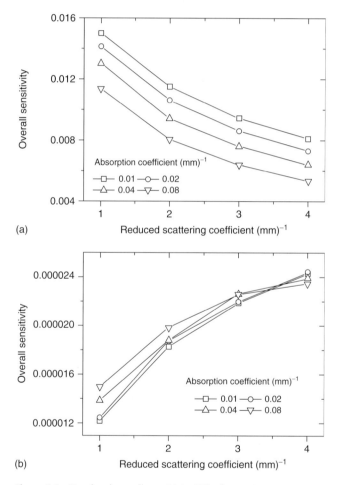

(a)

(b)

Figure 7.6 Simulated overall sensitivity [20] of scanning beam LDPI system with 1 mm beam diameter for a range of absorption and reduced scattering coefficients. (a) Based on photon statistics only. (b) Speckle effects included. (Source: Printed with permission of SPIE.)

photon statistics and the speckle effect. Both show a completely different picture. On the basis of photon statistics only, sensitivity decreases with both absorption and scattering level of the static medium, since both will reduce the path length of photons and therefore the probability of Doppler shifting. However, when the speckle effect is incorporated, the sensitivity increases with the level of scattering and absorption. Both can be explained, with reference to Figure 7.5, from the fact that increased absorption and/or scattering leads to a smaller effective detector, and therefore a larger value of N. These variations completely overrule the trends that are observed from photon statistics only.

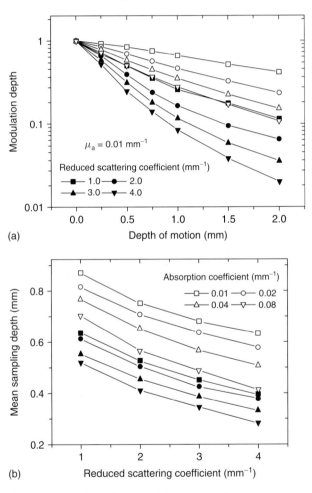

Figure 7.7 Simulated depth sensitivity [20]. (a) Sensitivity versus motion depth, for a range of reduced scattering coefficients. All results normalized to unit sensitivity at zero depth. (b) Mean sampling depth. White symbols: only photon statistics. Black symbols: speckle effects included. (Source: Printed with permission from SPIE.)

7.4.2
Depth Sensitivity

The same simulated medium as in the previous paragraph was used to analyze the sensitivity for motion at a certain depth. The result is shown in Figure 7.7a, which shows the sensitivity versus motion depth for a certain absorption coefficient and a range of scattering coefficients, and in Figure 7.7b, which shows the mean sampling depth. Results are based on photon statistics only (White symbols) and with inclusion of the speckle effect (black symbols). We observe that the effect of the factor $1/N$ in Eq. (7.8) is that the sampling depth is largely reduced. This can be explained by the fact that photons that penetrate deeper in the medium will drift further away from the point of injection and will therefore occupy a larger part of the detector. Our results show that the effect is a suppression of sensitivity to motion at a larger depth. An experimental verification of this behavior is described by in [20].

7.5
Consequences and Concluding Remarks

In this chapter, we surveyed the consequences of the speckled nature of light in LDPI. The analysis is limited to scanning beam LDPI devices that use a single collimated laser beam [12, 13]. This speckled character has a significant influence on the measurement characteristics of these devices. First, the overall sensitivity is affected, depending on the tissue optical properties. This effect, shown in Figure 7.6, is additional to the obvious influence of the optical properties on photon path length.

Second, the depth sensitivity is affected. Neglecting the speckle effect when analyzing the depth sensitivity may lead to an error by a factor of 2, as shown in Figure 7.6.

Finally, not shown in this chapter but demonstrated in reference [11] the speckle phenomenon has an influence on the shape of the power spectrum of photocurrent fluctuations and, therefore, on the estimated average Doppler shift. The effect is a reduction of the average Doppler shift of 10–30% compared to the unknown real value.

Generally, then, speckle leads to an additional cross talk between perfusion estimations and tissue optical properties. In principle, this cross talk can be suppressed by increasing the beam diameter. However, this will deteriorate both the signal level and the spatial resolution, and therefore cannot be considered as a fundamental solution of the problem. The tissue optical dependence of the system sensitivity on the tissue optical properties due to the speckle phenomenon is inevitable in scanning beam laser Doppler perfusion imagers.

References

1. Aizu, Y. and Asakura, T. (1991) Bio-speckle phenomena and their application to the evaluation of blood flow. *Opt. Laser Technol.*, **23** (4), 205–219.

2. Asakura, T. and Takai, N. (1981) Dynamic laser speckles and their application to velocity measurements of the diffuse object. *Appl. Phys.*, **25**, 179–194.

3. Fuji, H. *et al.* (1985) Blood flow observed by time-varying laser speckle. *Opt. Lett.*, **10** (3), 104–106.

4. Ruth, B. (1990) Blood flow determination by the laser speckle method. *Int. J. Microcirc. Clin. Exp.*, **9**, 21–45.

5. Nilsson, G.E., Tenland, T., and Oberg, P.A. (1980) Evaluation of a laser Doppler flowmeter for measurement of tissue blood-flow. *IEEE Trans. Biomed. Eng.*, **27** (10), 597–604.

6. Bonner, R. and Nossal, R. (1981) Model for laser Doppler measurements of blood-flow in tissue. *Appl. Opt.*, **20** (12), 2097–2107.

7. Goodman, J.W. (1976) Some fundamental properties of speckle. *J. Opt. Soc. Am.*, **66** (11), 1145–1150.

8. Goodman, J.W. (2007) *Speckle Phenomena in Optics – Theory and Applications*, Roberts & Company.

9. Serov, A., Steenbergen, W., and de Mul, F. (2001) Prediction of the photodetector signal generated by Doppler-induced speckle fluctuations: theory and some validations. *J. Opt. Soc. Am. A*, **18** (3), 622–630.

10. Born, M. and Wolf, E. (1985) *Principles in Optics*, 6th edn, Cambridge University Press, Cambridge.

11. Rajan, V. *et al.* (2006) Speckles in laser Doppler perfusion imaging. *Opt. Lett.*, **31** (4), 468–470.

12. Essex, T.J.H. and Byrne, P.O. (1991) A laser Doppler scanner for imaging blood-flow in skin. *J. Biomed. Eng.*, **13** (3), 189–194.

13. Wardell, K., Jakobsson, A., and Nilsson, G.E. (1993) Laser-Doppler perfusion imaging by dynamic light-scattering. *IEEE Trans. Biomed. Eng.*, **40** (4), 309–319.

14. Draijer, M. *et al.* (2009) Twente optical perfusion camera: system overview and performance for video rate laser Doppler perfusion imaging. *Opt. Express*, **17** (5), 3211–3225.

15. Gu, Q., Hayes-Gill, B.R., and Morgan, S.P. (2008) Laser Doppler blood flow complementary metal oxide semiconductor imaging sensor with analog on-chip processing. *Appl. Opt.*, **47** (12), 2061–2069.

16. Serov, A. and Lasser, T. (2005) High-speed laser Doppler perfusion imaging using an integrating CMOS image sensor. *Opt. Express*, **13** (17), 6416–6428.

17. Serov, A., Steenbergen, W., and de Mul, F. (2002) Laser Doppler perfusion imaging with a complimentary metal oxide semiconductor image sensor. *Opt. Lett.*, **27** (5), 300–302.

18. Serov, A., Steinacher, B., and Lasser, T. (2005) Full-field laser Doppler perfusion imaging and monitoring with an intelligent CMOS camera. *Opt. Express*, **13** (10), 3681–3689.

19. Rajan, V. *et al.* (2008) Influence of tissue optical properties on laser Doppler perfusion imaging, accounting for photon penetration depth and the laser speckle phenomenon. *J. Biomed. Opt.*, **13** (2), 024001.

20. Rajan, V. *et al.* (2007) Effect of speckles on the depth sensitivity of laser Doppler perfusion imaging. *Opt. Express*, **15** (17), 10911–10919.

8
Laser Speckle Contrast Analysis (LASCA) for Measuring Blood Flow

J. David Briers, Paul M. McNamara, Marie Louise O'Connell, and Martin J. Leahy

8.1
Introduction: Fundamentals of Laser Speckle

Laser speckle is a random interference pattern produced when laser light is scattered from an optically rough surface or a diffuse medium such as biological tissue [1]. Light from different parts of the surface within a resolution cell (the area just resolved by the optical system imaging the surface) traverses different optical path lengths to reach the image plane. The resulting intensity at a given point on the image is determined by the algebraic addition of all the wave amplitudes arriving at the point. If the resultant amplitude is zero, a dark speckle is seen at the point; if all the waves arrive at the point in phase, an intensity maximum is observed.

Laser speckle is a random phenomenon and can only be described statistically. One important result is an expression for the contrast of a speckle pattern. Assuming ideal conditions for producing a speckle pattern – highly coherent, single-frequency laser light and a perfectly diffusing surface with a Gaussian distribution of surface height fluctuations – it can be shown that the standard deviation of the intensity variations in the speckle pattern is equal to the mean intensity. In practice, speckle patterns often have a standard deviation that is less than the mean intensity: this is observed as a reduction in the contrast of the speckle pattern. It is customary to define speckle contrast as the ratio of the standard deviation to the mean intensity

$$\text{Speckle contrast} = \frac{\sigma}{\langle I \rangle} \leq 1 \tag{8.1}$$

Although a detailed account of laser speckle statistics [2] is outside the scope of this chapter, it is worth mentioning at this point that the size of the individual speckles has, in general, nothing to do with the structure of the surface producing them. It is entirely determined by the aperture of the optical system used to observe the speckle pattern. If the speckle pattern is being observed directly by the human eye, it is the pupil of the eye that determines the speckle size. More importantly, if a camera is used, it is the setting of the aperture stop that determines the speckle size. This can have a serious effect if the aperture is used to control the exposure of the photograph.

Microcirculation Imaging, First Edition. Edited by Martin J. Leahy.
© 2012 Wiley-VCH Verlag GmbH & Co. KGaA. Published 2012 by Wiley-VCH Verlag GmbH & Co. KGaA.

8.2
Time-Varying Speckle

When an object moves, the speckle pattern it produces changes. For small movements of a solid object, the speckles move with the object – that is, they remain correlated. For larger motions, the speckles "decorrelate" and the speckle pattern changes completely. Decorrelation also occurs when the light is scattered from a large number of individual moving scatterers, such as particles in a fluid. An individual speckle appears to "twinkle" like a star. This phenomenon has come to be known as *time-varying speckle*. It is frequently seen when living organisms are observed under laser light illumination.

It is reasonable to assume that the frequency spectrum of the fluctuations should be dependent on the velocity of the motion. It should therefore be possible to obtain information about the motion of the scatterers from a study of the temporal statistics of the speckle fluctuations. This analysis can be based on the techniques of either *photon correlation spectroscopy* or *laser Doppler velocimetry*. It is not intuitively obvious that time-varying speckle and Doppler-induced fluctuations are identical. The theory of time-varying speckle starts with the classical (though random) interference pattern produced when light beams of the same frequency interfere. The fluctuations are caused by the changes in optical path lengths of the interfering beams, which is caused by the movement of the scatterers. Doppler fluctuations, on the other hand, are explained by the beating effect that occurs when two waves of slightly different frequency are superimposed, the difference being due to the frequency shift induced by the Doppler effect when light is scattered by a moving object. Thus the speckle explanation is based on the superposition of waves of the *same* frequency, whereas in the Doppler explanation, the superimposed waves have *different* frequencies. Despite these apparent differences in approach, it can be shown mathematically that the two explanations lead to identical equations linking the fluctuations to the velocity distribution of the scatterers [3, 4]. Thus, the two approaches are merely different ways of looking at the same physical phenomenon.

8.3
Full-Field Speckle Methods

One problem with using the temporal statistics of time-varying speckle is that measurements are made at only one point in the speckle pattern (a single speckle). If an area is to be analyzed, it is necessary to scan the detector over the field. If a map of velocity distribution is required, some method of scanning the area of interest is necessary. Such a map is of particular importance if blood flow is to be used as a diagnostic tool. Fujii *et al.* [5] used a scanning technique in their application of time-differentiated speckle to measure skin capillary blood flow. They used a linear CCD array to monitor simultaneously a line of speckles and a scanning mirror to extend this to a two-dimensional area. They later applied the technique to the mapping of retinal blood flow [6–9]. They produced a microcirculation map of the retina by illuminating the retina with light from a diode laser, scanning and storing the speckle images, and then calculating the differences between successive images. The parameter they use is the ratio of the mean intensity to the intensity difference, a quantity they call "normalized blur" and which they use as a measure of velocity. Experiments on a rabbit eye showed good correlation with invasive methods [7].

Scanning has also been applied to the laser Doppler technique [8, 10, 11], and commercial scanning Doppler systems that can provide full-field monitoring of capillary blood flow over quite large areas of the body are now on the market. The problem of either processing or storing vast amounts of data demands a compromise between cost and performance, and the systems offered suffer from both long scanning times and a loss of spatial resolution [10, 12]. Nevertheless, they are useful as a diagnostic tool and offer easily interpreted false-color maps of blood velocity and/or flow.

The scanning necessary to apply time-varying speckle techniques to map velocity distributions results in the collection of a vast amount of data and usually takes an appreciable time (typically 5 min for 256×256 pixels). Ideally, a full-field technique would avoid the need for scanning. One such technique is the "global Doppler" method [13]. This directly converts velocity to intensity (or false color) by the ingenious device of measuring how much of the return light is absorbed by a substance of known absorption/frequency properties. Unfortunately, resolution problems limit the technique to fairly high velocities, and it is not suitable for biomedical applications. Further advances in this area are described in Chapter 6.

There is another way to avoid the need to scan – by using the *spatial* statistics (specifically the contrast) of time-integrated fluctuating speckle patterns. If the integration time is comparable with the period of the fluctuations, it is clear that the effect will be a reduction in the speckle contrast.

8.4
Single-Exposure Speckle Photography

The use of such *time-integrated speckle* led to a technique for flow visualization in the early 1980s that simultaneously achieved full-field operation (without scanning) and very simple data gathering and processing. It was originally called *"single-exposure speckle photography"* [14], to distinguish it from the then well-known technique of double-exposure speckle photography for measuring displacement and strain. Single-exposure speckle photography was developed primarily for the measurement of retinal blood flow [15, 16]. The basic technique is simply to photograph the retina under laser illumination using an exposure time that is of the same order as the decorrelation time of the intensity fluctuations. It is clear that a very short exposure time will "freeze" the speckle and result in a high-contrast speckle pattern, whereas a long exposure time will allow the speckles to average out, leading to a low contrast. In general, the velocity distribution in the field of view is mapped as variations in speckle contrast. In the original technique, high-pass optical spatial filtering of the resulting photographs converted these contrast variations to more easily seen intensity variations [17]. Later work introduced digital image processing of the speckle photographs, including a color coding of the velocities [18].

8.5
Laser Speckle Contrast Analysis (LASCA)

By 1990, digital techniques were sufficiently advanced to allow the photographic stage to be eliminated. By measuring the speckle contrast directly and converting the data to a false-color image, a fully digital, real-time technique for mapping skin capillary blood flow was developed [19]. The technique was called "laser speckle contrast analysis" or LASCA. Some researchers still use this name [20, 21], but others have introduced names such as laser speckle contrast imaging (LSCI) [22] or laser speckle imaging (LSI) [23]. For the sake of simplicity, we shall use the term *LASCA* in this chapter, as this was the name used in the original 1996 work [24].

In the past decade, there has been an accelerated adoption of LASCA technology as the neuroscience community has used it to measure blood flow in the brain. Over the past decade, there have been more than 100 publications on the topic, significantly advancing its theory and application. For example, Bandyopadhyay *et al.* [25] presented an important correction in the calculation of laser speckle contrast and its relation to temporal fluctuations. This was an important calibration procedure for handling static scattering from the skull, which would otherwise confuse the estimate of blood flow from spatial laser speckle contrast [26], while Li *et al.* [27] showed that temporal laser speckle contrast imaging, or TLSCI, is intrinsically less sensitive to static scattering. More recently, Kirkpatrick *et al.* [28] and Duncan *et al.* [2], presented important theoretical work quantifying the impact of speckle size and sampling windows on the statistics of laser speckle, while others have demonstrated more efficient algorithms for calculating speckle contrast to enable real-time visualization [29, 30]. The technique is also being incorporated into multimodal imaging schemes to obtain additional information about the tissue [31–34].

The experimental setup for LASCA is very simple, as shown in Figure 8.1. Diverging laser light illuminates the object under investigation, which is imaged by a CCD camera (or equivalent). The image is captured by a frame grabber (or equivalent), and the data is passed to a personal computer for processing by custom software. Usually, the operator has several options at his disposal. In the original LASCA technique [24], this included the exposure time, the number of pixels over which the local contrast was computed, the scaling of the contrast map, and the choice of colors for coding the contrast. The choice of the number of pixels over which to compute the speckle contrast is important: with too few pixels, the statistics will be compromised, whereas with too many pixels, the spatial resolution is sacrificed.

A survey of the literature indicates that the community has empirically settled on a window size of 7×7 pixels as a reasonable trade-off between spatial resolution

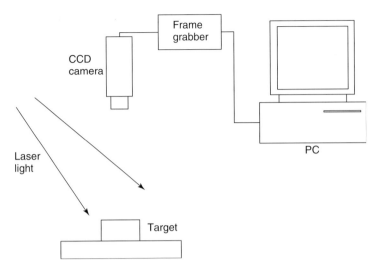

Figure 8.1 Basic setup for laser speckle contrast analysis (LASCA).

and uncertainty in the estimated speckle contrast, but all this depends on camera resolution, speckle size, and desired contrast resolution [35]. (A square with sides of an odd number of pixels was chosen so that the computed contrast could be assigned to the central pixel.) The speckle contrast is quantified by the usual parameter of the ratio of the standard deviation to the mean ($\sigma / \langle I \rangle$) of the intensities recorded for each pixel in the square (Eq. (8.1)). The pixel square is then moved along by 1 pixel and the calculation repeated: this overlapping of the pixel squares results in a much smoother image than would be obtained by using contiguous squares, and at little cost in terms of additional processing time. It must be remembered, though, that this overlapping of the squares does not lead to an increase in resolution, which is determined by the size of square used: there is a trade-off between spatial resolution and reliable statistics.

If the object under investigation contains moving scatterers, such as blood cells, each speckle will be fluctuating in intensity. A time-integrated image therefore shows a reduction in speckle contrast because of the averaging of the intensity of each speckle over the integration time. In practice, the exposure time can be very short, typically 0.02 s, and the processing time is less than 1 s for the whole frame [36], effectively making it a real-time technique. (Recent work has further reduced the processing time to milliseconds, making real-time video possible.)

8.6
The Question of Speckle Size

A complicating factor for the technique is that of speckle size. As mentioned in Section 8.1, this is determined entirely by the aperture of the imaging system used (in this case the camera). The pixels of the detector are effectively sampling the speckle pattern. If the speckles are smaller than the pixels, some averaging will occur and the technique rapidly becomes less effective. If the speckles are much larger than the pixels, only a few speckles will be sampled by the square of pixels used, and the statistics will become unreliable. It was previously thought that the best compromise was to arrange for the speckle size to be equal to the pixel size. However, recent studies have shown that an increased contrast is achieved when the minimum speckle size is twice the camera pixel size [2, 35]. Assuming that the Nyquist sampling criterion is met, it was determined that the variation of the estimated speckle contrast could be expressed by a dimensionless width parameter. The formulation reveals that the variation in the speckle contrast dramatically decreases as the window size is increased to 7×7, but then, diminishing returns are obtained for larger window sizes. Essentially, increasing the speckle size means that a given window of pixels is estimating the speckle contrast from fewer speckles. Ultimately, smaller window sizes resulted in an underestimation of the speckle contrast [2].

The speckle size can be easily set by choosing an appropriate setting for the aperture of the camera lens. However, this removes the possibility of using the aperture to control the amount of light reaching the detector, the usual function of a variable lens aperture. Further, the shutter speed cannot be used to do this, as it is determined by the need to match the velocities being measured, and some other method of controlling the amount of light reaching the detector must be found.

8.7
Theory

The principle of LASCA is very simple. A time-integrated image of a moving object exhibits blurring. In the case of a laser speckle pattern, this appears as a reduction in the speckle contrast, defined (and measured) as the ratio of the standard deviation of the intensity to the mean intensity. This occurs whatever be the "movement" of the speckle. For random velocity distributions, each speckle fluctuates in intensity. For lateral motion of a solid object, on the other hand, the speckles also move laterally and become "smeared" on the image, but a reduction in speckle contrast still occurs. For fluid flow, the situation might be a combination of both these types of "movement." In each case, the problem for quantitative measurements is the establishment of a relationship between speckle contrast and velocity (or velocity distribution).

It is clear that there must be a link between the flow velocity and the amount of blurring. The higher the velocity, the faster are the fluctuations and the more is the blurring that occurs in a given integration time. By making certain assumptions, the following mathematical relationship can be established between speckle contrast and the temporal statistics of the fluctuating speckle [14]:

$$\sigma_s^2(T) = \frac{1}{T} \int_0^T \tilde{g}_2(\tau)d\tau \tag{8.2}$$

where σ_s^2 is the *spatial* variance of the intensity in the speckle pattern, T is the integration time, and $\tilde{g}_2(\tau)$ is the autocovariance of the *temporal* fluctuations in the intensity of a single speckle. The autocovariance is a normalized version of the autocorrelation function and is defined as follows:

$$\tilde{g}_2(\tau) = \frac{\tilde{G}_2(\tau)}{\tilde{G}_2(0)} \tag{8.3}$$

where $\tilde{G}_2(\tau) = \langle \left(I(t) - \langle I \rangle_t \right) \left(I(t+\tau) - \langle I \rangle_t \right) \rangle_t$

Equation (8.3) defines the relationship between LASCA and those techniques that use the intensity fluctuations in laser light scattered from moving objects or particles. LASCA measures the quantity on the left-hand side of Eq. (8.3); photon correlation spectroscopy, laser Doppler, and time-varying speckle techniques measure the quantity on the right-hand side. (It is also worth noting that LASCA uses *image speckle*, whereas most of the temporal techniques use *far-field speckle*. However, this does not detract from the fundamental equivalence of the two approaches expressed in Eq. (8.3)).

Provided the assumptions made in establishing Eq. (8.3) are valid, LASCA is now on an equal footing with all the temporal techniques (photon correlation, Doppler, time-varying speckle) so far as linking the measurements to actual velocities is concerned. All the techniques now allow the correlation time τ_c to be determined. In the case of photon correlation, this parameter is measured directly. In the case of LASCA, some further assumptions must be made in order to link the measurement of speckle contrast (defined as $\sigma_s/\langle I \rangle$) with τ_c.

Various models can be used, depending on the type of motion being monitored. For the case of a Lorentzian velocity distribution, for example, the equation becomes [14]

$$\frac{\sigma_s}{\langle I \rangle} = \left[\frac{\tau_c}{2T} \left\{ 1 - \exp\left(\frac{-2T}{\tau_c} \right) \right\} \right]^{\frac{1}{2}} \tag{8.4}$$

Equation (8.4) (and similar equations for other types of scatterer motion) relates the speckle contrast, defined as the ratio of the standard deviation of the speckle pattern intensity to its mean intensity, to the ratio of correlation time τ_c to the integration time T. The relationship is plotted in Figure 8.2.

Figure 8.2 shows that the speckle contrast increases from near zero to near its maximum value of 1 over about 3 orders of magnitude of τ_c (and hence of velocity). (For a single exposure, of course, T is a constant.) For flow velocities corresponding to values of τ_c less than about $0.04T$, the speckle contrast is very low, that is, the speckles are completely blurred out by the motion. For velocities corresponding to values of τ_c greater than about $4T$, the speckle pattern has high contrast. Between these limits, flow velocity will be mapped as variations in speckle contrast. If a different velocity distribution is assumed, for example, a Gaussian or a uniform distribution, the curve is slightly different, but still shows this characteristic S-shape. The dynamic range – the range of velocities that can be covered – remains similar.

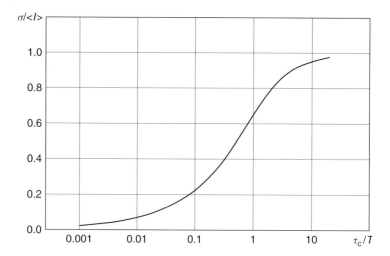

Figure 8.2 Variation of speckle contrast with the ratio decorrelation time to integration time for the Lorentzian model of LASCA.

8.8
Practical Considerations

From this point on, LASCA experiences the same problem as all the *temporal* frequency measurement techniques – photon correlation spectroscopy, laser Doppler, and time-varying speckle. This is the problem of relating the correlation time τ_c to the velocity distribution of the scatterers. It is not straightforward. Problems include the effects of multiple scattering, the size of the scattering particles (blood cells in the present case), the shape of the scatterers, non-Newtonian flow, non-Gaussian statistics resulting from a low number of scatterers in the resolution cell, spin of the scatterers, and so on. Much work is being done on these effects, and the question is far from settled. Because of the uncertainties caused by these factors, it is common in all of these techniques to rely mainly on ratiometric rather than on absolute measurements.

Another problem that occurs with LASCA is the difficulty in achieving the full range of contrasts that should theoretically be available. A stationary object should give a speckle contrast of one ($\sigma = \langle I \rangle$, in accordance with well-established speckle statistics theory and experiment). A fully blurred speckle pattern produced by rapidly moving scatterers should have zero contrast. The Lorentzian model of Eq. (8.4), for example, predicts the relationship between contrast ($\sigma/\langle I \rangle$) and the ratio τ_c/T presented in Figure 8.2. This suggests that, for a given integration time T, the dynamic range of the technique corresponding to contrasts between 0.1 and 0.9 should be about 3 orders of magnitude in τ_c (and hence in velocity). In practice, maximum contrasts of only 0.6 were being measured, even for stationary random diffusers [19]. One possible cause of this problem is the CCD camera. Most CCD cameras are designed to produce a DC offset from zero called the *pedestal*. This is to avoid cutting off the negative peaks produced during any processing. It is formed because of the dark current and other anomalies in the video circuitry of the camera. By carrying out some preprocessing on the data, it is possible to remove the effect of the dark current. When this was done [37], the measured speckle contrast on the image of a stationary diffusing surface rose to 0.95, very close to the theoretical value of 1.0 for a fully developed speckle pattern. Similarly, the measured contrast in the speckle pattern recorded from a hand increased from 0.33 to 0.68. This lower contrast (compared with the stationary diffuser) is due to the scatterers in the hand (the red blood cells) being in motion.

Other problems with the statistics occur as a result of effects such as the Gaussian profile of the laser beam and the nonlinearity of the CCD camera [37]. However, many of these problems also affect the laser Doppler, photon correlation, and other time-varying speckle techniques.

Other parameters can be varied. The effect of using different exposure times (integration times) has been investigated, and times as short as 1 ms have been used. Also, wavelengths other than 633 nm could be used. There is a need in some clinical situations, for example, eczema and other dermatological problems, to measure the superficial dermal blood flow [38]. This has prompted several groups to use other wavelengths with the laser Doppler technique [38–40]. Penetration of tissue is highly wavelength dependent, with infrared light penetrating the furthest (several millimeters) and green and blue hardly penetrating (typically 150 μm for green light).

8.9
Applications and Examples

The original LASCA technique was developed specifically for monitoring capillary blood flow in the skin. Figure 8.3 shows an example from the mid-1990s. It shows part of a forearm with a superficial hot-water burn. The increased perfusion around the burn is clearly visible.

Some researchers have continued this theme of using LASCA and related techniques to measure skin and other microcirculation blood flow [41–45]. Others have used it to characterize atherosclerotic plaques [46]. There has also been a return to the area that first prompted the development of single-exposure speckle photography in the 1980s – ophthalmology [7, 15, 47–49]. However, the most important application of the LASCA technique is currently in the area of neurological research, for monitoring cerebral blood flow [21, 31, 50–60]. A specific investigation was into the causes of migraine [61]. (It is stressed that these examples are just a selection from the large amount of work that is going on – the list is not meant to be exhaustive. We are aware of more than 40 groups in at least 18 countries who are working on or with the LASCA technique.)

The intensive activity involving the LASCA technique in recent years has, of course, been accompanied by improvements in the images produced. Two

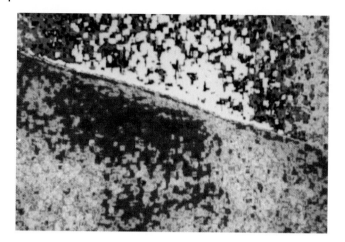

Figure 8.3 LASCA image of part of a forearm, showing increased perfusion around the site of a hot-water burn [24].

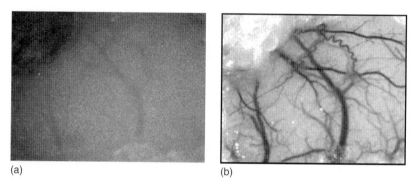

(a)   (b)

Figure 8.4 Raw image of part of a rat cortex (a), and its processed version (b). (Source: D. Boas, Harvard Medical School.)

examples are reproduced here. Figure 8.4 is from David Boas' group at the Harvard Medical School, and Figure 8.5 is from Andrew Dunn at the University of Texas. In both cases, the improvement in the quality of the images is clear.

8.10
Recent Developments

In general, researchers using LASCA have developed their own version of the technique. This has naturally led to some significant improvements. Developments include optimization of the exposure time [22], noise reduction [62], and some significant contributions to the theory [23, 63]. Optimal integration time varies from 1 ms for faster flow to 20 ms where the flow in smallest vessels

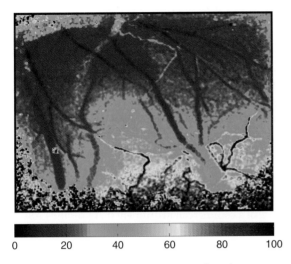

0   20   40   60   80   100

Figure 8.5 Blood flow changes during stroke: relative cerebral blood flow 10 min after occlusion of the middle cerebral artery in a rat, demonstrating the spatial gradient in the blood flow deficit due to the ischemia. (Source: A. K. Dunn, University of Texas.)

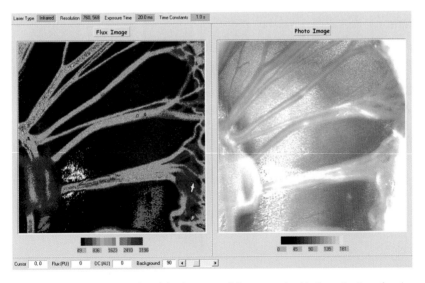

Figure 8.6 This image, produced by the Moor Instruments laser perfusion imager (FLPI), shows the mesenteric vessels in a frog. The area shown is approximately 1 cm², and the gut runs around the right periphery of the image. In this investigation, the user is assessing angiogenic growth in mesenteric vessels caused by a virus. This image was taken before injection of the virus. (Source: Moor Instruments Ltd: *www.moor.co.uk*.)

(with slower flow) is being studied [22, 35]. Issues such as the need to know the flow range *a priori* and the fact that the theoretical basis is not as rigorous have meant that laser speckle has a much slower uptake than LDPI. A proposal to use a multiple exposure version of LASCA has recently been made [64]. The authors show that this approach leads to a power spectral measurement that is exactly equivalent to the Doppler spectrum and therefore provides a more robust theoretical basis for the technique. This means that laser speckle contrast can be used to measure perfusion with the same assumptions that are required for Doppler perfusion measurements, but with the advantage of generating full-field images at video rates. Some workers [25] have identified errors in the original theoretical formulations (such as Eq. (8.4)). Some recent work, however, shows that the model still forms a reliable basis on which to quantify velocities from the contrast measurements [59].

In late 2006, a major development took place with the announcement by Moor Instruments Ltd, a UK company, of a commercial instrument that uses the LASCA technique. Moreover, it has a real-time video capability. For the first time, this allows the researcher or clinician to follow changes of blood flow in real time. Of course, some resolution is sacrificed in order to achieve the high-speed processing required, but the instrument also has a still facility for those cases where resolution must be maintained. Typical images from the instrument are shown in

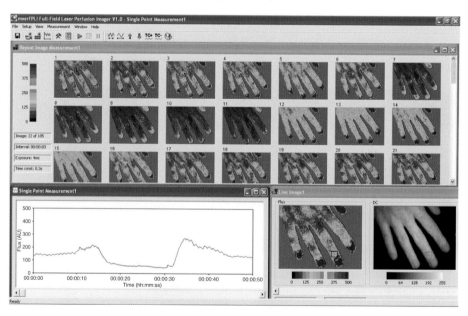

Figure 8.7 A composite image produced by the Moor Instruments laser perfusion imager (FLPI). The series of images of the hand shows the baseline blood flow, the changes during a partial occlusion using a pressure cuff, and the flow following pressure release. The images were taken at 3 s intervals. The single image window is from a video sequence taken at 25 frames per second with a time constant of 0.3 s. The single point measurement is taken from a finger tip. (Source: Moor Instruments Ltd: *www.moor.co.uk*.)

Figures 8.6 and 8.7. A second company, Perimed of Sweden, has recently launched their own version of LASCA.

8.11
Conclusions

Although in existence for more than two decades, very little has changed in LASCA technology other than the acronyms. LASCA (whether known as *laser speckle contrast imaging* or *laser speckle imaging*) offers a full-field, real-time, noninvasive, and noncontact method of mapping flow fields such as capillary blood flow. Sensitive to both the speed and morphological changes of the scattering particles, it is particularly suitable for *in vivo* blood flow cytometry as well as investigation into the evolutions of cell parameters. In its basic form, it uses readily available off-the-shelf equipment. Laser Doppler, photon correlation spectroscopy, and time-varying speckle are related techniques, but these work by analyzing the intensity fluctuations in scattered laser light. As they are essentially methods that operate at a single point in the flow field, some form of scanning must be used if a high resolution full-field velocity map of the flow area is required. Typical scanning laser Doppler systems take some minutes to complete this scan. LASCA achieves this goal in a single shot by utilizing the spatial statistics of time-integrated speckle. The technique produces a false-color map of blood flow in a fraction of a second, without the need to scan. Thus, LASCA is a truly real-time technique. In addition, the LASCA system is much more cost effective and very simple to operate. The main disadvantage of LASCA compared with the other techniques is the loss of resolution caused by the need to average over a block of pixels in order to produce the spatial statistics used in the analysis. In principle, at least, the time-domain techniques can operate on a single pixel. However, in practice, even this disadvantage is not always present, as many of the temporal methods use sampling in order to speed up the processing. In any case, the advantage of real-time operation without scanning probably outweighs the problem of loss of resolution, as demonstrated by the current global interest in the technique. Finally, a more complete account of the history and development of LASCA can be found in recent review papers [35, 65].

Acknowledgments

The authors are very grateful to David Boas of the Harvard Medical School, Andrew Dunn of the University of Texas, and Moor Instruments Ltd, for their cooperation and permission to use some of their images.

References

1. Goodman, J.W. (2006) *Speckle Phenomena in Optics: Theory and Applications*, Roberts & Company, Berlin, p. 384.

2. Duncan, D.D., Kirkpatrick, S.J., and Wang, R.K.K. (2008) Statistics of local speckle contrast. *J. Opt. Soc. Am. A*, **25** (1), 9–15.

3. Leahy, M.J. (1996) Biomedical instrumentation for monitoring microvascular blood perfusion and oxygen saturation. DPhil thesis. University of Oxford.

4. Briers, J.D. (1996) Laser Doppler and time-varying speckle: a reconciliation. *J. Opt. Soc. Am. A*, **13** (2), 345–350.

5. Fujii, H., Nohira, K., Yamamoto, Y., Ikawa, H., and Ohura, T. (1987) Evaluation of blood flow by laser speckle image sensing. *Appl. Opt.*, **26** (24), 5321–5325.

6. Fujii, H. (1994) Visualisation of retinal blood flow by laser speckle flowgraphy. *Med. Biol. Eng. Comput.*, **32** (3), 302–304.

7. Tamaki, Y., Araie, M., Kawamoto, E., Eguchi, S., and Fujii, H. (1994) Noncontact, two-dimensional measurement of retinal microcirculation using laser speckle phenomenon. *Invest. Ophthalmol. Vis. Sci.*, **35** (11), 3825–3834.

8. Konishi, N. and Fujii, H. (1995) Real-time visualization of retinal microcirculation by laser flowgraphy. *Opt. Eng.*, **34** (3), 753–757.

9. Watanabe, G., Fujii, H., and Kishi, S. (2008) Imaging of choroidal hemodynamics in eyes with polypoidal choroidal vasculopathy using laser speckle phenomenon. *Jpn. J. Ophthalmol.*, **52** (3), 175–181.

10. Essex, T.J. and Byrne, P.O. (1991) A laser Doppler scanner for imaging blood flow in skin. *J. Biomed. Eng.*, **13** (3), 189–194.

11. Nilsson, G.E., Jakobsson, A., and Wardell, K. (1992) Tissue perfusion monitoring and imaging by coherent light scattering. *Bioptics: Optics in Biomedicine and Environmental Sciences*, Proc. SPIE 1524, 90.

12. Wardell, K., Jakobsson, A., and Nilsson, G.E. (1993) Laser-Doppler perfusion imaging by dynamic light-scattering. *IEEE Trans. Biomed. Eng.*, **40** (4), 309–319.

13. Komine, H., Brosnan, S.J., Litton, A.B., and Stappaerts, E.A. (1991) Real-time Doppler global velocimetry. AIAA Aerospace Sciences Meeting, Nevada.

14. Fercher, A.F. and Briers, J.D. (1981) Flow visualization by means of single-exposure speckle photography. *Opt. Commun.*, **37** (5), 326–330.

15. Briers, J.D. and Fercher, A.F. (1982) Retinal blood-flow visualization by means of laser speckle photography. *Invest. Ophthalmol. Vis. Sci.*, **22** (2), 255–259.

16. Briers, J.D. and Fercher, A.F. (1982) Laser speckle technique for the visualization of retinal blood-flow. Proc. SPIE 369, 22–28.

17. Briers, J.D. (1983) Optical filtering techniques to enhance speckle contrast variations in single-exposure laser speckle photography. *Optik*, **63** (3), 265–276.

18. Fercher, A.F., Peukert, M., and Roth, E. (1986) Visualization and measurement of retinal blood-flow by means of laser speckle photography. *Opt. Eng.*, **25** (6), 731–735.

19. Briers, J.D. and Webster, S. (1995) Quasi real-time digital version of single-exposure speckle photography for full-field monitoring of velocity or flow fields. *Opt. Commun.*, **116** (1–3), 36–42.

20. Cheng, H.Y., Luo, Q.M., Zeng, S.Q., Chen, S.B., Cen, J., and Gong, H. (2003) Modified laser speckle imaging method with improved spatial resolution. *J. Biomed. Opt.*, **8** (3), 559–564.

21. Paul, J.S., Luft, A.R., Yew, E., and Sheu, F.S. (2006) Imaging the development of an ischemic core following photochemically induced cortical infarction in rats using laser speckle contrast analysis (LASCA). *NeuroImage*, **29** (1), 38–45.

22. Yuan, S., Devor, A., Boas, D.A., and Dunn, A.K. (2005) Determination of optimal exposure time for imaging of blood flow changes with laser speckle contrast imaging. *Appl. Opt.*, **44** (10), 1823–1830.

23. Zakharov, P., Völker, A., Buck, A., Weber, B., and Scheffold, F. (2006) Quantitative modeling of laser speckle imaging. *Opt. Lett.*, **31** (23), 3465–3467.

24. Briers, J.D. and Webster, S. (1996) Laser speckle contrast analysis (LASCA): a nonscanning, full-field technique for monitoring capillary blood flow. *J. Biomed. Opt.*, **1** (2), 174–179.

25. Bandyopadhyay, R., Gittings, A.S., Suh, S.S., Dixon, P.K., and Durian, D.J.

(2005) Speckle-visibility spectroscopy: a tool to study time-varying dynamics. *Rev. Sci. Instrum.*, **76**, 093110.

26. Parthasarathy, A.B., Tom, W.J., Gopal, A., Zhang, X.J., and Dunn, A.K. (2008) Robust flow measurement with multi-exposure speckle imaging. *Opt. Express*, **16** (3), 1975–1989.

27. Li, P.C., Ni, S.L., Zhang, L., Zeng, S.Q., and Luo, Q.M. (2006) Imaging cerebral blood flow through the intact rat skull with temporal laser speckle imaging. *Opt. Lett.*, **31** (12), 1824–1826.

28. Kirkpatrick, S.J., Duncan, D.D., and Wells-Gray, E.M. (2008) Detrimental effects of speckle-pixel size matching in laser speckle contrast imaging. *Opt. Lett.*, **33** (24), 2886–2888.

29. Liu, S.S., Li, P.C., and Luo, Q.M. (2008) Fast blood flow visualization of high-resolution laser speckle imaging data using graphics processing unit. *Opt. Express*, **16** (19), 14321–14329.

30. Tom, W.J., Ponticorvo, A., and Dunn, A.K. (2008) Efficient processing of laser speckle contrast images. *IEEE Trans. Med. Imaging*, **27** (12), 1728–1738.

31. Dunn, A.K., Devor, A., Bolay, H., Andermann, M.L., Moskowitz, M.A., Dale, A.M., and Boas, D.A. (2003) Simultaneous imaging of total cerebral hemoglobin concentration, oxygenation, and blood flow during functional activation. *Opt. Lett.*, **28** (1), 28–30.

32. Sakadzic, S., Yuan, S., Dilekoz, E., Ruvinskaya, S., Vinogradov, S.A., Ayata, C., and Boas, D.A. (2009) Simultaneous imaging of cerebral partial pressure of oxygen and blood flow during functional activation and cortical spreading depression. *Appl. Opt.*, **48** (10), D169–D177.

33. Luo, Z.C., Yuan, Z.J., Pan, Y.T., and Du, C.W. (2009) Simultaneous imaging of cortical hemodynamics and blood oxygenation change during cerebral ischemia using dual-wavelength laser speckle contrast imaging. *Opt. Lett.*, **34** (9), 1480–1482.

34. Obrenovitch, T.P., Chen, S.B., and Farkas, E. (2009) Simultaneous, live imaging of cortical spreading depression and associated cerebral blood flow changes, by combining voltage-sensitive dye and laser speckle contrast methods. *Neuroimage*, **45** (1), 68–74.

35. Boas, D.A. and Dunn, A.K. (2010) Laser speckle contrast imaging in biomedical optics. *J. Biomed. Opt.*, **15** (1), 011109.

36. He, X.W. and Briers, J.D. (1998) Laser speckle contrast analysis (LASCA): a real-time solution for monitoring capillary blood flow and velocity. Proc. SPIE 3337, 98–107.

37. Briers, J.D., Richards, G., and He, X.W. (1999) Capillary blood flow monitoring using laser speckle contrast analysis (LASCA). *J. Biomed. Opt.*, **4** (1), 164–175.

38. Obeid, A.N., Boggett, D.M., Barnett, N.J., Dougherty, G., and Rolfe, P. (1988) Depth discrimination in laser Doppler skin blood-flow measurement using different lasers. *Med. Biol. Eng. Comput.*, **26** (4), 415–419.

39. Duteil, L., Bernengo, J.C., and Schalla, W. (1985) A double wavelength laser Doppler system to investigate skin microcirculation. *IEEE Trans. Biomed. Eng.*, **32** (6), 439–447.

40. Gush, R.J. and King, T.A. (1991) Discrimination of capillary and arterio-venular blood-flow in skin by laser Doppler flowmetry. *Med. Biol. Eng. Comput.*, **29** (4), 387–392.

41. Cheng, H., Luo, Q., Liu, Q., Lu, Q., Gong, H., and Zeng, S. (2004) Laser speckle imaging of blood flow in microcirculation. *Phys. Med. Biol.*, **49** (7), 1347.

42. Choi, B., Kang, N.M., and Nelson, J.S. (2004) Laser speckle imaging for monitoring blood flow dynamics in the in vivo rodent dorsal skin fold model. *Microvasc. Res.*, **68** (2), 143–146.

43. Forrester, K.R., Stewart, C., Tulip, J., Leonard, C., and Bray, R.C. (2002) Comparison of laser speckle and laser Doppler perfusion imaging: Measurement in human skin and rabbit articular tissue. *Med. Biol. Eng. Comput.*, **40** (6), 687–697.

44. Gonik, M.M., Mishin, A.B., and Zimnyakov, D.A. (2002) Visualization of blood microcirculation parameters in human tissues by time-integrated dynamic speckles analysis. *Ann. N.Y.*

Acad. Sci., **972**, 325–330. (Visualization and Imaging in Transport Phenomena).

45. Forrester, K.R., Tulip, J., Leonard, C., Stewart, C., and Bray, R.C. (2004) A laser speckle imaging technique for measuring tissue perfusion. *IEEE Trans. Biomed. Eng.*, **51** (11), 2074–2084.

46. Nadkarni, S.K., Bouma, B.E., Helg, T., Chan, R., Halpern, E., Chau, A., Minsky, M.S., Motz, J.T., Houser, S.L., and Tearney, G.J. (2005) Characterization of atherosclerotic plaques by laser speckle imaging. *Circulation*, **112** (6), 885–892.

47. Flammer, J., Orgul, S., Costa, V.P., Orzalesi, N., Krieglstein, G.K., Serra, L.M., Renard, J.P., and Stefansson, E. (2002) The impact of ocular blood flow in glaucoma. *Prog. Retin. Eye Res.*, **21** (4), 359–393.

48. Nagahara, M., Tamaki, Y., Araie, M., and Umeyama, T. (2001) The acute effects of stellate ganglion block on circulation in human ocular fundus. *Acta Ophthalmol. Scand.*, **79** (1), 45–48.

49. Yaoeda, K., Shirakashi, M., Funaki, S., Funaki, H., Nakatsue, T., Fukushima, A., and Abe, H. (2000) Measurement of microcirculation in optic nerve head by laser speckle flowgraphy in normal volunteers. *Am. J. Ophthalmol.*, **130** (5), 606–610.

50. Dunn, A.K., Bolay, T., Moskowitz, M.A., and Boas, D.A. (2001) Dynamic imaging of cerebral blood flow using laser speckle. *J. Cereb. Blood Flow Metab.*, **21** (3), 195–201.

51. Atochin, D.N., Murciano, J.C., Gursoy-Ozdemir, Y., Krasik, T., Noda, F., Ayata, C., Dunn, A.K., Moskowitz, M.A., Huang, P.L., and Muzykantov, V.R. (2004) Mouse model of microembolic stroke and reperfusion. *Stroke*, **35** (9), 2177–2182.

52. Ayata, C., Dunn, A.K., Gursoy-Ozdemir, Y., Huang, Z.H., Boas, D.A., and Moskowitz, M.A. (2004) Laser speckle flowmetry for the study of cerebrovascular physiology in normal and ischemic mouse cortex. *J. Cereb. Blood Flow Metab.*, **24** (7), 744–755.

53. Dunn, A.K., Devor, A., Dale, A.M., and Boas, D.A. (2005) Spatial extent of oxygen metabolism and hemodynamic changes during functional activation of the rat somatosensory cortex. *Neuroimage*, **27** (2), 279–290.

54. Durduran, T., Burnett, M.G., Yu, G.Q., Zhou, C., Furuya, D., Yodh, A.G., Detre, J.A., and Greenberg, J.H. (2004) Spatiotemporal quantification of cerebral blood flow during functional activation in rat somatosensory cortex using laser-speckle flowmetry. *J. Cereb. Blood Flow Metab.*, **24** (5), 518–525.

55. Kharlamov, A., Brown, B.R., Easley, K.A., and Jones, S.C. (2004) Heterogeneous response of cerebral blood flow to hypotension demonstrated by laser speckle imaging flowmetry in rats. *Neurosci. Lett.*, **368** (2), 151–156.

56. Murari, K., Li, N., Rege, A., Jia, X., All, A., and Thakor, N. (2007) Contrast-enhanced imaging of cerebral vasculature with laser speckle. *Appl. Opt.*, **46** (22), 5340–5346.

57. Shin, H.K., Dunn, A.K., Jones, P.B., Boas, D.A., Moskowitz, M.A., and Ayata, C. (2006) Vasoconstrictive neurovascular coupling during focal ischemic depolarizations. *J. Cereb. Blood Flow Metab.*, **26** (8), 1018–1030.

58. Strong, A.J., Bezzina, E.L., Anderson, P.B.J., Boutelle, M.G., Hopwood, S.E., and Dunn, A.K. (2006) Evaluation of laser speckle flowmetry for imaging cortical perfusion in experimental stroke studies: quantitation of perfusion and detection of peri-infarct depolarisations. *J. Cereb. Blood Flow Metab.*, **26** (5), 645–653.

59. Wang, Z., Hughes, S., Dayasundara, S., and Menon, R.S. (2007) Theoretical and experimental optimization of laser speckle contrast imaging for high specificity to brain microcirculation. *J. Cereb. Blood Flow Metab.*, **27** (2), 258–269.

60. Weber, B., Burger, C., Wyss, M.T., von Schulthess, G.K., Scheffold, F., and Buck, A. (2004) Optical imaging of the spatiotemporal dynamics of cerebral blood flow and oxidative metabolism in the rat barrel cortex. *Eur. J. Neurosci.*, **20** (10), 2664–2670.

61. Bolay, H., Reuter, U., Dunn, A.K., Huang, Z.H., Boas, D.A., and Moskowitz, M.A. (2002) Intrinsic brain

activity triggers trigeminal meningeal afferents in a migraine model. *Nat. Med.*, **8** (2), 136–142.

62. Volker, A.C., Zakharov, P., Weber, B., Buck, F., and Scheffold, F. (2005) Laser speckle imaging with an active noise reduction scheme. *Opt. Express*, **13** (24), 9782–9787.

63. Serov, A., Steenbergen, W., and de Mul, F. (2001) Prediction of the photodetector signal generated by Doppler-induced speckle fluctuations: theory and some validations. *J. Opt. Soc. Am. A*, **18** (3), 622–630.

64. Thompson, O.B. and Andrews, M.K. (2010) Tissue perfusion measurements: multiple-exposure laser speckle analysis generates laser Doppler-like spectra. *J. Biomed. Opt.*, **15** (2), 027015.

65. Briers, J.D. (2007) Laser speckle contrast imaging for measuring blood flow. *Opt. Appl.*, **37** (1–2), 139–152.

9
Tissue Viability Imaging

Jim O'Doherty, Martin J. Leahy, and Gert E. Nilsson

9.1
Introduction

There is a constantly growing need for reliable and user-independent assessment of the skin microcirculation and other skin parameters not only in medical applications but also in the development and evaluation of pharmaceuticals, skin care products, and cosmetics. Owing to the essential link between microcirculation function and adequate tissue oxygen delivery and thus organ function, the tissue blood supply has been noted as a crucial indicator of injury and disease [1, 2]. Given that many of the parameters of interest vary spatially over the skin surface, these needs are generally better served by the use of imaging technologies than by single-point measurement devices. Since the most superficial microvascular network of the skin resides in the papilla just under the epidermal layer, the measurement depth of the technology of choice must be compatible with these dimensions. Methods based on photonics operating in the visible and near-infrared regions possess a depth sensitivity that fulfills these requirements. To attain a high productivity in skin testing, such methods should also incorporate software for effective processing of the large amount of data generated and should preferably be able to reduce image information to numbers and indexes suitable for statistical testing. Furthermore, the methods should be easy to apply in a reproducible way in clinical settings as well as at the skin test laboratory and work site. Among the suitable candidates based on photonics principles available for fulfillment of these requirements, capillary video microscopy [3], laser Doppler imaging [4], and subsurface spectroscopic imaging [5] are currently the most promising. Owing to the variability in tissue optical parameters from one tissue to another, these technologies deliver arbitrary values that scale linearly with the parameter of interest rather than absolute quantities. In this chapter, tissue viability imaging (TiVi) based on wideband spectroscopy of backscattered light is described in further detail.

Microcirculation Imaging, First Edition. Edited by Martin J. Leahy.
© 2012 Wiley-VCH Verlag GmbH & Co. KGaA. Published 2012 by Wiley-VCH Verlag GmbH & Co. KGaA.

9.2
Operating Principle

Since the digital camera was introduced in the 1990s, they have developed quickly and are increasingly used as part of advanced imaging systems in a variety of medical and other applications. Skin observations through perpendicularly oriented linear polarization filters to reduce surface glare first transpired in 1991 [6]. Owing to research carried out in the mid-1990s, which stated that reflection-based polarized light imaging in skin would not suffer significant blurring [7] and also the accelerated arrival of high-resolution charge coupled devices (CCDs), led to increased use of the technique. To reduce the influence of direct reflections of the light from the flash in the surface of the object and capture a "subsurface" photo based on diffusely backscattered and depolarized photons, cross-polarization filter techniques are frequently used. Alternatively, if information about the surface structure of the skin is of primary interest, copolarization filter techniques that suppress the influence of the diffusely backscattered and depolarized photons remitted from inside the tissue while direct surface reflection is enhanced can be used [8]. The group's work improves image contrast based on light scattering in the superficial layers of the skin, which can visualize the disruption of the normal texture of the papillary and upper reticular dermis of the skin. The group expanded the work to be used in Mohs surgery, whereby the images may be used to guide clinical excision of skin cancers, and shows promise in the assessment of skin topography. An example image is shown in Figure 9.1, where the borders of a burn wound are significantly enhanced. They also expanded the system to a handheld prototype camera and refined the image processing to include data from two CCDs, while investigating the characteristics of the texture and surface appearance of a range of skin conditions [9].

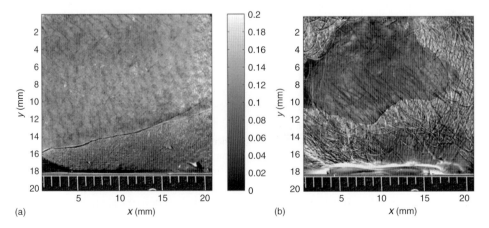

Figure 9.1 Polarization images of normal (a) and a burn scar (b), showing clearly defined boundaries of the wound. (Source: Figure after Ref. [8], reproduced with permission.)

In the cross-polarized mode, the polarization filters in front of the flash and the detector array have orthogonal polarization directions. Linearly polarized white light from the flash is partly reflected by the upper layer of the skin and partly diffusely scattered in the deeper dermal layers where the microvascular network is located (Figure 9.1). Most of the directly reflected light (7% in total) preserves its state of linear polarization, while the light diffusely scattered in the tissue (93%) becomes randomly polarized. About 53% of the light is directly absorbed in the tissue, while the remaining portion emerges from the tissue as diffusely reflected light, is almost completely depolarized, and can be considered to consist of two 20% fractions of parallel and perpendicular polarizations with respect to the direction of the original filter. A portion of the randomly polarized light emanating from deeper tissue layers, however, passes through this filter and reaches the detector. This light is filtered through a set of red, green, and blue filters integrated in the camera photodetector array, and the corresponding photo is stored electronically in the camera or the computer as three matrixes representing the red (600–700 nm), green (500–600 nm), and blue (400–500 nm) color planes, respectively. These three combined color planes constitute the true color photo. This gating of photons is based on the assumption that weakly scattered light (the surface reflections) retains its polarization state, whereas strongly scattered light will successively depolarize with each scattering event. A schematic is shown in Figure 9.2 where the difference in generation of copolarized images (CO) and cross-polarized images (CR) can be observed.

The effect is clearly seen in materials that reflect the majority of light impinging on them. As an example, Figure 9.3 shows that the intensity reflected by the metal key occurs from surface reflections only, hence the larger change in intensity when progressing in filter angle degrees from a cross-polarized image to a copolarized image. The resulting curves were fitted with a standard sinusoid, since rotating the polarizer further would cause a repeating pattern. It is interesting to note that the full width half maximum for skin (84°) is less than that for the metal key (124°), which may be caused by subsurface scattering and absorption in the skin tissue (Figure 9.4). There is also a larger dynamic range when examining the back-reflections from the key because the returning light is attributed to surface reflections only (≈90%); thus, minimum intensity (only 10% of incident light)

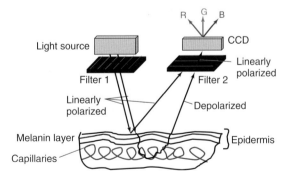

Figure 9.2 Schematic showing the operating principle of subsurface spectroscopic imaging.

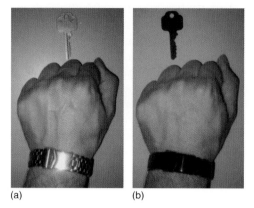

(a)   (b)

Figure 9.3 Copolarized (a) and cross-polarized (b) images of directly reflecting objects. The surface skin tissue is suppressed in the cross-polarized image, and information from the deeper layers reached the CCD as is indicated from the more red color of the subjects hand. The metallic objects serve as extremes as all light from them will retain its linear polarization.

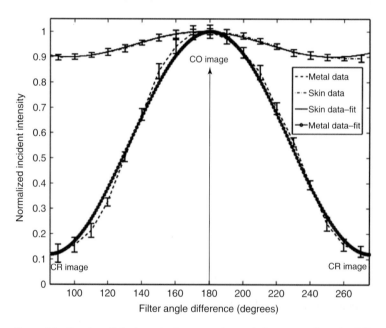

Figure 9.4 Resultant light intensity by rotation of a detecting linear polarizing filter from 90° (CR image) to 180° (copolarized image) and 270° (cross-polarized image) for a metal key and Caucasian skin (Figure 9.3b). Note the higher intensity variation of surface reflections from the key. Maximal surface reflections for the metal key and skin occur when the difference between the filters is 180°, leading to a CO image. Minimal reflections occur when the filters are crossed. The shape of light intensity with polarization angle variation for the tissue and key closely follows a sinusoidal shape.

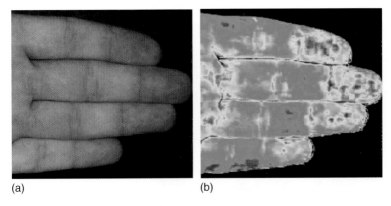

(a)   (b)

Figure 9.5 (a) Acquired cross-polarized image and (b) the
associated TiVi image showing the concentration of RBCs in
the microvasculature.

is reached when the surface reflections are blocked. This is not the case for the
skin sample, and it can be noticed that the surface reflections represent only a
small fraction of the returning light ($\approx$10%) due to the penetration into the deeper
compartments of the tissue. Reflections from the metal key reduce from 100% of
detected intensity to ~10%, while for the skin sample, the reflections are reduced
from 100 to 90% of detected intensity.

The green component of the light reaching the detector is attenuated due to
a high absorption in the red blood cells (RBCs), while the red component is
virtually unaltered because of its relatively low absorption in the RBCs. Surrounding tissue absorbs green and red light to approximately the same amount
[10]. Subsurface imaging of the skin RBC concentration takes advantage of this
wavelength-dependent absorption in the hemoglobin molecule of the RBC. By
applying an algorithm in which the value of each picture element in the green
color matrix is subtracted from the corresponding value in the red color matrix, an
output matrix representing the local RBC concentration is generated. This output
matrix is displayed as a color-coded map of the local RBC concentration of the
skin microvascular network, an example of which is shown in Figure 9.5. Further
images are provided as to the applicability of TiVi in the large and narrow fields
of view, with Figure 9.6 showing the human nail fold in the index finger, with the
concentration of RBCs visible in individual vessels. This builds on the technique
of nail fold capillaroscopy where blood velocity can be determined by direct visual
observation of the flowing RBCs in the capillary loops to a system where the
concentration may be quantified.

It should be noted that the spectral signature between the light source used for
microscopy and the standard TiVi system are not consistent; with changing a light
source, a recalibration should be performed to ensure that system output scales
linearly with RBC concentration. This linearity is discussed further in Section 9.2.2.
Figure 9.7 shows a wide field of view of a burn wound that may allow detailed
comparison of different areas of the wound concurrently. Brain hemodynamics

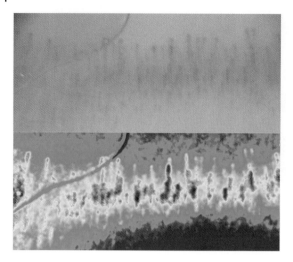

Figure 9.6 A cross-polarized image acquired of the nail fold plexus acquired with a standard digital microscope and its associated TiVi image showing the concentration of RBCs in the individual vessels (magnification at ×400).

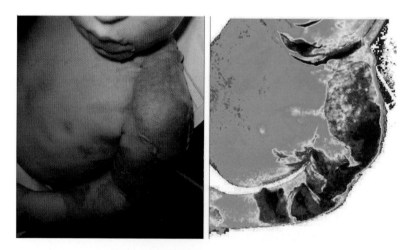

Figure 9.7 An example image showing the capability for wide field burn wound assessment. Different parts of the wound may be assessed concurrently and, over time, providing a reproducible setup of the patient.

may also be investigated as shown in Figure 9.8, where TiVi images of an exposed mouse brain show the individual blood vessels. The image shows that brain hemodynamics may be performed on the exposed brain. With the system operating in photo mode, a new photo can be captured every 5 s with a maximum image size of 5184 × 3456 pixels, limited by the recharge time of the flash (∼5 s).

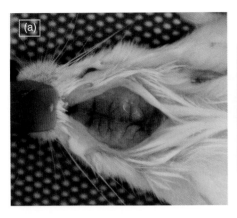
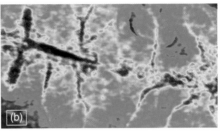

Figure 9.8 (a) Image showing an exposed mouse brain and (b) corresponding TiVi image of a section of the brain. The TiVi visualization of the brain allows the hemodynamics of single vessels to be assessed over time, and dynamic studies may be performed with the high-speed system.

The theoretical basis of the TiVi system is based on Kubelka–Munk theory of diffuse reflection. The wavelength-dependent intensity of backscattered light with a perpendicular polarization to the incident-polarized light is described by the equation [11]

$$I_{\text{per}}(\Delta\lambda) \propto k_0 (\Delta\lambda) \, I_0 T_{\text{epid}}(\Delta\lambda) R_{\text{d}}(\Delta\lambda) \tag{9.1}$$

where $k_0(\Delta\lambda)$ represents the fraction of the total emitted light intensity I_0 within the wavelength interval $\Delta\lambda$, impinging on the skin, $T_{\text{epid}}(\Delta\lambda)$ represents the transmission properties of the epidermal layer, and $R_{\text{d}}(\Delta\lambda)$ represents diffusely reflected light in the area of the reticular dermis. An algorithm is suggested which is sensitive to the concentration of RBCs in the tissue and does not depend on the total light intensity. Using Eq. (9.1) above, the algorithm is stated as

$$\text{RBC}_{\text{conc}} = k_{\text{gain}} \left(\frac{T_{\text{epid}} (\Delta\lambda_{\text{r}}) \, R_{\text{d}} (\Delta\lambda_{\text{r}}) - k T_{\text{epid}} (\Delta\lambda_{\text{g}}) \, R_{\text{d}} (\Delta\lambda_{\text{g}})}{T_{\text{epid}} (\Delta\lambda_{\text{r}}) \, R_{\text{d}} (\Delta\lambda_{\text{r}})} \right) \tag{9.2}$$

An assumption is made where $T_{\text{epid}}(\Delta\lambda_{\text{r}})$ and $T_{\text{epid}}(\Delta\lambda_{\text{g}})$ are approximated to 1 on the basis of mathematical observations by regarding the melanin layer as a modulating filter. Using Kubelka–Munk and associated diffusion theory, it can be shown that

$$R_{\text{d}}(\Delta\lambda) = 1 + \frac{8\mu_{\text{a}}(\Delta\lambda)}{3\mu_{\text{s}}(\Delta\lambda)} - \left(\frac{(8\mu_{\text{a}}(\Delta\lambda))^2}{(3\mu_{\text{s}}(\Delta\lambda))^2} + 2\frac{8\mu_{\text{a}}(\Delta\lambda)}{3\mu_{\text{s}}(\Delta\lambda)} \right)^{\frac{1}{2}} \tag{9.3}$$

Where the absorption (μ_{a}) and scattering (μ_{s}) coefficients are composed of two parts; one relating directly to the RBC itself ($\mu_{\text{RBC}}(\Delta\lambda)$) and the other part relating to background tissue ($\mu_{\text{TISSUE}}(\Delta\lambda)$). Thus,

$$\mu_{\text{s}} (\lambda) = \text{RBC}_{\text{f}}\mu_{\text{sRBC}} (\lambda) + (1 - \text{RBC}_{\text{f}}) \, \mu_{\text{sTISSUE}} (\lambda) \tag{9.4a}$$

$$\mu_{\text{a}} (\lambda) = \text{RBC}_{\text{f}}\mu_{\text{aRBC}} (\lambda) + (1 - \text{RBC}_{\text{f}}) \, \mu_{\text{aTISSUE}} (\lambda) \tag{9.4b}$$

Table 9.1 Average absorption (μ_a) and scattering (μ_s) coefficients (cm^{-1}) for the relevant biological chromophore in the red ($\Delta\lambda_r$) and green ($\Delta\lambda_g$) wavelength regions.

Absorber	Red (600–700 nm)		Green (500–600 nm)	
	$\mu_a(\Delta\lambda_r)$	$\mu_s(\Delta\lambda_r)$	$\mu_a(\Delta\lambda_r)$	$\mu_s(\Delta\lambda_r)$
Tissue	2.7	187	3	223
RBCoxy	3.5	861	177	920
RBCdeoxy	25	861	201	920
Epidermis	35	450	40	535

where RBC$_f$ represents the volume fraction of RBCs in the tissue volume. Table 9.1 represents the coefficients for the chromophores of interest in the determination of μ_a and μ_s. In practice, Eq. (9.5) is applied to an image by way of mathematical operations on the color planes that constitute the image, namely

$$\mathbf{M} = k_{gain} \frac{\mathbf{M}_{red} - k\mathbf{M}_{green}}{\mathbf{M}_{red}} \tag{9.5}$$

And further processing in order to linearize the relationship between RBC$_{conc}$ and RBC$_f$ by

$$\mathbf{M}_{out} = \mathbf{M}e^{-pM} \tag{9.6}$$

The matrix produced, $\mathbf{M}_{out}$, is a 2D array of RBC$_{conc}$ values.

9.3
Validation

9.3.1
Monte Carlo Modeling

The average penetration depth of red and green photons in skin tissue returning to the skin surface was investigated by adaptation of a Monte Carlo simulation model that incorporated the polarization properties of the photons [12]. Previous codes have established the fundamentals of polarized light propagation in turbid media [13]. Gating of the photons by monitoring the Stokes vector of the photon on detection was performed in order to compare the sampling depth of total detected photons with the sampling depth-detected CR photons. Optical properties of the relevant biological chromophores in tissue used in these simulations are shown in Table 9.1. Their results in Figure 9.9 showed that by using cross-polarized detection, the average penetration depth increased from 345 to 482 µm for red wavelengths and from 316 to 387 µm for green wavelengths [5]. This implies that the measurement volume (the volume from which the bulk of the signal is

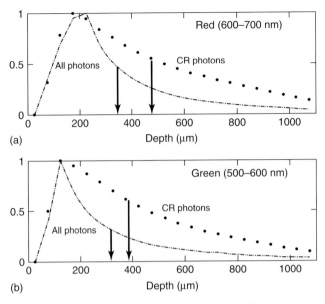

Figure 9.9 (a,b) Probability density functions of the Monte Carlo simulation in the red and green wavelength regions. The vertical arrows represent the average sampling depth of the "all photons" (unpolarized) simulation and the "CR photons" simulation where only linearly polarized photons are accepted. (Source: After Ref. [5], reproduced with permission.)

acquired) is located well into the reticular dermis in most skin sites. Owing to the epidermal layer thickness of ~50–100 μm being unaccounted for in this model, the total depth of detected photons as stated above will be marginally larger than the Monte Carlo depth, that is, on the order of 400–500 μm. This increase in depth sensitivity has been confirmed also in enhanced visual scoring of skin erythema using a polarized light visualization system [14].

9.3.2
Experimental Modeling

The linear relationship between the output matrix values (TiVi$_{index}$-values) generated and the actual concentration of RBCs was verified by way of a fluid model composed of tightly wound latex tubing simulating the blood vessels of the microcirculations. The system was perfused by fresh human blood mixed with saline to produce RBC concentrations ranging from 0 to 4% in steps of 0.2%, which was considered to cover the physiological range of skin tissue. Maximal oxygen saturation (~100%) of the mixture was provided by stirring and exposure to ambient air, while minimal oxygen saturation (~0%) was attained by bubbling N$_2$ gas through the blood samples. Five photos were captured for each RBC fraction and cropped to a region of interest (ROI) covering the center of the fluid model. The average TiVi$_{index}$-values were then plotted as a function of the actual

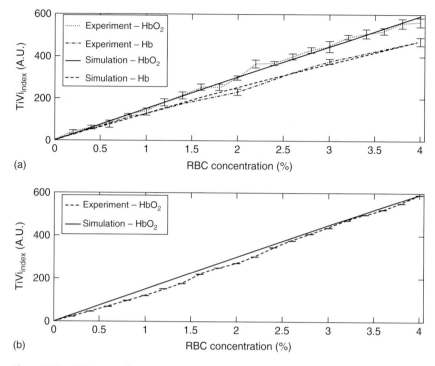

Figure 9.10 TiVi output from experiments with oxygenated and deoxygenated blood, along with linearized Kubelka–Munk theoretical fits from theory. (a) Data from high-resolution imager. Error bars represent the average value of five images ± one standard deviation. (b) Data from high-speed video imager used for research purposes. Error bars represent the average of 25 frames ± 1 standard deviation.

RBC fraction from 0 to 4%, as shown in Figure 9.10. For 0 and 100% oxygen saturation, the correlation coefficient was calculated to 0.998 ($n = 4$) and 0.997 ($n = 20$), respectively. The average $TiVi_{index}$-value calculated for the lower oxygen saturation was on average 91.5% of that calculated for the higher oxygen saturation, corresponding to a deviation of <3.9% within the physiological range (70–100% oxygen saturation) well in accordance with theory. TiVi images can therefore be considered to be virtually independent of the state of tissue oxygen saturation for both the high-resolution commercial system and the research-based high-peed system.

9.4
Technology

The principle of subsurface mapping of local RBC concentration has been implemented in the Tissue Viability Imager (TiVi) TiVi600 brought to market by WheelsBridge AB, Linkoping, Sweden (*http://www.wheelsbridge.se*). The complete TiVi600 system composed of a Canon EOS system camera (Canon Inc. Lake Success, MA, USA) equipped with polarization filters to generate cross- or copolarized photos and remotely controlled by a USB-connected interface with a portable PC. Camera control, photocapturing, further image processing of TiVi images, and result generation are made via the dedicated TiVi600 system software. In many applications, photos are recorded in sequence, thereby allowing studies of dynamic skin reactions following topical or systemic application of substances that cause vasodilatation (increased RBC concentration) or vasoconstriction (reduced RBC concentration) in the skin. By use of the integrated wizards and statistic measures, erythema (vasodilatation) and blanching (vasoconstriction) can be visualized and quantified. The entire process of assessing a specific skin reaction by, for example, naked eye observation thereby becomes increasingly independent of the individual investigator. To use the integrated wizards effectively, the object in a sequence of photos must appear in the same position in all photos. When photos are recorded at different points in time, the first photo can be used as the *Reference Photo*. When successive photos are to be captured, actual test photos are displayed superimposed on the *Reference Photo* and the object is repositioned until there is an acceptable overlap of the object in the *Reference Photo* and that of the actual test photo, where after the next photo in the sequence is captured. Alignment of the object in successively captured photos can thus be attained. To further align the objects in the different photos of a sequence, an integrated preprocessor performs photo alignment automatically as a first step in the image processing procedure. These arrangements prepare a sequence of photos to be analyzed by use of the integrated wizards. An example of such a procedure is demonstrated in Figure 9.11. Following topical application of methyl nicotinate (50 mmol) in patches on the skin of the back to produce vasodilatation, photos were captured in sequence for 20 min with a frequency of 12 photos per min. In the analysis, regions of interests were drawn around the patches and combined with a set threshold to produce the *Erythema Area Chart* and the *Erythema Intensity Chart* displaying the dynamic development of the erythema area and intensity as the drug penetrated the top layer of the skin to produce vasodilatation in the superficial microvascular network. Data reduction is thereby attained by reducing images to time traces that, in turn, can be reduced to indexes (e.g., the time at which 50% of the top level is reached) describing the entire experiment. The maximum resolution of the images is 18 million pixels, thereby rendering it possible to zoom in on a small area with still adequate resolution.

Figure 9.12 displays the result of the same experiment using the integrated *Cross Section Visualizer*. This image displays the development of erythema along a user-selected cross section in the photos as a function of the time elapsed. The cross section shows that, during the first 5 min, the vasodilatation occurs mainly within the individual patches, while toward the end of the experiment, the drug diffuses laterally to produce vasodilatation also in the skin sites between the individual patches.

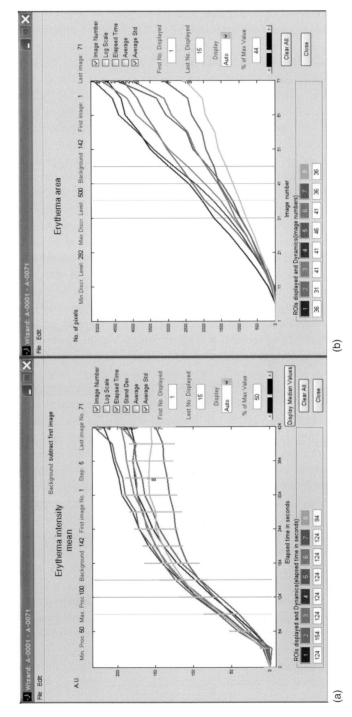

(a)

(b)

Figure 9.11 Development of (a) *Erythema Intensity* and (b) *Erythema Area* following topical application of metyl nicotinate in eight patches on the skin of the back.

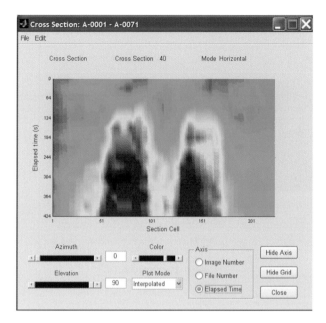

Figure 9.12 Cross section along two patches following topical application of methyl nicotinate (time along the dependent axis). After about 2 min following application of the substance, the erythema appears inside the patches. After 7 min, the erythema has spread outside the patches.

9.4.1
Software Toolboxes

To address specific applications and needs, dedicated toolboxes have been developed that can be integrated with the TiVi system software.

9.4.1.1 Skin Damage Visualizer
In general, the *Skin Damage Visualizer* toolbox was developed for direct assessment of skin damage at the work site or in occupational medicine applications. Skin damage at the work site can occur as a consequence of exposure to aggressive chemicals (skin irritation causing erythema) or following the use of vibrating tools (vasospasm causing vasoconstriction). By displaying the fraction of, for example, a hand that possesses erythema (RBC concentration above a user-selected threshold value) in red color, the healing process and/or progressions of contact dermatitis can be evaluated over time, using the integrated library and trend monitor functions. This is shown in Figure 9.13.

9.4.1.2 Skin Color Tracker
The color of the skin changes over time in many diseases and conditions and can thus be a useful indicator for assessment of the development and progression of

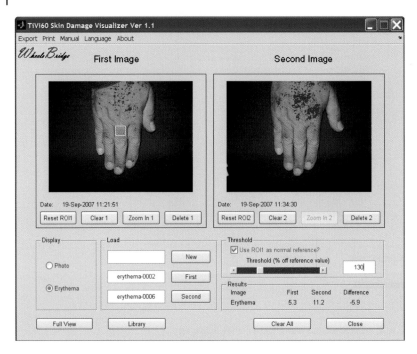

Figure 9.13 Skin areas with erythema above a set threshold level before (left) and after (right) the exposure to a skin irritating agent.

skin disease or a healing process. What is generally referred to as *skin color* is the spectral content of backscattered light following illumination by a broadband light source. Consequently, the skin color observed is not only dependent on the optical properties of the skin but also dependent on the spectral signature of the illuminating light. If a digital camera is used to capture a photo of the skin, the spectral sensitivity of the photodetector array further influences the color of the photos recorded. Consequently, skin color can not be regarded as an absolute quantity. However, changes in spectral content of the diffusely backscattered light from the skin under illumination by a light source with a fixed spectral signature, carry useful information about changing skin conditions. The *Skin Color Tracker* toolbox makes it possible to follow a preselected color (or a range of colors) and thereby to track the progressive development of, for example, scaling tissue in psoriasis. These color changes are minute and cannot be readily verified by naked eye observation alone.

9.4.1.3 Spot Analyzer
Facial spots including acne appear most frequently during puberty with a varying degree of severity. About 90% of the adolescent population is believed to be affected by this skin disease. Numerous skin care products are commercially available for treatment of spots, and new and more effective products are continuously released

on the market. To evaluate the performance of these skin care products, the product candidates are generally tested using a panel of volunteers with spots of varying severity. The result is assessed by naked eye observation at which both the intensity and the extension of the spot erythema are evaluated. These evaluations are generally performed by a skillful dermatologist, and a severity score on a scale from one to five may be used to quantify the findings. Because of the unavoidable investigator-dependent element of these naked eye inspection procedures, results vary among observers and interlaboratory comparison of data may be difficult to perform. The *Spot Analyzer* toolbox renders this process fully automatic and investigator independent. Results are delivered in terms of diagrams displaying the intensity and extension of the spot erythema. The results from individual sessions can be integrated into a project window that displays the overall result of a test panel project.

9.4.1.4 Wrinkle Analyzer

Wrinkles frequently appear on the parts of the body where there has been extensive sun exposure. Wrinkles can appear as fine structures or deep furrows. Smoking, skin type, heredity occupational, and recreational habits are factors that all promote wrinkling of the skin. Many products have been developed for the reduction of wrinkles or rather their appearance, but few cost-effective techniques are to date available for quantitative analysis of wrinkle appearance. The *Wrinkle Analyzer TiVi90* is a software package that analyzes several features of wrinkles based on photos captured by polarization spectroscopy camera technology.

9.4.1.5 Surface Analyzer

Most women and some men show signs of cellulite where the skin of the lower limbs, abdomen, and the pelvic region becomes dimpled. The causes of cellulite are not fully understood, but hormonal components are thought to play a dominant role in its formation. Several genetic factors promote the development of cellulite as do lifestyle factors. A number of therapies for treatment of cellulite are available, but empirical evidence of the efficacy of these treatment regimes is limited, mainly due to lack of methods for quantification of cellulite appearance. The *Surface Analyzer TiVi95* is a software package that analyzes important features of cellulite and associated skin dimples based on photos captured by polarization spectroscopy camera technology.

Both the basic TiVi system software and all toolboxes are supported by an on-line and interactive Demo Assistant that guides the user through the different steps of photocapturing and image analysis.

9.5
Evaluation

The basic operation principles and practical use of many commercially available instruments for assessment of the skin have been thoroughly evaluated, and Guidelines regarding their effective use have been published [15–18]. Standardization reports regarding assessment of critical performance parameters such as deviation in sensitivity and reproducibility for a batch of presumably identical instruments are, however, frequently limited or nonexistent. Data recorded in different laboratories and/or at different points in time are therefore difficult to compare, which hampers the use of these instruments on a broader scale. The TiVi600 system has been evaluated with respect to these performance parameters [19]. The average systematic drift in TiVi system sensitivity over a three-month time period, while the systems were moved in between laboratories, is reported to be 0.27% and discrepancy in sensitivity between different units is limited to 4.1%, due to offset rather than gain deviation when measurements were performed using a paper of uniform pink color as a object. Spatial variation in image uniformity is below 3.08 and 1.93% in the corners and the center of an individual image, respectively. Since the intensity of the flash is generally much higher than that of ambient light, virtually no influence on the image of ambient light can be demonstrated under ordinary daylight conditions. The distance dependence was assessed by recording images alternatively at a distance of 15–25 cm and calculating the $TiVi_{index}$-values produced by erythema-inducing methyl nicotinate in forearm skin. No significant difference in the average $TiVi_{index}$-values at the two distances could be demonstrated ($n = 25$). In contrast to what is the case with laser Doppler devises, TiVi is further not sensitive to movement artifacts because no Doppler components are recorded. Since all image points are recorded simultaneously, there is no interpretation ambiguity regarding spatial and temporal variations in skin microcirculation, as may be the case with raster scan laser Doppler perfusion imaging (LDPI) devices. On the other hand, since TiVi is based on spectroscopy, it is sensitive to all objects of a specific color. Consequently, heavily pigmented skin results in higher TiVi values than nonpigmented skin due to an offset in the TiVi value. The sensitivity of the TiVi value parameter is, however, less affected by the degree of skin pigmentation. Alterations in skin RBC concentration as recorded by TiVi over a short period of time (in comparison with the timescale under which pigmentation changes) are therefore comparable also for skin types with different degree of pigmentation. However, it has been observed that skin freckles may mimic skin erythema [20]. Day-to-day variations of normal values of skin response on the dorsal side of the hand were estimated at 5–7%, with short-term variation (i.e., within 70 s) of <2%. Studies into the reproducibility and detection ability of the postocclusive reactive hyperemia (PORH) test showed up to 60% increase in local RBC concentration, remaining 18% above preocclusion level 30 min posttesting [20].

9.5.1
Iontophoresis

The TiVi device has also been used to map changes in cutaneous microvascular concentrations of RBCs during the iontophoresis of vasoactive substances (namely, noradrenaline (NA) and phenylephrine (Phe) for vasoconstriction and acetylcholine (ACh) and sodium nitroprusside (SNP) for vasodilatation). As the TiVi output variable is only dependent on the concentration of RBCs, studies of iontophoresis of vasoactive agents using both TiVi and LDPI were shown to be

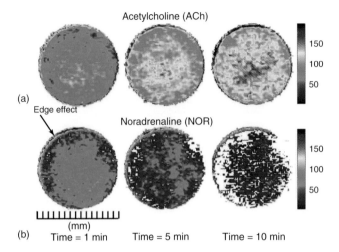

Figure 9.14 The effects of the iontophoresis of (a) a vasodilating and (b) vasoconstricting agent. Both the increase and decrease in local perfusion can be quantified.

able to separate the concentration and velocity components of the skin response fit to an experimental model [21]. Example images of the iontophoresis procedure of such substances are shown in Figure 9.14 with analysis carried out by the method of "dose–response" curves, as shown in Figure 9.15. The 50% response level (ED 50) variable has been shown to be a reliable method to quantify the physiological response of the microvasculature to various drugs, and values determined by TiVi technology are similar to those previously determined by laser Doppler systems. "Islands" of perfusion can be seen in the region, thus displaying the heterogeneous structure of the skin microcirculation, the effect of which can influence the transdermal delivery of drugs. The onset of vasoconstriction and vasodilation can be observed graphically as shown in Figure 9.16. Epidermal thickness, resistance to charged particle movement [22], and variation in the underlying microvascular network [23] may also influence the appearance of islands.

Recent work has also independently quantified the effects of topical vasoconstrictive agents, providing an operator-independent assessment of skin blanching. Studies were compared to Minolta chromameter CR 200, which was used as an independent color reference measurement. The application of the corticoid Desoximetasone gel (0.05%) was assessed after 6 h and showed that the relative uncertainty in the blanching estimate produced by the TiVi system was about 5% and similar to that of the chromameter operated by a single user [24].

9.5.2
Lipid Studies

Using the TiVi technology, changes in erythema following application of 0.5% benzyl nicotinate in formulations with different lipid content were investigated

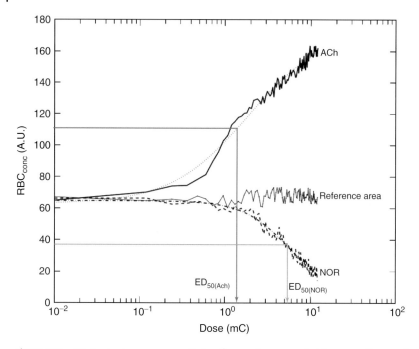

Figure 9.15 Dose–response curves outlining the reaction presented by vasoactive agents.

[25]. They observed that benzyl nicotinate containing 10% fat had the effect of inducing erythema more rapidly and with higher intensity than the formulations with fat content >10%. They also investigated the blanching agent betamethasone valerate, showing that efficacy was increased with lower fat content formulation. They concluded that the rate of penetration of the active ingredients was inversely related to the lipid content; thus, simple changes of the cosmetic properties by modifications of the lipid content may affect the efficacy of a formulation. These results can be summarized in Figure 9.17, whereby the response of the TiVi system can be observed for benzyl nicotinate formulations with various lipid concentrations. These results have an impact on the formulations of dermatological treatments, where the physical and dermatopharmacological actions of the active ingredients may be changed to suit the patient (i.e., for appearance, odor, etc.).

9.5.3
UV-B Studies

Recent research expanded the use of the TiVi technology to study UV-B (280–320 nm) phototesting, using a radially attenuating beam of characterized dosimetry [26]. Previously, LDPI was used to give quantitative evaluation to doses above the minimal erythemal dose (MED – the lowest dose of UV light that produces an identifiable erythematous reaction). This improves on current practice for UV-B phototesting whereby single exposures of increasing dose are made over

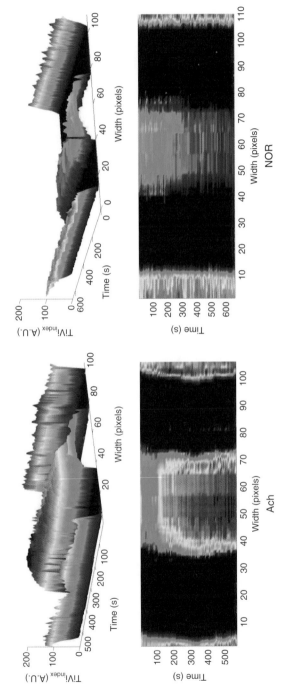

Figure 9.16 Profiles of a cross section of the reacting area undergoing iontophoresis showing the vasodilation and vasoconstriction process. The area affected can be assessed spatially and temporarily with TiVi technology.

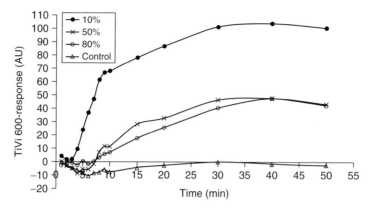

Figure 9.17 Relationship between TiVi output and three different lipid concentrations of benzyl nicotinate (representing different formulations). (Source: After Ref. [25], reproduced with permission.)

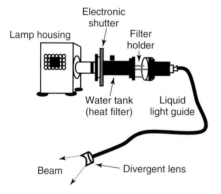

Figure 9.18 Instrumentation for wide field UV-B provocation. The water tank removes heat, and optical filters limit the light to UV-specific wavelengths. A liquid light guide transmits the UV-B radiation to the conical applicator with a lens diverging the beam. (Source: After Ref. [26], reproduced with permission.)

an area of the skin and are subject to a visual assessment scoring scale. The radial UV-B methodology has been validated by way of evaluating the anti-inflammatory effects of topically applied substances [27]. The instrumentation for provoking the UV-B reactions is shown in Figure 9.18.

Visually assessed diameters were also determined to match LDPI determined reaction diameters within a 95% confidence interval [28] and allowed the plotting of dose–response curves using the quantitative response data of the LDPI images against the corresponding dosimetry data. It has also been recently determined that if naked eye readings are to be used to assess UV-B reaction diameters and then advantages are shown by the use of a sharp-edged reaction, whereas the use of an

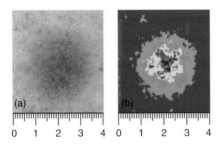

Figure 9.19 (a) Six hour delay photograph and (b) corresponding LDPI image. (Source: After Ref. [29], reproduced with permission.)

assessment technology such as LDPI (or perhaps TiVi) is advocated if the borders between the reaction and normal tissue is diffuse (as in the radial provocation) [29] (Figure 9.19).

The improved spatial resolution of TiVi over LDPI allows a more accurate visualization of the increased concentration of RBCs, as is shown by the delayed reaction in Figure 9.20. The group determined the reaction diameter by using the

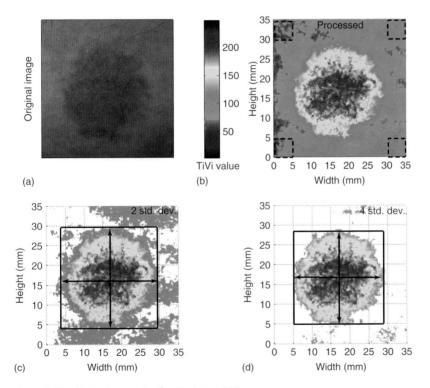

Figure 9.20 (a) A photograph of a 6 h delay UV-B provocation, (b) standard processed image showing background regions (dashed), and (c,d) the thresholded image using two times the standard deviation of the background regions and also by four times the standard deviation. (Source: After Ref. [26], reproduced with permission.)

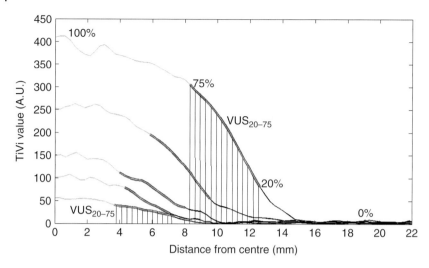

Figure 9.21 Plot of five responses to provocations by radial analysis. The volume under different parts of the curve reflects the "amount" of erythema under the surface of the skin at the test site and can be used as a method of comparison between responses. It should be noted that the same provocation dose does not elicit the same intensity of reaction in each individual. (Source: After Ref. [26], reproduced with permission.)

method of thresholding the image by two and four times the standard deviation of the four regions of background, a method well used with thresholding of LDPI images [27]. They compared these results to the values provided by a radial analysis tool, which divided the reaction into concentric isodose rings centered on the reaction. Each ring is averaged to produce an intensity at a distance from the reaction center. Figure 9.21 details the dose–response of five test subjects 6 h postexposure to the volar forearm. The group used a linear fit between 20 and 75% of the reaction maximum (at the center) to estimate the reaction radius and used calculations of the area under the curve that estimates the volume under the surface of the skin reaction. The group also describe how the mismatch of the clinician and TiVi technology may be due to the polarization detection of the system, which is effectively seeing a deeper range of returning photons from the tissue than the clinician detects. Owing to the known effects of TiVi response variation of 10% on imaging a curved area such as the forearm [19], efforts should be made to standardize testing, and other work is geared toward dewarping the images of the forearm, to effectively "flatten out" the image for a more reproducible analysis [26].

9.5.4
Temporal Studies

Research studies have developed the wide field imaging system further to include a video mode, applicable to the same instrumentational setup as the high-resolution imager with some modifications [30]. Two systems were developed, one with a light emitting diode (LED) ringlight using a three CCD video camera with direct streaming of data to a PC for processing [31] and another portable system which replaced the flash light source with a continuous light source of a similar shaped spectrum [32]. This system has been tested using the PORH test, a test that has previously been employed to study microvascular reactivity functionality [33]. Their results show that greater significance may be placed on the pattern or trend of behavior in these responses over a defined time period rather than an absolute measurement of peak reaction or the time to peak reaction. The group also examined the capillary refilling manoeuvre, a quick physical exam used clinically that provides important information regarding skin perfusion. Abnormal perfusion of the skin can indicate a number of medical conditions; for example, dehydration, hypothermia, and many types of shock cause a prolonged capillary refill time that is >2 s. The pressure on the arteriolar capillaries blanches or whitens the skin by a clinician pressing on the tissue, so that when the skin is uncompressed this allows blood to flow back into the vessels and the skin returns to a normal color. The amount of time it takes for the skin to return to normal is the capillary refill time. An example of the increase in RBC concentration in the nail fold during an occlusion maneuver known as the *postocclusive reactive hyperemia* can be observed in Figure 9.22. This test was performed with sphygmomanometer occlusion of the brachial artery with a pressure of 80 mmHg (which inhibits venous return flow but allows arterial inflow) for 30 s. The increase in concentration during occlusion can clearly be observed. The vasculature has not returned to normal 90 s postocclusion.

Despite the simplicity of occlusion tests, especially the capillary refilling test, they are often performed incorrectly thus yielding useless results. The group attempted standardization of the test maneuver and also quantified its effects using high-speed TiVi, rather than relying on visual observation. An example time trace

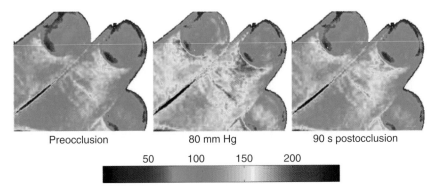

Preocclusion   80 mm Hg   90 s postocclusion

50   100   150   200

Figure 9.22 TiVi video frame images at various stages during the PORH cycle. The resulting RBC concentration in the nail fold is observed to be higher than the preocclusion level. (Source: After Ref. [31], reproduced with permission.)

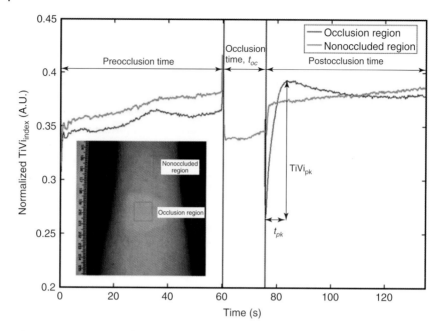

Figure 9.23 Time traces from a reactive hyperemia test using a blunt tool, showing the increase in local RBC concentration in the volar forearm. Statistics such as the time to peak, t_{pk}, and peak TiVi value, TiVi$_{pk}$, are used to characterize the response. (Source: After Ref. [32], reproduced with permission.)

of the reaction is shown in Figure 9.23, using an ROI over the reaction area and a similar sized area located a distance away from the primary reaction. The influence of the capillary refilling can be seen in the nonoccluded region, indicating the far-reaching effects of a local decrease in skin perfusion. The group proved by correlation functions that longer occlusion times lead to larger differences between the occluded and nonoccluded time series, although failed to prove any distinction between men and women and between smokers and nonsmokers. This may be a result of the small sample size of subjects and the large inter- and intrasubject variation in TiVi responses [32].

Limitations of the video imaging method with the high-speed imager are the same as those shared with many noninvasive imaging technologies (i.e., capillary microscopy, LDPI), with the largest effect being patient motion causing the subject area to move outside of the imaging frame. Slight patient motion in this method can be compensated for by the aligning function included in the TiVi600 main code, and larger motion can be compensated for by zooming out of the area and refocusing the camera on the new area. This will, of course, cause the loss of data but provided the new area is refocused, the frames can be aligned. For experiments using maximum temporal resolution, this may lead to hundreds of iterations of marking and alignment, even over a time of <20 s.

9.6
Comparison with Other Instrumentation

LDPI and laser speckle perfusion imaging (LSPI) represent well-established modern approaches to the investigation of microcirculatory function. The principles of laser Doppler and laser speckle technology are available from other sources [34–38], and here, it suffices to say that both LDPI and LSPI are sensitive to both the concentration and velocity of the RBCs in the skin's blood vessels, whereas TiVi technology is sensitive only to the concentration of RBCs in the tissue. Table 9.2 outlines the differences between the TiVi, a commercial LDPI system (known as laser Doppler line scanner – LDLS) and a commercial LSPI system (known as full field laser perfusion imager).

In order to evaluate the effect of vasoconstrictive agents on the skin microvasculature involves the measurement of signals below the normal biological zero for a subject. The use of LDPI for this test requires an increase in background flow to enhance contrast, usually achieved by local warming of the area [39]. The use of TiVi systems to allow vasoconstriction studies without the need for predilation as required by LDPI studies has been shown to represent an advantage in the reduction of confounding factors [21]. Other experiments recently performed corroborate the inability of LDPI and LSPI to measure below the biological background in the

Table 9.2 A comparison table outlining the mechanical and operational specifications of the LDPI (LDLS), LSPI (FLPI) speckle, and TiVi imaging devices.

Property	LDLS	FLPI	TiVi
Principle	Doppler effect	Reduced speckle contrast	Polarization spectroscopy
Variable recorded	Perfusion (speed × concentration)	Perfusion (speed × concentration)	Relative concentration
Measurement sites	16 384	431 680	Up to 18 million
Best resolution (μm)	~500	~100	~50
Measurement depth	~1 mm	~ 300 μm	~ 500 μm
Repetition rate (s)	6 (50 × 64)	4 (568 × 760)	5 (5184 × 3456)
Best capture time (s)	6	4	1/60
Zoom function	No	Yes	Yes
Video rate	None	25 fps	30 fps
Video size	–	113 × 152	up to 760 × 1080
Pixel resolution (cm^{-2})	100	40 000	900 000
View angle	Top only	Top only	User selectable
Weight (kg)	Scanner 3.2	2	3
Calibration	Motility standard	Motility standard	None
Ambient light sensitivity	Intermediate	Substantial	Negligible

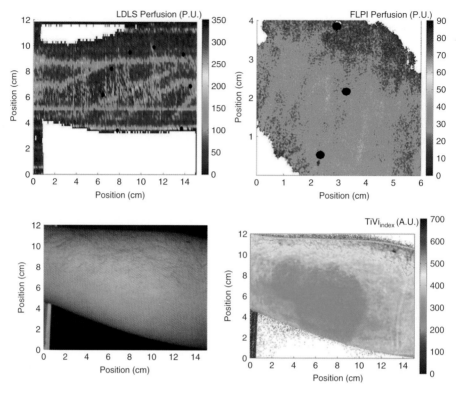

Figure 9.24 Skin blanching due to a vaso-constricting corticosteroid by the three systems. The black dots in the FLPI and LDLS images bound the area affected by the drug. The FLPI image is shown over a smaller scale due to background level; hence, the border between affected and unaffected tissue is shown. (Source: After Ref. [40], reproduced with permission.)

volar forearm, as shown for all three devices in Figure 9.24 [40]. An example of a vasoconstriction as detected by the three systems is shown in Figure 9.25, showing that the measurement depth of the LDPI system does not determine the superficial pattern produced in skin. This is due to the longer wavelength used in the LDPI as opposed to the FLPI and TiVi systems. These experiments also highlighted the variation in response with increasing pressure applied to a tourniquet on the upper arm. The increased spatial resolution of TiVi imaging is also apparent in this work. Other work in the literature compares and contrasts further the advantages and disadvantages between the use of the main microcirculation imaging modalities [41].

9.7
Other Technology for Polarization Imaging

Other forms of polarization imaging have also been used with various degrees of success. The technique of optical polarization spectroscopy (OPS) uses

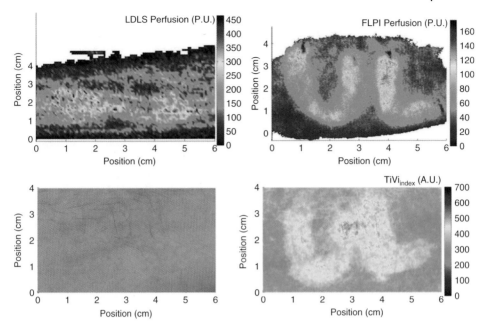

Figure 9.25 Comparison of a topical application of a common analgesic "Deep Heat" as assessed by the LDLS, FLPI, and TiVi imaging technologies. The cross-polarized image from the TiVi system can also be used as a visual aid. Neither LDPI of FLPI offers a standard color image. (Source: After Ref. [40], reproduced with permission.)

cross-polarized filters at a single wavelength (at 548 nm – the isobestic point of hemoglobin) employed in a video microscope designed to image in gray scale a 1×1 mm area of the microvasculature of many various types of tissue [42, 43]. It has been shown to provide better image quality than standard capillary microscopy in the nail fold [44] and has been applied to study superficial and deep burns to the skin [45, 46], adult brain microcirculation [42], and also preterm infant skin microcirculation [47]. Other uses include colon microcirculation [48] and studies in patients with sepsis [49]. Image resolution is stated as 1 CCD pixel $\approx 1\,\mu$m, using a 1 MP CCD. Flow velocity measurements are 20 mm s^{-1} – 1 maximum, and there is no direct contact between the probe head and the tissue surface. Major advantages are the devices small size and portability for bedside use, while also avoiding the need for transillumination and dyes for contrast enhancement [47]. Limitations of the device include the small imaging area, with motion artifacts making a stable set of images from the area difficult to acquire, thus making RBC velocity difficult to measure and limiting the reproducibility of results [50].

Using combinations of copolarized and cross-polarized images, other research instrumentation previously discussed in Section 9.2 has shown that differentiation between freckles, melanocytic nevi, and malignant tumors is possible [11], contrast of burn scars is improved [8], and visibility of squamous cell carcinomas is greatly enhanced. The determination of fundamental scattering parameters of turbid media via the use of backscattered polarization images is also possible [51]. In anisotropic media such as tissue, the achievable resolution and contrast of polarization-gated transillumination imaging are significantly influenced by the refractive index of scatterers in the medium [52].

9.8
Discussion

This chapter deals with an emerging technology – TiVi – intended for quantitative analysis of skin erythema (vasodilatation) and blanching (vasoconstriction). TiVi was designed with ease of use in mind and productive in gaining investigator-independent data in terms of images visualizing the spatial distribution of RBC concentration in tissue. TiVi can be said to quantify what can be observed by the naked eye and take the subjectivity out of skin testing. Preliminary results also point to the fact that alterations in skin RBC concentration can be detected at an earlier stage by TiVi than what is possible by naked eye observation, mainly due to the use of a cross-polarized detection technique. By reducing data from a sequence of images to curves and indexes, TiVi is a versatile tool in skin testing including evaluation of new skin care products, assessment of pharmaceuticals, and grading the performance of sensitive skin to various kinds of challenges. In contrast to what is the situation with Laser Doppler technology, TiVi measures only the concentration of RBCs and not their velocity, thereby making the images closer related to what can be observed by the naked eye. TiVi is not sensitive to movement artifacts and distance to the object but the amount of melanin in the epidermal layer modulates the output signal. This disadvantage can be effectively eliminated by recording only alterations in skin RBC concentration, since these generally appear on a timescale much shorter than that at which the melanin content of the skin is altered.

References

1. Vincent, J.L. and DeBacker, D. (2005) Microvascular dysfunction as a cause of organ dysfunction in severe sepsis. *Crit. Care*, **4** (Suppl. 9), 9–12.
2. Spronk, P.E., Zandstra, D.F., and Ince, C. (2004) Bench-to-bedside review: sepsis is a disease of the microcirculation. *Crit. Care*, **8**, 462–468.
3. Nagy, Z. and Czirják, L. (2004) Nail-fold digital capillaroscopy in 447 patients with connective tissue disease and Raynaud's disease. *J. Eur. Acad. Dermatol. Venereol.*, **18**, 62–68.
4. Wårdell, K., Jakobsson, A., and Nilsson, G.E. (1993) Laser Doppler perfusion imaging by dynamic light scattering. *IEEE Trans. Biomed. Eng.*, **40**, 309–316.
5. O'Doherty, J., Henricson, J., Anderson, C., Leahy, M.J., Nilsson, G.E., and Sjöberg, F. (2007) Sub-epidermal imaging using polarized light spectroscopy for assessment of skin microcirculation. *Skin Res. Technol.*, **13**, 472–484.
6. Anderson, R.R. (1991) Polarized-light examination and photography of the skin. *Arch. Dermatol.*, **127**, 1000–1005.

7. Ostermeyer, M.R., Stephens, D.V., Wang, L., and Stephens, D. (1996) in *OSA Topics on Biomedical Optical Spectroscopy and Diagnostics*, OSA Trends in Optics and Photonics Series, Vol. **3** (eds E. Sevick-Muraca and E. Benaron), *Optical Society of America*, Washington, DC, p. SP2.

8. Jacques, S.L., Roman, J., and Lee, K. (2002) Imaging skin pathology with polarized light. *J. Biomed. Opt.*, **7**, 329–340.

9. Ramella-Roman, J.C., Lee, K., Jacques, S.L., and Prahl, S.A. (2004) Design and testing of a clinical hand-held polarisation camera. *J. Biomed. Opt.*, **9**, 1305–1310.

10. Cheong, W.F., Prahl, S.A., and Welch, A.J. (1990) A review of the optical properties of biological tissues. *IEEE J. Quantum Electron.*, **26**, 2166–2185.

11. Jacques, S.L., Roman, J.R., and Lee, K. (2000) Imaging superficial tissues with polarized light. *Lasers Surg. Med.*, **26**, 119–129.

12. Ramella-Roman, J.C., Prahl, S.A., and Jacques, S.L. (2005) Three Monte Carlo programs of polarized light transport into scattering media: Part I. *Opt. Express*, **13**, 4420–4438.

13. Wang, X. and Wang, L.V. (2002) Propagation of polarized light in birefringent turbid media: a Monte Carlo study. *J. Biomed. Opt.*, **7**, 279–290.

14. Farage, M. (2008) Enhancement of visual scoring of skin irritant reactions using cross-polarized light and parallel-polarized light. *Contact Dermat.*, **58**, 147–155.

15. Pinnagoda, J., Tupker, R.A., Agner, T., and Serup, J. (1990) Guidelines for transepidermal water loss (TEWL) measurement. A report from the standardization group of the European society of contact dermatitis. *Contact Dermat.*, **22**, 164–178.

16. Bircher, A., De Boer, E.M., Agner, T., Wahlberg, J.E., and Serup, J. (1994) Guidelines for measurement of cutaneous blood flow by laser Doppler flowmetry. A report from the standardization group of the European society of contact dermatitis. *Contact Dermat.*, **30**, 65–72.

17. Serup, J. (1994) Bioengineering and the skin: from standard error to standard operating procedure. *Acta Derm. Venereol. (Stockholm)*, **185** (Suppl.), 5–8.

18. Fullerton, A., Stucker, M., Wilhelm, K.P., Wardell, K., Anderson, C., Fischer, T., Nilsson, G.E., and Serup, J. (2002) Guidelines for visualization of cutaneous blood flow by laser Doppler perfusion imaging. A report from the tandardization group of the European society of contact dermatitis based upon the HIRELADO European community project. *Contact Dermat.*, **46**, 129–140.

19. Nilsson, G.E., Zhai, H., Chan, H.P., Farahmand, S., and Maibach, H.I. (2009) Cutaneous bioengineering instrumentation standardization: the tissue viability iImager. *Skin Res. Technol.*, **15**, 6–13.

20. Zhai, H., Chan, H.P., Farahmand, S., Nilsson, G.E., and Maibach, H.I. (2009b) Tissue viability imaging: mapping skin erythema. *Skin Res. Technol.*, **15**, 15–19.

21. Henricson, J., Nilsson, A., Tesselaar, E., Nilsson, G., and Sjoberg, F. (2009) Tissue Viability imaging: microvascular response to vasoactive drugs induced by iontophoresis. *Microvasc. Res.*, **78**, 199–205.

22. Ramsay, J.E., Ferrel, W.R., Greer, I.A., and Sattar, N. (2002) Factors critical to iontophoretic assessment of vascular reactivity: Implications for clinical studies of endothelial dysfunction. *J. Cardiovasc. Pharmacol.*, **39**, 9–17.

23. Gardner-Medwin, J.M., Taylor, J.Y., Macdonald, I.A., and Powell, R.J. (1997) An investigation into variability in microvascular skin blood flow and the response to transdermal delivery of acetylcholine at different sites in the forearm and hand. *Br. J. Pharmacol.*, **43**, 392–397.

24. Zhai, H., Chan, H.P., Farahmand, S., Nilsson, G.E., and Maibach, H.I. (2009) Comparison of tissue viability imaging and colorimetry: skin blanching. *Skin Res. Technol.*, **15**, 20–23.

25. Wiren, K., Fritihof, H., Sjoqvist, C., and Loden, M. (2009) Enhancement of bioavailability by lowering of fat content in topical formulations. *Br. J. Dermatol.*, **160**, 552–556.

26. O'Doherty, J., Henricson, J., Enfield, J., Nilsson, G.E., Leahy, M.J., and Anderson, C.D. (2011) Tissue viability imaging (TiVi) in the assessment of divergent beam UV-B provocation. *Arch. Dermatol. Res.*, **303** (2), 79–87.

27. Falk, M., Ilias, M.A., Wårdell, K., and Anderson, C. (2003) Phototesting with a divergent UVB beam in the investigation of anti-inflammatory effects of topically applied substances. *Photodermatol. Photomed.*, **19**, 195–202.

28. Ilias, M.A., Wårdell, K., Falk, M., and Anderson, C. (2001) Phototesting based on a divergent beam – a study on normal subjects. *Photodermatol. Photomed.*, **17**, 189–196.

29. Falk, M., Ilias, M., and Anderson, C. (2008) Inter-observer variability in reading of phototest reactions with sharply or diffusely delineated borders. *Skin Res. Technol.*, **14**, 397–402.

30. O'Doherty, J., Henricson, J., Nilsson, G.E., Anderson, C., and Leahy, M.J. (2007) Real time diffuse reflectance polarisation spectroscopy imaging to evaluate skin microcirculation. *Proc. SPIE*, **6631**, 66310.

31. O'Doherty, J., McNamara, P., Fitzgerald, B., and Leahy, M.J. (2010) Dynamic microvascular responses with a high speed TiVi imaging system, accepted for publication. *J. Biophotonics.*, **4**, 7–8, August 2011, 509–513.

32. McNamara, P., O'Doherty, J., O'Connell, M.L., Fitzgerald, B.W., Anderson, C.D., Nilsson, G.E., Toll, R., and Leahy, M.J. (2010) Tissue viability (TiVi) imaging: temporal effects of local occlusion studies in the volar forearm. *J. Biophotonics*, **3**, 66–74.

33. Yvonne-Tee, G.B., Rasool, A.H.G., Halim, A.S., and Rahman, A.R.A. (2005) Reproducibility of different laser Doppler fluximetry parameters of postocclusive reactive hyperemia in human forearm skin. *J. Pharmacol. Toxicol.*, **52**, 286–292.

34. Leahy, M.J., de Mul, F.F.M., Nilsson, G.E., and Maniewski, R. (1999) Principles and practice of the laser-Doppler perfusion technique. *Technol. Health Care*, **7**, 143–162.

35. Nilsson, G.E., Salerud, E.G., Stromberg, T., and Wardell, K. (2004) Laser doppler perfusion monitoring and imaging, *Biomedical Photonics Handbook*, Chapter 15, CRC Press, Boca Raton, FL, 15-1 to 15–23.

36. Draijer, M., Hondebrink, E., van Leeuwen, T., and Steenbergen, W. (2009) Review of laser speckle contrast techniques for visualizing tissue perfusion. *Lasers Med. Sci.*, **24**, 639–651.

37. Briers, J.D. (2001) Laser Doppler, speckle and related techniques for blood perfusion mapping and imaging. *Physiol. Meas.*, **22**, R35–R66.

38. Briers, J.D. (2007) Laser speckle contrast imaging for measuring blood flow. *Appl. Opt.*, **XXXVII**, 139–152.

39. Drummond, P.D. (2002) Prior iontophoresis of saline enhances vasoconstriction to phenylephrine and clonidine in the skin of the human forearm. *Br. J. Clin. Pharmacol.*, **54**, 45–50.

40. O'Doherty, J., McNamara, P., Clancy, N.T., Enfield, J.G., and Leahy, M.J. (2009) Comparison of instruments for investigation of microcirculatory blood flow and red blood cell concentration. *J. Biomed. Opt.*, **14**, 034025.

41. Leahy, M.J., Enfield, J.G., Clancy, N.T., O'Doherty, J., McNamara, P., and Nilsson, G.E. (2007) Biophotonic methods in microcirculation imaging. *Med. Laser Appl.*, **22**, 105–126.

42. Groner, W., Winkelman, J.W., Harris, A.G., Ince, C., Bouma, G.J., Messmer, K., and Nadeau, R.G. (1999) Orthogonal polarisation spectral imaging: a new method for study of the microcirculation. *Nat. Med.*, **5**, 1209–1213.

43. DeBacker, D. (2005) Orthogonal polarisation spectral imaging: principles, techniques, human studies, *Anaesthesia, Pain, Intensive Care and Emergency Medicine*, Chapter 48, Springer, 535–542.

44. Mathura, K.R., Vollebregt, K.C., Boer, K., De Graaff, J.C., Ubbink, D.T., and Ince, C. (2001) Comparison of OPS imaging and conventional capillary microscopy to study the human microcirculation. *J. Appl. Physiol.*, **91**, 74–78.

45. Milner, S.M. (2002) Predicting early burn wound outcome using orthogonal polarization spectral imaging. *Int. J. Dermatol.*, **41**, 715.

46. Milner, S.M., Bhat, S., Gulati, S., Gherardini, G., Smith, C.E., and Bick, R.J. (2005) Observations on the microcirculation of the human burn wound using orthogonal polarization spectral imaging. *Burns*, **31**, 316–319.

47. Genzel-Boroviczeny, O., Strotgen, J., Harris, A.G., Messmer, K., and Christ, F. (2002) Orthogonal polarization spectral imaging (OPS): a novel method to measure the microcirculation in term and preterm infants transcutaneously. *Pediatr. Res.*, **51**, 386–391.

48. Biberthaler, P. and Langer, S. (2002) Comparison of the new OPS imaging technique with intravital microscopy: analysis of the colon microcirculation. *Eur. Surg. Res.*, **34**, 124–128.

49. De Backer, D., Creteur, J., Preiser, J.C., Dubois, M.J., and Vincent, J.L. (2002) Microvascular blood Flow is altered in patients with sepsis. *Am. J. Respir. Crit. Care Med.*, **166**, 98–104.

50. Lindert, J., Werner, J., Redlin, M., Kuppe, H., Habazetti, H., and Pries, A.R. (2002) OPS imaging of human microcirculation: a short technical report. *J. Vasc. Res.*, **39**, 368–372.

51. Jaillon, F. and Saint-Jalmes, H. (2005) Scattering coefficient determination in turbid media with backscattered polarized light. *J. Biomed. Opt.*, **10**, 034016.

52. Shukla, P., Sumathi, R., Gupta, S., and Pradhan, A. (2007) Influence of size parameter and refractive index of the scatterer on polarization-gated optical imaging through turbid media. *J. Opt. Soc. Am. A*, **24**, 1704–1713.

10
Optical Microangiography: Theory and Application

Ruikang K. Wang and Hrebesh M. Subhash

10.1
Introduction

In physiology, the term *microvascular blood perfusion* refers to the process involved in the nutritive blood delivery to the tissue's capillary bed, which is vital for homeostasis, and thereby the survival of an organ. Noninvasive and chronic imaging of blood flow within microcirculatory tissue beds is required in many basic research and clinical circumstances including cancer diagnosis and therapy, arteriosclerosis, therapeutic angiogenesis, vasospastic conditions, reconstructive surgery and also the for development and implementation of antivascular strategies. Over the past decade, a number of emerging technologies have become available for the study of microvascular blood flow, including photoelectric plethysmography [1, 2] thermal [3] and radioisotope [4, 5] clearance, orthogonal polarization spectral imaging [6, 7], videophotometric capillaroscopy [8, 9], and Doppler ultrasound [10]. Some of these methods traumatize the tissue, which may seriously disturb the microcirculation; others have practical limitations in clinical use. None of these methods, however, have fulfilled the requirements of being noninvasiveness and applicable to a large number of tissues as well as offering the possibility of recording the tissue perfusion continuously or visualizing the results in terms of three-dimensional perfusion maps. Methods for clinical studies of the blood flow in small vessels should therefore preferably be noninvasive, versatile, and easy to use.

In general, microvasculature imaging is a challenging task because of the requirement of relatively high spatiotemporal resolution and sensitivity to image small diameter of the blood vessels. Most of the available methods that fulfill these conditions are based on optical measurement technologies such as intravital confocal microscopy, laser Doppler technique, infrared thermography, optical intrinsic signal imaging, photoacoustic imaging (PAI) and phase-resolved Doppler optical coherence tomography (PRDOCT), and so on. Intravital confocal microscopy uses a fluorescence microscope to image various molecular and cellular processes *in vivo* with high resolution. However, intravital microscopy is a time-consuming invasive procedure, and the imaging depth is limited to a few hundred microns in highly scattering specimens [11–13]. The laser Doppler technique uses the

Microcirculation Imaging, First Edition. Edited by Martin J. Leahy.
© 2012 Wiley-VCH Verlag GmbH & Co. KGaA. Published 2012 by Wiley-VCH Verlag GmbH & Co. KGaA.

frequency shift produced by the Doppler effect to measure blood flow. This technique is capable of noninvasive and continuous recording of blood perfusion in tissue. A major limitation of laser Doppler technique is its inability to image tissue deeper than 1 mm [14, 15]. Moreover, laser Doppler is not able to measure flow in absolute units (i.e., milliliters per minute), thus it often uses the arbitrary unit of flux, which is the product of concentration of moving blood cells and the mean velocity of those blood cells. Infrared thermography graphically depicts temperature gradients over a given body surface area. Generally, an increase in the blood flow can be related to a rise in temperature due to increased metabolic activity in the highly vascular region [16, 17]. This approach has lower sensitivity because a number of physiological changes involved with increased blood flow do not necessarily indicate pathology [16]. Infrared thermography is generally used in conjunction with other imaging techniques such as laser Doppler technique and mammography [16]. Optical intrinsic signal imaging is another imaging modality with very high spatial and temporal resolution, but which is limited to superficial two-dimensional mapping and is invasive in nature [18]. PAI, based on thermoacoustic phenomena resulting from the strong light absorption of blood and the subsequent thermoelastic expansion, has been reported to map vascular structures deep within the brain of small animals [19, 20]. However, the spatial ($\sim$100 µm) resolution of this approach is limited by the viscoelastic filtering of higher acoustic frequencies by the tissue. Moreover, obtaining blood flow information is difficult, if not impossible, with this method. PRDOCT is an alternative low-coherence interferometric (LCI) technique to extract depth-resolved velocity information of blood flow in functional vessels within the tissue beds. Although this method is of high resolution and high sensitivity to the blood flow, its imaging performance is greatly deteriorated by the characteristic texture pattern artifact, which is caused by optical heterogeneity of the sample [21], and the phase instability that is caused by the sample motion as well as system noise artifacts [22].

Optical microangiography (OMAG) [23] is a recently developed imaging method, capable of resolving 3D distribution of dynamic blood perfusion at the capillary level within microcirculatory beds *in vivo*. The imaging contrast of blood perfusion is based on the endogenous light scattering from the moving blood erythrocytes in the blood vessels; thus no exogenous contrasting agents are necessary. This is achieved by efficient separation of the moving scattering elements from the static scattering ones within tissue through the OMAG hardware associated with mathematical analysis of the optical scattering signals emerging from an illuminated tissue sample. The basic principle of OMAG is based on Fourier domain optical coherence tomography (FDOCT) [24], an LCI technique, which is now becoming a noninvasive clinical tool for high-resolution ophthalmic imaging of the human eye.

10.2
Optical Coherence Tomography

The development of OMAG has its origin in FDOCT, which is a variant of optical coherence tomography (OCT), a well-established LCI technique for imaging biological tissues. LCI is a powerful technique for measuring the magnitude and echo-time delay of backscattered light with very high sensitivity, which was first described by Sir Isaac Newton. In principle, OCT is an optical analog to clinical ultrasound. In OCT, the temporally gated optical pulse remitted from scattering sites within the sample is localized by LCI [25–30]. This is typically achieved with a Michelson interferometer. The sample rests in one arm of the interferometer, and a scanning reference optical delay line is in the other arm. In LCI, light interferes at the detector only when light reflected from the sample has an optical path length that matches with that of light reflected from the scanning reference mirror (RM). A single scan of the RM thus provides a one-dimensional depth reflectivity profile of the sample. Two-dimensional cross-sectional images are formed by laterally scanning the incident probe beam across the sample. The reconstructed OCT image is essentially a map of the changes of reflectivity that occurs at internal interfaces, similar to the discontinuities in acoustic impedance in ultrasound images.

10.2.1
Principle of OCT

A schematic of a time domain fiber optics based OCT setup is shown in Figure 10.1. The OCT system comprises a broadband light source emitting light of high spatial and low temporal coherence, which is coupled into a 2 × 2 fiber optics based Michelson interferometer. The Michelson interferometer divides the light beam and directs it into two arms of the interferometer. The sample arm beam directs into the object to be analyzed. It usually contains collimating optics, enabling formation of a narrow beam, which penetrates the object. In order to reconstruct two-dimensional cross-sectional images of the object, the beam is galvanometrically scanned across the sample surface. Light backscattered or reflected from the various structures returns to the interferometer and is brought to interference with light reflected back from the RM, which scans back and forth through the required depth of imaging. The standard fiber-optics Michelson interferometer is not the most efficient design for practical implementation, because a major disadvantage of this configuration is that the DC signal and intensity noise generated by the light from the reference arm add to the interference signal. In order to eliminate this problem, an alternative configuration called *balanced heterodyne* configurations as shown in Figure 10.1a has been commonly used, in which these background noise components are canceled by subtracting the photocurrents generated by two photodetectors. Then the resulting interfering light is detected by a photodiode (PD). Figure 10.1b shows the relative target positions in the eye, and Figure 10.1c shows the raw interferograms (A-scan) that are obtained by scanning the RM and correspond to the different structural features of the ocular medium. Figure 10.1d shows the reference-arm-signal-subtracted interference signal from the output of the balanced detector. In the preceding step, the interferograms are amplified and backed up with a band pass filter tuned to the Doppler frequency, often called the *"carrier frequency,"* which is related to the scanning speed of the RM. This

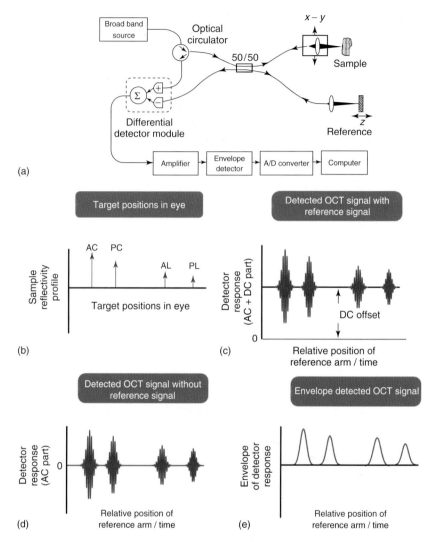

Figure 10.1 (a) Schematic of a typical fiber-optics-based time domain OCT setup, (b) reflectivity profile of target in the ocular medium, assuming there exists 4 interfaces: AC, PC, AL, and PL (c) detected interference signal by the photodetector, (d) detected signal with reference signal filtered out, and (e) demodulated and envelop-detected OCT signals.

procedure helps to eliminate extraneous signals arising from background light. Then, for the next scan of the RM, the probing beam is shifted to an adjacent position, and so on, to yield a set of consecutive A-scans. These A-scans are then combined into a single picture to form a cross-sectional image of the object, the B-scan. Three-dimensional, volumetric data sets can be generated by acquiring sequential cross-sectional images by scanning the incident optical beam in a raster pattern.

In contrast to standard microscopy, OCT can achieve fine axial resolution independent of the beam focusing and spot size. The axial image resolution in OCT is determined by the measurement resolution for echo-time delays of light. The axial resolution of an OCT is an important specification of an OCT system, and in many biomedical applications, high axial resolution is often required to distinguish different cellular ultrastructures. The axial resolution of OCT is defined as the full width half maximum (FWHM) of the source coherence length l_c. For a source with a Gaussian spectral distribution, the axial resolution is given by

$$\Delta z = \frac{2 \ln 2}{\pi} \frac{c}{\Delta \nu} = \frac{2 \ln 2}{\pi} \frac{\lambda^2}{\Delta \lambda} \approx 0.44 \frac{\lambda^2}{\Delta \lambda} \tag{10.1}$$

where Δz and $\Delta \lambda$ are the FWHM of the autocorrelation function and spectral width, respectively, and λ_0 is the central wavelength of the light source [31]. It can be seen that broadband light sources are required to achieve high axial resolution, as the axial resolution is inversely proportional to the spectral width of the light source. The transverse resolution in OCT imaging is the same as in optical microscopy and is determined by the diffraction-limited spot size of the focused optical beam. The diffraction-limited minimum spot size is inversely proportional to the numerical aperture (NA) or the focusing angle of the beam. The lateral resolution Δx can be written as

$$\Delta x = \frac{4\lambda}{\pi} \left(\frac{f}{d} \right) \tag{10.2}$$

where f is the focal length of the objective lens and d is the $1/e^2$ Gaussian beam wrist at the objective lens. It can be seen from the above equation that high lateral resolution can be achieved by using a large NA to decrease the spot size. However, for the selection of optics, there is a trade-off between the lateral resolution and the imaging depth. A higher lateral resolution leads to a decrease in the depth of focus, or confocal parameter b, which is twice the Rayleigh range

$$2\Delta z_R = b = \frac{\pi \Delta x^2}{2\lambda} \tag{10.3}$$

The Rayleigh range gives the distance from the focal point to the point where the light beam diameter has increased by a factor of $\sqrt{2}$. This effectively limits the scanning range of the OCT, different from the working range of the scanning reference delay line, as it is the range over which lateral resolution is maintained.

In OCT, the coherence-gated information about the elementary volume of the scatters within the obscuring scattering specimen can be obtained from either the time domain measurement (TD-OCT) or the frequency domain (FD-OCT) [24, 31] measurement. As a variant of coherence domain variant interferometric imaging modality, FD-OCT has been widely attracted in the biomedical imaging field because of its higher sensitivity and imaging speed compared to conventional TD-OCT. The principle of FD-OCT relies on the transformation of the OCT time-varying signal along the optical axis, termed the *A-scan*, into the frequency domain.

10.2.2
Frequency Domain OCT (FD-OCT)

The basic physics of FD-OCT is based on the inverse scattering theorem. According to Wiener–Khintchine theorem, the spectral power amplitude of the backscattered wave equals the Fourier transform (FT) of the axial distribution of the object scattering potential. FD-OCT has the advantage that the full sample depth information is obtained in a parallel manner such that no moving parts are necessary. On the basis of implementation, the FDOCT can be divided into two classes, spectral domain optical coherence tomography (SD-OCT) and swept-source optical coherence tomography (SS-OCT) [32]. In SD-OCT, the optical frequency components are captured simultaneously with a dispersive element and linear detector; on the other hand, in SS-OCT, the optical frequency components are captured by a single detector in a time-encoded sequence by sweeping the frequency of the optical source. Recent studies have shown that FD-OCT can provide signal-to-noise ratio (SNR) that is more than 20 dB better than that provided by the conventional TD-OCT.

The OMAG imaging modality can be implemented either using the SS-OCT or the SD-OCT technique. However, at present, we implemented the OMAG imaging modality based on the SD-OCT technique. A typical implementation of fiber optics based SD-OCT setup is shown in Figure 10.2a. The backscattered low-coherence light is mixed with a reference beam by the 2×2 fiber-optics-based Michelson interferometer, then the grating-based spectrometer at the output of the interferometer separates each spectral component detected using a linear array detector. The interference signal detected by the linear detector is expressed as

$$I(k) = I_S(k) + I_R(k) + 2\sqrt{I_S(k)I_R(k)} \sum_n \alpha_n \cos\left(2kz_n\right) \tag{10.4}$$

where $I_R(k)$ and $I_S(k)$ are the wavelength-dependent intensities reflected from the reference and sample arms, respectively, and k is the wave number. The third term on the right-hand side of Eq. (10.4) represents the interference between the backreflected lights from the sample and reference arm. α_n is the square root of the sample reflectivity at depth z_n. In order to reconstruct the depth information, the spectrum is inverse Fourier transformed, which yields the following convolution:

$$\left|FT^{-1}[I(k)]\right|^2 = \Gamma^2(z) \otimes \left[I_R\delta(z) + \sum_n I_{S,n}\delta(z) + \sum_n \alpha_n^2\delta(z - z_n) \right.$$

$$\left. + \sum_n \alpha_n^2\delta\left(z + z_n\right) \right] \tag{10.5}$$

where $\Gamma(z)$ represents the envelope of the coherence function. The first and second terms on the right-hand side of the Eq. (10.42) describe the autocorrelation (or self-interference) of the reference signal and sample signal, respectively. The third and fourth terms are due to the interference of backreflected beam from the reference and sample surfaces and its complex conjugates. The SD-OCT detects the spectrally resolved interference signal with a spectrometer that consists of a

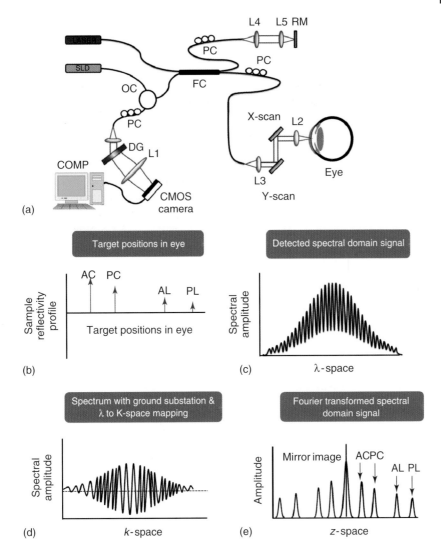

Figure 10.2 (a) Experimental schematic of a FDOCT setup, (b) reflectivity profile of anterior chamber of an eye, (c) detected spectral interferogram by the camera (A-scan), (d) remapped spectral interferogram in *k*-space with background subtraction, and (e) Fourier transformed spectrum.

high-efficiency diffraction grating (DG) and a high-speed line camera. Figure 10.2b shows the reflectivity profile of the different target positions in the ocular medium, and Figure 10.2c shows the intensity spectrum detected by the camera. In order to suppress autocorrelation, self-cross-correlation, and camera noise artifacts, all the spectral interferograms in each slice along the *x*-direction (B-scan) were first ensemble-averaged at each wavelength to obtain a reference spectrum. This back ground spectrum was then subtracted from each A-scan. However, since the FT relates the physical distance (z) with the wave number ($k = 2\pi/\lambda$), the spectra obtained with the SD-OCT spectrometer are not necessarily evenly spaced in k-space. In order to obtain a proper depth profile, the subtracted spectral interferograms are then remapped from λ-space to k-space by using the spline interpolation method, as shown in Figure 10.2d. Owing to the Fourier relation (Wiener–Khintchine theorem between the autocorrelation and the spectral power density), the depth-resolved information can be immediately reconstructed by a Fourier transformation from the remapped spectra, without movement of the reference arm, as shown in Figure 10.2e.

For a Gaussian source centered at λ_0 with a FWHM bandwidth $\Delta\lambda$, the complex coherence function is described by Eq. (10.1). The depth range that can be probed with an SD-OCT is dependent on the spectrometer resolution and the detector size (number of pixels). For a conventional SD-OCT system, the maximum imaging depth is defined as

$$l_{max} = \frac{1}{4n} \frac{\lambda_0^2}{\Delta\lambda_S} N \tag{10.6}$$

Where n is the refractive index of the medium, λ_0 is the center wavelength of the detected spectrum, $\Delta\lambda_S$ is the spectrometer bandwidth, and N is the number of pixels of the camera. For ambiguity-free image, this depth range should be doubled. The term $(\Delta\lambda_S/N)^{-1}$ can be seen as the inverse of the spectral resolution power $\delta\lambda^{-1}$ of the detecting spectrometer and is proportional to the coherence length of the detected spectral channel, which is responsible for one of the main drawbacks of SD-OCT, which is the signal decay observed for structures far away from the relative zero-delay.

10.2.3
Doppler OCT

Doppler optical coherence tomography (DOCT) or optical Doppler tomography (ODT) is the functional extension of OCT, which can permit quantitative imaging of fluid flow in highly scattering specimens [33–38]. The technique is similar to Doppler velocimetry. However, Doppler velocimetry suffers from imprecise imaging due to the long coherence length of the light source used, which causes interference of the static and Doppler-shifted components of light over a long optical path. The low-coherence gating property of OCT overcomes this problem, permitting quantitative imaging of fluid flow in highly scattering media, such as monitoring *in vivo* blood flow beneath the skin. In DOCT, the velocity resolution depends on detection electronics, scan angle, and acquisition time. Reported flow velocity resolutions are in the region 10–100 μm s^{-1}; however, recent development in Fourier domain Doppler optical coherence tomography (FD-DOCT) has shown that a velocity resolution of just a few micrometers per second may be achieved [39–46]. The DOCT can provide 3D tomographic map and velocity profile of blood flow in tissue, which attracted a number of biomedical applications, for example, determination of the depth of burns and determination of tissue perfusion to ensure adequate oxygenation of the tissue after injury, wound closure, grafting, and so on. Other applications include distinguishing between arterial and venous blockages in tissue after injury and monitoring the effect of pharmaceuticals on blood transport in the tissues.

10.2.3.1 Principle of Doppler OCT (DOCT)

The Doppler effect describes the shift in frequency of waves reflected from moving objects. This frequency shift can be used to determine object-moving velocity. For electromagnetic waves such as light, derivation of the Doppler-shifted frequency from a moving object requires the application of special relativity. The result for a Doppler-shifted frequency f_d is

$$f_d = \sqrt{\frac{c+u}{c-u}} f_0 \tag{10.7}$$

where f_0 is the initial frequency of the electromagnetic wave, c the speed of light, and u is the speed of the moving object. Here it is assumed that u is positive when the object is moving toward the observer. In this case, it is seen that the Doppler-shifted frequency, Δf, must be greater than the initial frequency

$$\Delta f = f_d - f_0 \tag{10.8}$$

It can be shown that when u is much less than c, the velocity of the moving sample is given by

$$\Delta f = \frac{u}{c} f_d \tag{10.9}$$

In the practical DOCT system, Figure 10.3, the interferometer sample arm is angled relative to the direction of flow by an amount θ. Detected light is scattered from a moving particle in the sample, undergoing a double Doppler shift – once from the source to the particle, and once again from the particle back to the objective. These two factors are taken into account by expressing Eq. (10.9) in terms of initial source and scattered wave vectors k_0 and k_d, respectively. The Doppler shift can then

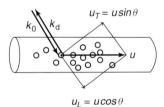

Figure 10.3 Schematic for optical Doppler tomography. The sample arm beam is held at some angle θ to the direction of flow. Therefore, an optical signal with wave vector k_0 falls on a particle moving with velocity u. The light scattered back into the sample objective is Doppler shifted and has wave vector k_d.

be written as

$$\Delta f = \frac{1}{2\pi} \left(k_d - k_0 \right) u \tag{10.10}$$

Therefore, the velocity of moving particles can be determined from the measurement of the Doppler shift and the knowledge of the relative angle between the optical signal and the flow [42]

$$u = \lambda_0 \frac{\Delta f}{2 \cos(\theta)} \tag{10.11}$$

Structural information about the sample is obtained by either conventional TD-OCT or the more recent FD-OCT [24]. However, to retrieve data regarding the flow of particles within submerged capillary, extra measurements of the Doppler-shifted frequency must be made. To do this in the time domain, the RM of the interferometer is scanned to match the path length within the capillary. At each spatial point within the capillary, the detector intensity is sampled at a rate not less than two samples per time period of the source. The time-varying result is then Fourier transformed to give the Doppler frequency shift due to moving particles within the capillary. By doing this at a number of points within the capillary, a profile of particle flow is determined.

The axial resolution of DOCT is again dependent on the source temporal coherence length and the lateral scan resolution on the beam spot size. Velocity resolution depends on the detection electronics, the scan angle, and the acquisition time. Reported flow velocity resolutions are in the region $10{-}100\,\mu m\,s^{-1}$; however, recent developments in FD-DOCT have shown a velocity resolution of just a few micrometers per second. FD-DOCT has also shown greater sensitivity in the region of $90{-}115\,dB$ and may, therefore, lend itself to ocular flow imaging where ANSI laser safety standards require optical powers to be below $1\,mW$. DOCT has been applied to a number of medical situations. Not least of these, imaging *in vivo* blood flow in both the skin [47] and retina [40] has been demonstrated. The capability of DOCT to measure flow within a scattering sample also has potential in new areas of research such as micro-fluidics [48].

10.2.3.2 An Overview of DOCT-Based Flow Imaging Modalities

The original development of DOCT was based on spectrogram method. The spectrogram method uses the short time fast Fourier transform (STFFT) analyses on the time domain interferograms signals [33, 35] that are formed between the reference light and the light that is backscattered from tissue. It was quickly realized that STFFT method has severe limitation on real-time *in vivo* imaging of blood flow, largely due to the coupling issue between the flow imaging resolution and the short time Fourier window size that can be used for flow analyses [42]. This limitation was then removed by an innovative use of the phase-resolved technique in DOCT [47, 49, 50], which was initially developed in the field of ultrasound imaging of blood flow [51]. This use of the phase-resolved technique in DOCT is now commonly referred to as *phase-resolved DOCT*. By evaluating the phase difference between adjacent axial OCT scans (A-scan), PRDOCT greatly improves the detection sensitivity for imaging the flow velocity. Recent development of FDOCT has made an important step further for PRDOCT from laboratory research into visualization and monitoring of the dynamic blood flow within living tissue *in vivo*. This is largely due to the reason that FDOCT has a significant advantage in detection sensitivity over its time domain counterpart [52–54], leading to increased imaging speed that is essential for any *in vivo* imaging application. PRDOCT has seen successful developments in many *in vivo* imaging applications [40, 52, 53, 55], especially in visualizing microvasculatures within the human retina [39, 40, 46, 55].

Although the PRDOCT method could potentially achieve high spatial resolution and high sensitivity for imaging blood flow, its practical *in vivo* imaging performance has so far being disappointing. The following are the factors that degrade *in vivo* imaging performance of PRDOCT. (i) The biological tissue is generally optically heterogeneous. This heterogeneous property of the sample imposes a characteristic texture pattern artifact overlaid onto the PRDOCT flow images [21] that masks the slow blood flow signals that would otherwise be detected by the method. (ii) *In vivo* sample is always in constant motion, for example, due to heart beat. Thus, the motion artifacts in the PRDOCT blood flow images are inevitable [56]. Several methods have been developed to overcome these problems. One most straightforward method is to increase the axial scan density (A-scan density) over a single B-scan. Although successful, this method drastically increases the experimental time, which is not acceptable for *in vivo* imaging situations. Another method was proposed by Wang and Ma [21], which uses a reverse scan pattern for the probe beam to eliminate the texture pattern artifact. For the same purpose, Ren *et al.* [50] used a delay line filter to minimize the artifacts produced by the heterogeneous properties of tissue sample. Although these methods can reduce the texture pattern artifact and increase the velocity sensitivity, they are still based on the phase-resolved method, which has strong dependence on system SNR [57, 58]. On the basis of spatial distribution of the flow velocity, Wojtkowski *et al.* proposed a method called *joint spectral* and *time domain OCT* [58], which has shown to increase the velocity sensitivity, especially in the low SNR regions within a scanned tissue volume. Still, this method needs a high-A-scan-density B-scan, which is time consuming for *in vivo* experiments. To minimize the phase instability caused by the sample movement during the *in vivo* experiments, resonant Doppler imaging [59] was proposed. This method could directly extract the flow velocity information from the intensity distribution without the evaluation of phase distribution. However, this method requires an additional phase modulation in the reference arm, which no doubt increases the complexity of the whole system.

10.3
Optical Microangiography (OMAG)

As described in the earlier section, the OMAG is a functional extension to FDOCT imaging modality, which uses the spectral domain configuration capable of resolving 3D distribution of dynamic blood perfusion at the capillary level within microcirculatory beds *in vivo*. The key difference between OMAG and FDOCT is that in OMAG the interferogram in the lateral direction (B-scan) is spatially modulated with a carrier frequency, which can separate the moving and static scattering components within the sample. This carrier modulation frequency can be introduced either by mounting the RM in the reference arm onto a linear piezotranslation stage, which moves the mirror at a constant velocity across the B-scan (i.e., *x*-direction scan), or an off-pivot scanning beam. In the earlier version of OMAG system [23, 60], this was achieved by mounting the RM in the reference arm onto a linear piezotranslation stage that moved the mirror at a constant velocity across the B-scan (i.e., *x*-direction scan). However, the latest version of OMAG utilizes the spatial modulation frequency provided by the inherent blood flow modulation rather than reference arm modulation [61].

10.3.1
Optical Instrumentation

The schematic of a typical OMAG setup is shown in Figure 10.4 as an example. In this particular setup, the light source was a broadband, superluminescent diode

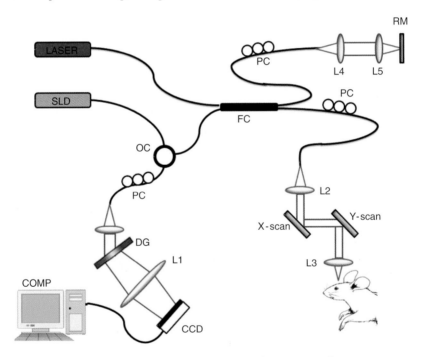

Figure 10.4 Experimental setup of ultrahigh speed full range SD-OCT setup: SLD – superluminescent diode, OC – optical circulator, FC – 50 : 50 fiber coupler, PC – polarization controller, NDF – neutral density filter, DC – dispersion compensator, L1–L5 – lenses, RM – reference mirror, laser-pilot laser for beam guiding, DG – diffraction grating, CCD – line-scan camera, COMP – computer. (Source: Image is reproduced from Ref. [61].)

(SLD) with FWHM of 56 nm centered at 1.3 μm. The total output power was 10 mW. This light source yielded a measured axial resolution of 13 μm in air. The light source was coupled into a fiber-based Michelson interferometer, via an optical circulator. A pilot laser was also coupled into the interferometer for beam guiding and aiming. In the reference arm, the light was delivered onto a stationary mirror; and in the sample arm, the light was focused into a sample via an objective lens. The zero-delay line of the system was set at ~0.5 mm above the focus spot of the sample beam. With a 50 mm focal length of the objective lens in the sample arm, the lateral resolution of the system was ~16 μm. The light backscattered from the sample and reflected from the RM were recombined by a 2 × 2 optical fiber coupler and was then routed to a home-built high-speed spectrometer via the optical circulator. The spectrometer consisted of a collimator of 30 mm focal length, a 1200 lines mm^{-1} transmitting grating, an achromatic lens with 100 mm focal length, and a 14-bit, 1024 pixels InGaAs line scan camera. The maximum line scan rate of the camera was ~47 kHz. This spectrometer setup had a designed spectral resolution of 0.141 nm, which gave a measured imaging depth of ~3.0 mm on the each side of the zero-delay line.

To achieve 3D imaging, we used two galvoscanners to raster-scan the focused beam spot across the sample, with one scanner for the x-direction (lateral) scan and another for the y-direction (elevation) scan. For the experiments presented in this study, the camera integrating time was set at 31 μs for imaging, allowing 1 μm for downloading the spectral data from CCD (1024 pixels, A-scan) to the host computer via CameraLink™ and a high-speed frame grabber board (PCI 1428, National Instruments, USA). This configuration determined a line scan rate of ~31 kHz for the camera. The imaging rate was set at 20 frames (B-scan) per second. Each B-scan had 2.5 mm span over the sample, consisting of 1500 A-lines. This represents an oversampling factor of ~10, because the lateral resolution of the system is ~16 μm. In the elevation direction, there were 500 discrete points along ~2.5 mm, that is, 500 B-scans. Hence the data cube of each 3D image (C-scan) was composed of 1024 × 1500 × 500 (z-x-y) voxels, which took ~25 s to acquire. The operations for probe beam scanning, data acquisition, data storage, and handshaking between them were controlled by a custom software package written in C++ language. Note that 500 B-scans for a C-scan represented oversampling in the elevation direction. In practice, however, 200 B-scans would be sufficient to obtain the volumetric images, leading to a temporal resolution of ~10 s for 3D OMAG imaging using the current setup.

10.3.2
First-Generation OMAG

As described in the earlier section, in the first-generation OMAG, the static and moving scatterers were separated by modulating the reference arm with a modulation frequency. The schematic of the experimental setup for the first-generation OMAG is shown in Figure 10.5. The reference arm modulation is done by incorporating a delay line at the reference arm. If we consider the spectral domain

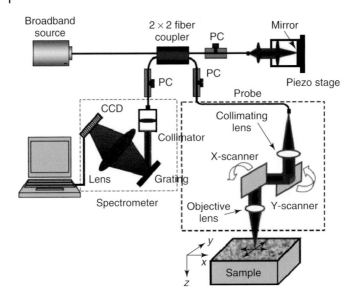

Figure 10.5 Schematic of the earlier version of the OMAG system used to collect the 3D spectral interferogram data cube to perform the 3D angiogram of thick tissue *in vivo*. CCD, charge coupled device, PC, polarization controller. (Source: Image is reproduced from Ref. [60].)

interferogram, which is formed between the light backscattered from the sample and that reflected from the mirror at each lateral (*x*-direction), positions captured by a spectrometer at each wavelength λ can be expressed as a function of two time variables t_1 and t_2 as show below [62]

$$B\left(t_1, t_2\right) = \cos\left(2\pi f_0 t_1 + 2\pi\left(f_M - f_D\right) t_2 + \varphi\right) \tag{10.12}$$

where f_0, f_M, and f_D are the frequency components, respectively and ϕ is a random phase term. In connection with the discussion below, we assume here that f_0 and f_M are two modulation frequency components whereas f_D is the Doppler frequency component. We also assume that there is no correlation between t_1 and t_2 and that when t_1 varies, t_2 is constant and vice versa.

In practice, at each scanning position, the interference spectrum is discretized by N segments, corresponding to the number of pixels in the camera in SD-OCT. For each B-scan, the object is sampled M times in the *x*-direction, which will produce a data matrix with a size of (N,M), as shown in Figure 10.6a.

The analytic function of Eq. (10.12) against t_2 can be constructed through the well-known Hilbert transformation if the Bedrosian theorem holds [63, 64], which states that if the modulation frequency $f_M - f_D$ does not overlap the signal bandwidth caused by the random phase fluctuation term ϕ. Under this condition, the Hilbert transform of Eq. (10.12) is equal to its quadrature representation. Bear in mind that the function $B(t_1, t_2)$ is modulated by the frequency $f_M - f_D$, and $2\pi f_0 t$ is a constant phase term. Therefore, if $f_M - f_D > 0$, the analytic function of

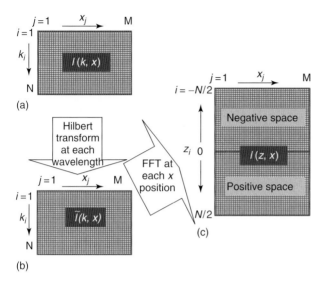

Figure 10.6 Flow chart of signal processing steps in OMAG
(a) Data matrix of single B-frame, (b) data matrix that is
Hilbert transformed at each wavelength, and (c) FFT along
the z-direction at each x-position. (Source: Image is reproduced from Ref. [62].)

Eq. (10.12) can be written as

$$\tilde{H}(t_1, t_2) = \cos\left(2\pi f_0 t_1 + 2\pi\left(f_M - f_D\right) t_2 + \varphi\right) + j\sin\left(2\pi f_0 t_1 + 2\pi\left(f_M - f_D\right) t_2 + \varphi\right) \tag{10.13}$$

where $j = \sqrt{-1}$; whereas if $f_M - f_D < 0$, it is

$$\tilde{H}(t_1, t_2) = \cos\left(2\pi f_0 t_1 + 2\pi\left(f_M - f_D\right) t_2 + \varphi\right) - j\sin\left(2\pi f_0 t_1 + 2\pi\left(f_M - f_D\right) t_2 + \varphi\right) \tag{10.14}$$

Equation (10.14) is clearly the complex conjugate of Eq. (10.13). Now we perform the Fourier transformation against the time variable t_1 (Note that t_2 is now constant). It is obvious that the frequency component f_0 of Eq. (10.13) is placed in the positive space in the entire Fourier plane, while it sits on the negative space for Eq. (10.14), which is shown in Figure 10.6a,b. This is the key element that allows OMAG to image the microvascular flow within tissue.

Consider the case of OMAG. If we assume that the RM mounted on the piezostage moves at a velocity $\vec{v}_{ref}$, with the probe beam proceeding in the B-scan (x-scan) at a velocity of v_x (scalar), and if we further assume that reflecting particles that are detected by OMAG also move, but with its directional velocity projecting onto the probe beam direction being $\vec{v}_s$, then for simplicity, we can state the spectral interferogram in the wavelength, λ, domain as

$$B\left(\frac{1}{\lambda}, x\right) = \cos\left(\frac{4\pi\left(z_s + \left(\vec{v}_{ref} + \vec{v}_s\right)\frac{x}{v_x}\right)}{\lambda} + \phi(x, z, \lambda)\right) \tag{10.15}$$

Note here that we use vector representations for velocities, with the movement toward the incident beam being positive and those opposite being negative. The term z_s is the initial depth position of the reflecting particle (e.g., the red blood cell) at the lateral position x, and $\vec{v}_s$ is the velocity of that reflecting particle, such that the path length difference between sample arm and reference arm is

$$2\left(z_s + \left(\vec{v}_{ref} + \vec{v}_s\right)t_x\right) \tag{10.16}$$

where $t_x = x/v_x$ is the scanning time of the probe beam in the B-scan and the factor of 2 accounts for the round trip of the sampling light scattered from the sample back into the interferometer. The term $\varphi(x, z, \lambda)$ is a random phase function that relates to the phases of the optical heterogeneous sample. The time $t_x = 0$ would be the start of a B-scan. Hence, $B(1/\lambda, x)$ is a sinusoidal oscillation function versus x for each $1/\lambda$ value. It is clear that Eqs. (10.12) and (10.15) are identical if the following substitutions are used

$$f_0 = z_s, \quad t_1 = \frac{2}{\lambda}, \quad f_M = \frac{2\vec{v}_{ref}}{\lambda}, \quad f_D = -\frac{2\vec{v}_s}{\lambda}, \quad t_2 = t_x \tag{10.17}$$

Thus, the values of $\vec{v}_{ref}$ and $\vec{v}_s$ determine whether the analytic function of Eq. (10.15) constructed through the Hilbert transformation is turned into Eq. (10.13) or (10.14). The analytic function is sequentially constructed through the Hilbert transformation to the B-scan along the x-axis at each $1/\lambda$. During the operation, the factor $4\pi z_s/\lambda$ is simply a constant phase since it does not vary with x (Figure 10.6c).

If $\vec{v}_s = 0$, positive velocities (v_{ref}) would modulate the signal with positive frequencies in the x-space and negative v_{ref} with negative frequencies. The Hilbert transformation converts the information of the modulated signal versus x into a complex number $\tilde{H}(1/\lambda, x)$, but now, any subsequent fast Fourier transform (FFT) toward $2/\lambda$, $FFT\{\tilde{H}(1/\lambda, x)\}|_{2/\lambda}$, of the Hilbert-encoded information would map positive frequency components into the positive-frequency space and negative frequency components into the negative-frequency space of the FFT result, allowing the full-range frequency space to be utilized for imaging [27]. This is in contrast to simply taking $FFT\{B(1/\lambda, x)\}|_{2/\lambda}$, which always maps both positive and negative frequencies into both the positive- and negative-frequency spaces of the transform, resulting in only half of the space being useful for imaging.

Now, consider the effect of a moving particle, $v_s \neq 0$. The particle movement will modify the modulation frequency through the velocity mixing, $\vec{v}_{ref} + \vec{v}_s$, similar to the frequency mixing in the signal processing discipline. An opposite movement of the particle, for example, blood cells, relative to the movement of the RM results in a decrease in the difference in photon path length between sample and reference arm and decreases the effective frequency of the modulation. If the value of v_s is sufficiently large, the value $\vec{v}_{ref} + \vec{v}_s$ will change its sign. Consequently, after the operations of Hilbert transform and FT, the corresponding signal due to the particle movement will map into the frequency space opposite to that with $v_s = 0$. However, any small particle movement that is not strong enough to change the sign of the value of $\vec{v}_{ref} + \vec{v}_s$ will still map to the frequency space when $v_s = 0$. Hence, the signals from the perfused blood cells and the bulk static tissue can be separated in the frequency space of the FT, with the background noise due to small tissue movements rejected in the space that represents the image of blood perfusion.

10.3.2.1 *In Vivo* Experimental Demonstration of OMAG

Figure 10.7 shows an example that was obtained through the OMAG method by imaging a mouse brain cortex with the skull left intact. Figure 10.7b shows the image obtained from the raw spectral B-scan interferograms (Figure 10.7a). Its entire Fourier space is separated into two equal regions. The bottom region is the positive-frequency space containing the normal OCT cross-sectional, static image, within which the histologically important layers such as cranium and cortex

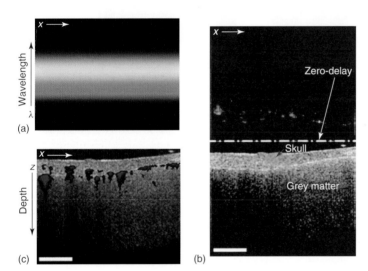

Figure 10.7 A cross section (slice) of an adult mouse brain with the skull intact was imaged with OMAG *in vivo*. (a) The data set representing the slice contains 2D real-valued spectral interferogram in $x - \lambda$. (b) The imaging result obtained from (a) by OMAG. It is separated by the zero-delay line into two equal spaces. The normal OCT image is located in the bottom region (2.2 by 1.7 mm) showing microstructures. The signals from the moving blood cells are located in the upper region (also 2.2 by 1.7 mm). (c) Folded and fused final OMAG image (2.2 by 1.7 mm) of the slice showing the location of moving blood (red color) within the cortex and meninges where there are more blood vessels than in the skull bone. The scale bar in (b) and (c) represents 500 µm [30]. (Source: Images are reproduced from Ref. [23].)

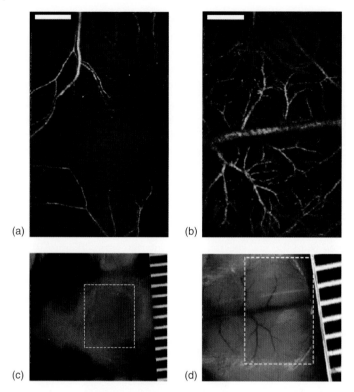

(a)   (b)

(c)   (d)

Figure 10.8 The head of an adult mouse with the skin and skull intact was imaged with OMAG *in vivo*. (a,b) The projection views of blood perfusion from within the skin and the brain cortex, respectively. (c) Photograph taken right after the experiments with skin and skull intact. (d) Photograph showing blood vessels over the cortex after the skin and skull of the same mouse were carefully removed. The scale bar indicates 1.0 mm [32]. (Source: Image is reproduced from Ref. [61].)

may be clearly demarcated. On the other hand, the moving signals from all blood vessels, including capillaries, can be precisely localized in the negative space, that is, the perfusion image (upper region, Figure 10.7b) in OMAG. As the positive and negative spaces are exactly mirrored, they can be folded to fuse into a single image to localize the blood vessels within the tissue with high precision (Figure 10.7c).

Figure 10.8a shows the result of OMAG method of mapping of blood flows within the skin of the mouse, while the cerebrovascular blood perfusion is given in Figure 10.8b. For comparison, the photograph of the head right after the OMAG imaging and the photograph of the brain cortex after removal of the skin and skull bone are shown in Figure 10.8c,d, respectively. From Figure 10.8c, seeing the blood vessels through the skin is almost impossible. Comparing Figure 10.8b,d, excellent agreement on the major vascular network over the brain cortex is achieved. Furthermore, the smaller blood vessels not observed in Figure 10.8d can be seen in the OMAG images, indicating the capability of OMAG to delineate the capillary-level vessels.

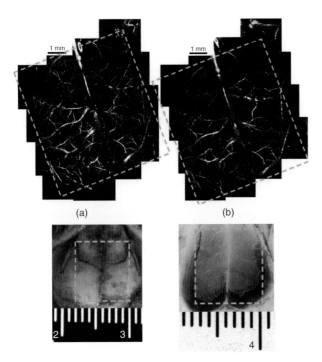

Figure 10.9 The entire cerebrovascular flow over the cortex of an adult mouse with the skull intact was imaged with OMAG *in vivo*. (a,b) The projection views of blood perfusion before and after the right carotid artery was blocked. (c) Photograph of the skull with the skin folded aside, taken right after the experiments. (d) Photograph showing blood vessels over the cortex after the skull and the meninges of the same mouse were carefully removed. (Source: Images are reproduced from Ref. [23].)

Figure 10.9 shows another OMAG imaging result obtained from an ischemic thrombotic stroke experiment on a mouse model. Figure 10.9a shows the blood flow in the cerebral cortex of a mouse with the skull intact. Occlusion of one carotid artery does not cause cerebral infarction or neurological deficits in the mouse. Figure 10.9b is taken from the same animal while the right carotid artery was blocked for 5 min. It is apparent that the blood flow in the cortex, rather than in the right hemisphere only, is reduced as compared to Figure 10.9a. This is consistent with the well-known collateral circulation between brain hemispheres, leading to a total reduction in cortical blood volume due to the occlusion of one common carotid artery. The capacity of OMAG to achieve such high-resolution imaging of the cerebral cortex – within minutes and without the need for dye injections, contrast agents, or surgical craniotomy, – makes it an extremely valuable tool for studying the hemodynamics of the brain.

10.3.2.2 Directional Flow Imaging in OMAG

The base model of first-generation OMAG is capable of resolving 3D distribution of dynamic blood perfusion at the capillary level within microcirculatory beds *in vivo*.

However, this base method does not give the capability to image the directional flow, which seriously limits the applications for OMAG, because the blood flow information regarding its direction is often important in a number of investigations, for example, in the study of complex flow dynamics in the microfluidic mixers and in the investigation of blood flow involvement in cerebrovascular diseases such as ischemia, hemorrhage, vascular dementia, traumatic brain injury (TBI), and seizure disorders. To overcome this drawback, Wang [65] proposed a method that forces the RM to move back and forth. However, this would significantly increase imaging complexity. For example, the OMAG imaging speed is reduced by half and the computational load on OMAG is doubled to obtain meaningful blood flow images, because OMAG needs to acquire two three-dimensional volumetric spectrogram data sets. It was then quickly realized that a digital modulation frequency (DMF) method can be used to manipulate the modulated interferograms so that the directional flow information can be obtained from one 3D volumetric spectrogram data set [66], without resorting to the hardware approach in [65].

Following the OMAG method described in the earlier section, assume the frequency modulation in the interferograms is f_M, which is a constant frequency. Here f_M can be provided by a number of approaches, for example, moving the RM at a constant velocity in one direction [23, 60, 65] or offsetting the sample beam at the scanner that gives the B-scan image [67]. For simplicity, the real function of a spectral interferogram can be expressed by Eq. (10.12). If we construct the analytic function of Eq. (10.12) by performing the Hilbert transform in terms of t_1 (note that t_2 is constant), then this analytic function is always Eq. (10.13), because f_0 is always >0, which is guaranteed by placing the sample surface below the zero-delay line. In this case, if we digitally multiply Eq. (10.13) with a complex function $\exp(-j4\pi f_M t_2)$ and then take the real part of the results, we can simply transfer Eq. (10.12) into

$$B'(t_1, t_2) = \cos\left(2\pi f_0 t_1 - 2\pi \left(f_M + f_D\right) t_2 + \varphi\right) \tag{10.18}$$

It is feasible because f_M is known *a priori*. Now, we can construct the analytic function of Eq. (10.18) by considering t_2 as a variable, while t_1 to be constant. Then, if $f_M + f_D < 0$, the analytic function is

$$\tilde{H}(t_1, t_2) = \cos\left(2\pi f_0 t_1 - 2\pi (f_M + f_D) t_2 + \varphi\right) + j\sin\left(2\pi f_0 t_1 \right.$$
$$\left. - 2\pi (f_M + f_D) t_2 + \varphi\right) \tag{10.19}$$

but if $f_M + f_D > 0$, the analytic function becomes

$$\tilde{H}(t_1, t_2) = \cos\left(2\pi f_0 t_1 - 2\pi (f_M + f_D) t_2 + \varphi\right) - j\sin\left(2\pi f_0 t_1 \right.$$
$$\left. - 2\pi (f_M + f_D) t_2 + \varphi\right) \tag{10.20}$$

Consequently, Eqs. (10.18–10.20) simulate the exact situation of the mirror moving in a direction opposite to that as described in Section 10.3.1. This derivation of the analytic function provides a solid mathematical basis for obtaining information on the directions of blood flow from only one 3D spectrogram data set captured by OMAG. As a result, the directional blood flow imaging can be obtained by the following approach: the analysis detailed in the previous section is used to give one

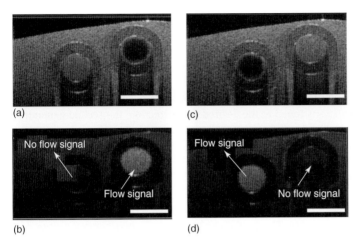

Figure 10.10 (a,b) The OMAG structural and flow images calculated from the spectrograms captured when $f_M = 400$ Hz. (c,d) Corresponding results computed from the digital frequency modulation (DFM) approach applied to the same data set. Scale bar = 500 μm. (Source: Images are reproduced from Ref. [66].)

image of blood flow direction when the RM moves toward the incident beam, and the analysis described here is used to give an image of blood flow in the opposite direction, as if the mirror moved away from the incident beam.

Figure 10.10 shows the imaging results obtained through the OMAG method and DMF approach. Two microtubes, within which scattering particles are flowing with flow directions against each other, were buried under a scattering phantom. Figure 10.10a,b are the microstructure and flow images respectively, which were directly obtained from the OMAG algorithm. Applying the DMF approach, different direction flow and microstructure images are present in Figure 10.10c,d. It is shown that the directional flow images can be successfully achieved by OMAG and DMF algorithms.

10.3.3
Second-Generation OMAG

In the first-generation OMAG, as explained in the earlier section, the moving and static scatters were separated by introducing a carrier frequency, and this carrier frequency is generated by adding a phase delay to each A-scan using a moving reference arm or an off-pivot scanning beam. However, these techniques rely on precise synchronization of reference arm modulation and B-scan acquisition, which require expensive or cumbersome modulators, and are unable to detect bidirectional flow in a single B-scan. In order to overcome this drawback, a modified Hilbert transform without the use of spatial frequency modulation is introduced in the OMAG. No frequency modulations are required, and a new

OMAG signal-processing algorithm based on a modified Hilbert transform is applied to the spatial frequency content across a single B-scan to obtain volumetric perfusion map with directional information. The new second-generation OMAG is applicable for both spectrometer-based OCT and SS-OCT systems, provided they have comparable B-scan acquisition rates. Unlike previously described techniques [23, 66], which require two separate B-scans to detect positive and negative flow, each with modulations tuned to the desired flow direction, the second-generation OMAG is able to resolve bidirectional flow in a single B-scan pass across the sample.

10.3.3.1   Theoretical Overview

If we consider the OMAG imaging of blood flow within the microcirculation tissue beds, under a B-scan condition, the static scatterers and the moving scatterers are illustrated in Figure 10.11a. The depth-encoded spectral interferogram captured by the linear detector is a real function, $B(z, t)$ and can be written as

$$B(z, t) = A(z) \cos(k_0 z) \tag{10.21}$$

where $A(z)$ is the reflective coefficient of the scatterer, k_0 is the wave vector of the detected light, and z relates to the detecting depth. In order to simplify the problem, we do not consider the random phase arising from the refractive index float and assume that the reflective coefficient $A(z)$ of the scatter is a constant along the B-scan direction; t is the B-scan time corresponding to the different lateral position.

According to Eq. (10.21), if we consider the nonmoving scatterers at a depth z, as shown in Figure 10.11a,b, the signal $B(z, t)$ does not vary with the B-scan time, t. So the corresponding signal can be viewed as a rectangular function, that is, $\mathrm{rect}\,(t/\tau_0) = F\,(t - \tau_0/2) - F\,(t + \tau_0/2)$, as shown in Figure 10.12a. On the other, for the moving scatterer, the signal is a rectangular enveloped cosine signal, that is, $\mathrm{rect}\,(t/\tau_0)_{\cos} = \cos\,(2\pi u_0 t)\,F\,(t - \tau_0/2) - F\,(t + \tau_0/2)$, which is illustrated

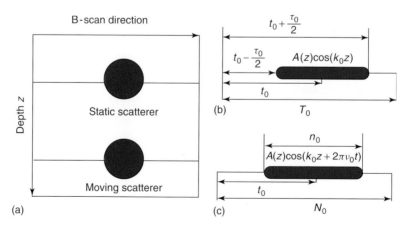

(a)   (b)   (c)

Figure 10.11   (a–c) Schematic of moving and nonmoving scattering structure under B-scan condition in SD-OCT.

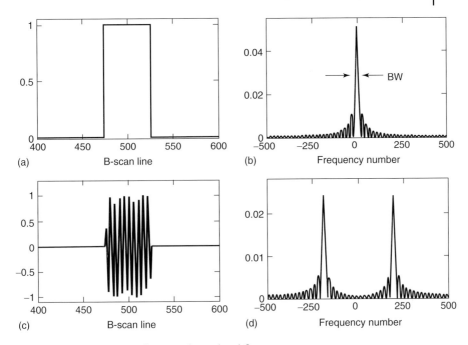

Figure 10.12 Comparison of structural signal and flow signal with N_0 and $N_0 = 1000$. (a) The structural signal, (b) the absolute FFT of the structural signal, (c) the flow signal, and (d) the absolute FFT of the flow signal.

in Figure 10.12c, where u_0 is the modulation frequency generated by the flow speed.

10.3.3.1.1 Frequency Domain Representation of Static Scatterer

If we consider the above assumption, according to Figure 10.11b,c, the total time required for a single B-scan is T_0, which corresponds to a total of N_0 A-lines in a B-scan frame. The scanning time for the scatterer (moving or static), τ_0, depends on the number of A-lines in the B-frame, n_0, to image the structure, which corresponds to the physical dimension of the imaged structure within a B-scan frame, and t_0 is the B-scan time required at the center of the scattering structure as illustrated in Figure 10.11c. According to the above parameters, the FT $R(z, u)$ of the lateral dimension (i.e., B-scan at time t) can be shown as

$$R(z, u) = \frac{A(z) \cos\left(k_0 z\right)}{T_0} \int_{t_0 - \frac{\tau_0}{2}}^{t_0 - \frac{\tau_0}{2}} e^{-i2\pi ut} \, dt \qquad (10.22)$$

where u is the FT frequency of B-scan at time t. This corresponds to the spatial frequency along the B-scan direction. After simplification, the result of Eq. (10.22) can be presented as

$$R(z, u) = A(z) \cos\left(k_0 z\right) \frac{\sin\left(\pi u\tau_0\right)}{\pi u T_0} e^{-i2\pi ut_0} \qquad (10.23)$$

If we consider the OMAG spectral detection section, the acquisition time of the linear detector is $1/f_0$ (sampling rate), that is, the time required to acquire each A-scan in a B-scan frame. Then the total acquisition time T_0 required for one B-scan can be expressed as: $T_0 = N_0/f_0$. The B-scan time for the scattering structure is $\tau_0 = n_0/f_0$. In frequency domain, the total frequency is f_0 and the frequency step is f_0/N_0. The variable frequency u can be expressed as $u = nf_0/N_0$, where n is the frequency number. Since the spectral signal detected by the camera is a real signal and therefore its FT is Hermitian, it has both positive and negative frequency components. Then Eq. (10.22) can be modified and represented as

$$R_{\pm}(z, n) = A(z) \cos\left(k_0 z\right) \frac{n_0}{N_0} \sin c \left(\frac{n_0 n}{N_0}\right) e^{-i2\pi n t_0 \frac{f_0}{N_0}} \tag{10.24}$$

where $\pm$ denotes the positive and negative frequencies. In Eq. (10.24), the range of the nonmoving scatterer, that is, n_0/N_0 determines the oscillation frequency and the amplitude of $\sin c$ function. The depth-encoded information is retained in $\cos\left(k_0 z\right)$, which is independent of the FT along the B-scan direction. Owing to the Hermitian symmetry of the FT, the frequency ranges from $-f_0/2$ to $f_0/2$; accordingly, the frequency number n ranges from $-N_0/2$ to $N_0/2$, with the max value of the $\sin c$ function $\sin c(x)$ centered at $n = 0$. This means that the main signal energy concentrates at the zero frequency. Figure 10.12a shows the absolute frequency signal of the nonmoving structural (static) signal. For example, we set the total B-scan lines N_0 to 1000, and the total B-scan lines of nonmoving scatterer n_0 to 50 (between 475 and 525). The reflectivity of the signal is assumed to unity, that is, $B(z, t) = 1$. The absolute frequency signal $\left|R_{\pm}(z, n)\right|$ is shown in Figure 10.12b; the amplitude of $\left|R_{\pm}(z, n)\right|$ has a maximum value of 0.05 ($n_0/N_0 = 0.05$), which is located at the zeroth frequency position with a frequency span of $\Delta n = 2N_0/n_0$, and the other consequent peaks on the either sides of the zeroth peak have a frequency span of $\Delta n = N_0/n_0$. This is because the biological tissue is often optically heterogeneous in nature, which means the magnitude of the backscattered light and the refractive index are functions of time variable. So the intensity captured by the linear detector will be modulated by the heterogeneous properties of the sample along each B-scan. The spatial frequency components of a static tissue sample, which we call the heterogeneous frequencies, will exhibit as a randomly distributed function around zero frequency with a bandwidth of BW, which is indicated in Figure 10.12b. This spatial frequency bandwidth depends on the heterogeneity of the static scatterers and is called *heterogeneous frequency*.

10.3.3.1.2 Frequency Domain Representation of Moving Scatterers

For the moving scatterers under the B-scan condition, the corresponding schematic is shown in Figure 10.11c. The depth-encoded real spectral interference signal recorded by the SD-OCT system can be written as

$$B(z, t) = A(z) \cos\left(k_0 z + 2\pi u t\right) \tag{10.25}$$

where t is the B-scan time corresponding to the lateral position across B-scan direction, u is the modulation frequency generated by the flow speed, where

$u = 2u_0 \cos\theta_d/\lambda$ and u_0 is the absolute velocity of moving scatterers, and λ is the wavelength of detected light. Here, the flow speed u can be viewed as a carrier frequency, and the flow associated with the moving scatterers include the negative flow (scatterers moving away from the sample beam) and the positive flow (scatterers moving forward to the sample beam). Then the FT of the spectral signal $B(z,t)$ can be expressed as

$$H(z,u) = \frac{A(z)}{T_0} \int_{t_0-\frac{\tau_0}{2}}^{t_0+\frac{\tau_0}{2}} \cos\left(k_0 z + 2\pi u t\right) e^{-i2\pi u_0 t} dt$$

$$= \frac{A(z)e^{ik_0 z}}{2T_0} \int_{t_0-\frac{\tau_0}{2}}^{t_0+\frac{\tau_0}{2}} e^{-i2\pi(u-u_0)t} dt + \frac{A(z)e^{-ik_0 z}}{2T_0} \int_{t_0-\frac{\tau_0}{2}}^{t_0+\frac{\tau_0}{2}} e^{-i2\pi(u+u_0)t} dt$$

(10.26)

This equation includes positive and negative frequency components

$$H(z,u) = H_+(z,u) + H_-(z,u) \tag{10.27}$$

where $H_+(z,u)$ is the positive frequency and $H_-(z,u)$ is the negative frequency. Then Eq. (10.26) can be split up as

$$H_+(z,u) = \frac{A(z)e^{ik_0 z}}{2T_0} \frac{\sin[\pi\tau_0(u-u_0)]}{\pi(u-u_0)} e^{-i2\pi(u-u_0)t_0} \tag{10.28}$$

$$H_-(z,u) = \frac{A(z)e^{-ik_0 z}}{2T_0} \frac{\sin[\pi\tau_0(u+u_0)]}{\pi(u+u_0)} e^{-i2\pi(u+u_0)t_0} \tag{10.29}$$

According to the assumption described in Section 10.2.1, Eq. (10.8) can also be expressed as

$$H_+(z,n) = A(z)e^{ik_0 z} \frac{n_0}{2N_0} \operatorname{sinc}\left(\frac{n_0}{N_0}\left(n - \frac{u_0 N_0}{f_0}\right)\right) e^{-i2\pi\left(\frac{n f_0}{N_0} - u_0\right)t_0} \tag{10.30}$$

$$H_-(z,n) = A(z)e^{-ik_0 z} \frac{n_0}{2N_0} \operatorname{sinc}\left(\frac{n_0}{N_0}\left(n + \frac{u_0 N_0}{f_0}\right)\right) e^{-i2\pi\left(\frac{n f_0}{N_0} + u_0\right)t_0} \tag{10.31}$$

If we consider Eqs. ((10.28)–(10.31)) with Eqs. (10.23) and (10.24), the nonmoving scatterers are centered at the zeroth frequency (DC) region (heterogeneous frequency) and the moving scatterers are shifted away from the zeroth frequency $n = 0$ to $n = \pm u_0 N_0/f_0$. This shifting distance in the frequency domain can be directly related to the velocity u_0 of the moving scatterers, total B-scan lines, N_0, and the acquisition rate of CCD, f_0. Since the max frequency number is $n_{max} = \pm N_0/2$, the maximum detectable velocity with OMAG is $v_{max} = \pm\lambda f_0/4$, which is the same as that with DOCT. Figure 10.12c,d illustrates a simulated signal for the moving scatterer and the corresponding frequency shift for the signal in the frequency domain, respectively. The two shifted sin c function peaks in Figure 10.12d correspond to Eqs. (10.28) and (10.29). The simulated illustration in Figure 10.12c,d clearly shows how the OMAG separates the moving scatterers from nonmoving scatterers by flow speed modulation.

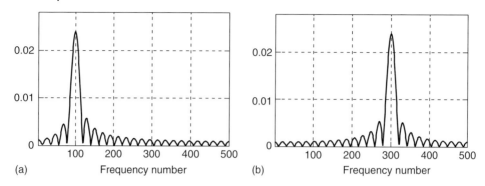

(a)   (b)

Figure 10.13 (a) The flow frequency signal with $v_0 = 2$ mm s^{-1} and shift distance $n = 101$. (b) The flow frequency signal with $v_0 = 6$ mm s^{-1} and the shift distance $n = 302$.

10.3.3.1.3 Parameters That Influence the Flow Signal Detection

Flow Velocity The frequency shift induced by the flow modulation can directly relate to the flow velocity of the moving scatterers, which is illustrated in Figure 10.13a,b. For example, we consider a B-scan condition at $\lambda = 840$ nm, with a sampling frequency $f_0 = 47$ kHz and sampling density of, $N_0 = 1000$ (A-lines in a B-scan) for a moving scatterer that covers A-lines of $n_0 = 50$. Figure 10.13a shows the signal in positive-frequency space, where the flow velocity $v_0 = 2$ mm s^{-1} by assuming that the Doppler angle, $\theta_d = 0$. Based on Eqs. (10.29) and (10.30), the shifting frequency number can be calculated by $n = \pm 2v_0 N_0 / \lambda f_0 = 101$, which is shown in Figure 10.13a. In case of velocity $v_0 = 6$ mm s^{-1}, the shifting frequency number is $n = 302$, which is shown in Figure 10.13b. As the flow speed increases, the frequency shift also increases, and at low flow speed, it is hard to separate moving scatterers from the static scatterer.

Size of the Moving Scatterer For a specific scan density, for example, $N_0 = 1000$, the size of the moving scatterer also influences the detected flow signal. For example,

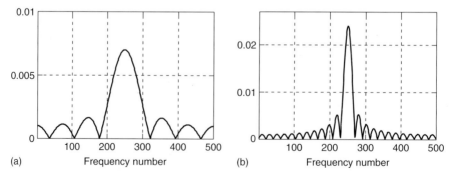

(a)   (b)

Figure 10.14 (a) The flow frequency signal with the flow size $n_0 = 15$ and (b) the flow frequency signal with the flow size $n_0 = 50$.

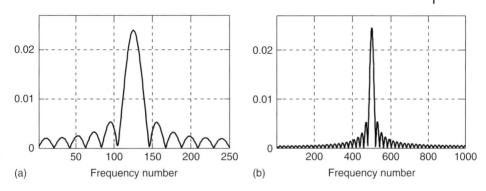

Figure 10.15 (a) The flow frequency signal with the total B-scan line $N_0 = 500$ and (b) the flow frequency signal with the total B-scan line $N_0 = 2000$.

we consider a moving scatterer with a flow size (oscillation cycle) of $T = N_0/n_0$ with a span of $2N_0/n_0$. Figure 10.14a,b shows the flow signals with a size of $n_0 = 15$ and $n_0 = 50$, respectively, for a flow velocity of $v_0 = 2.5$ mm s^{-1}, the imaging parameters are the same as mentioned above. It is obvious that the span of the first peak in Figure 10.14a is broader than that of the first peak in Figure 10.14b.

Sampling Line Density The influence of scan density N_0 along the lateral scan direction (B-scan density) on the flow signal is shown in Figure 10.15. If we consider a B-scan with a sampling rate of $f_0 = 47$ kHz and a moving scatterer with velocity $v_0 = 2.5$ mm s^{-1} and size $n_0/N_0 = 0.025$, the flow signal detected with scan densities $N_0 = 500$ and $N_0 = 2000$ are shown in Figure 10.15a,b, respectively. For a moving scatterer, high B-scan density shifts the flow signal away from the zero frequency regions more than low B-scan density does. Thus, by increasing the B-scan density, it is possible to effectively separate flow signal from structural signal, that is, the heterogeneous frequency noise should be reduced. On the other hand, the imaging speed would be sacrificed.

10.3.3.1.4 Flow Extraction in OMAG

A schematic of the OMAG signal processing flow chart is illustrated in Figure 10.16. Figure 10.16a shows a B-scan frame, which includes the static and moving scatterers. According to Eqs. (10.21) and (10.25), if we consider the nonmoving scatterers at a depth z, the signal $B(z, t)$ does not vary with the B-scan time t. Therefore, the corresponding signal can be viewed as a rectangular function. On the contrary, for the moving scatterers, the signal under B-scan condition is a rectangular envelope cosine signal, which is shown in Figure 10.16a. By applying a Fourier transformation along the B-scan direction, the spatial frequency components of a static tissue sample, which we call the heterogeneous frequencies, will exhibit as a randomly distributed function around zero frequency with a bandwidth of BW, which is indicated in Figure 10.16b. On the other hand, the moving scatterers produce a frequency shift, which is caused by the Doppler effect of the moving particles,

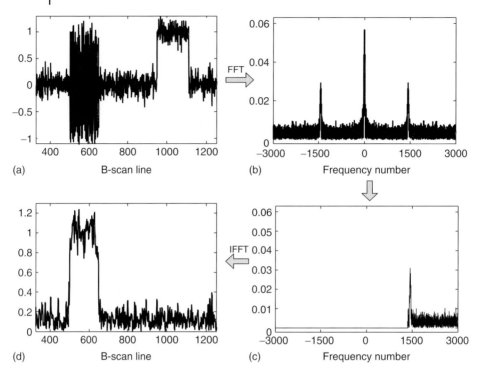

Figure 10.16 The flow chart of signal processing steps in OMAG. (a) The flow signal and structural signal, (b) the flow signal and structural signal in the frequency domain, (c) filtering of the structural signal and negative frequency of the flow signal, and (d) the flow signal inverting from the frequency domain.

and shifts it away from the heterogeneous frequencies due to static scatterers. This is illustrated in Figure 10.13b. Next, for extracting the flow information, the structural signal is filtered out in the frequency domain. This was accomplished by introducing the modified Hilbert transform algorithm. To achieve this, one of the conjugate terms was windowed out and the heterogeneous frequency was centered at the zeroth frequency region (DC) using a frequency-shifted Heaviside function. The cutoff frequency shift of the Heaviside function depends on the heterogeneity of the static scatterers. Then, an inverse FT is applied; the inverse FT has positive and negative frequency. After inverse transforming from frequency domain, and then applying the conventional spectral FT along the depth direction, the strength of the flow signal will be retrieved. This is illustrated in Figure 10.16c,d. For the flow signal, the inverse FT has positive and negative frequency, which retrieves the directional flow information and can be expressed as

$$iFFT\left(H_+\left(z,n\right)\right) = \frac{A(z)e^{i\left(k_0 z + 2\pi u_0 t\right)}}{2} \tag{10.32}$$

$$iFFT\left(H_-\left(z,n\right)\right) = \frac{A(z)e^{-i\left(k_0 z + 2\pi u_0 t\right)}}{2} \tag{10.33}$$

Figure 10.16d shows the inverse Fourier transformed signal. The absolute amplitude of the flow signal obtained by taking the FT can be expressed as

$$A(z) = 2\left|I\,\text{fft}[H\left(z,n\right)]\right| \tag{10.34}$$

From Eq. (10.34), it is evident that the imaging contrast is a result that represents the optical reflectance scattered from the flow particles and that it does not relate to the flow velocity. The amplitude of the flow signal $A(z)$ can be used to reconstruct the flow, just like that in the conventional OCT.

10.3.3.1.5 Directional Flow Imaging

Based on the above signal processing, the real flow signal is transformed to an analytical signal by Hilbert transform, which enables the bidirectional flow configuration, that is, the positive flow and the negative flow to be separated in different imaging plane. Figure 10.17 shows the Hilbert-transformed analytical flow signal, which is obtained by filtering out the negative frequency components and the structural signals and then taking the inverse FT as shown below [62]

$$iFFT[H\left(z,n\right)] = \frac{A(z)e^{ik_0 z}}{2}\left(\cos\left(2\pi\,|u_0|\,t\right) \pm i\sin\left(2\pi\,|u_0|\,t\right)\right) \tag{10.35}$$

where u_0 is the modulation frequency, which relates to the flow direction. If $u_0 > 0$, the Fourier transformation along the depth direction resolves the positive flow

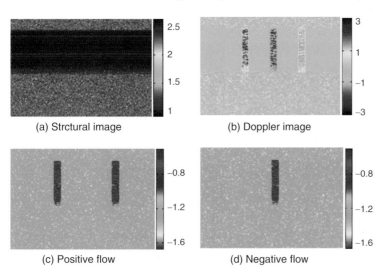

(a) Strctural image

(b) Doppler image

(c) Positive flow

(d) Negative flow

Figure 10.17 Bidirectional image with OMAG: (a) the structure image; (b) the Doppler image, left $v_0 = 7.5$ mm s^{-1} (red color), middle $v_1 = -7.5$ mm s^{-1} (blue color), right $v_2 = 4.5$ mm s^{-1} (orange color); (c) the positive flow image; and (d) the negative flow image.

components in the positive image plane, and if $u_0 < 0$, it resolves the negative flow components in the negative imaging plane.

10.3.3.1.6 Motion Compensation in OMAG

The sample movement during *in vivo* imaging conditions is an inevitable artifact in OMAG and which is particularly very dominant for imaging of the human eye or skin. The relative sample motion represents as a Doppler shift in the light frequency between the light it emits and that it receives. This shift is imparted when the light strikes an object that is moving relative to the probe. For the OMAG system, the Doppler frequency due to the sample motion is depicted as an additional modulation frequency, f_O, in the interferogram. Therefore, the decisive frequency mixing in the interferogram, as outlined in the previous section, will now become $f_M - f_D + f_O$, which determines whether the Hilbert transform of Eq. (10.18) is turned into Eq. (10.19) or (10.20). In addition, the sample movement is directional when the OMAG system sees it and it is not predictable. As such, if f_O is larger than f_M, the structural signals will appear in the flow image plane, giving severe artifacts on the blood flow measurement. As an example to illustrate the effect of subject motion on the OMAG results, Figure 10.18 shows a typical *in vivo* B-scan of the posterior part of the human eye from a volunteer. Figure 10.18a is the conventional OCT image in which the important physiological layers, such as the retina and choroids, can be delineated. Figure 10.18b is the corresponding OMAG flow image in which it can be seen that although the blood flow signals from retinal and choroidal layers are evident, the subject movement deteriorates the blood flow image, particularly in the right part of the image. Further analysis from Figure 10.18b implies that the motion is not uniform, even during one single

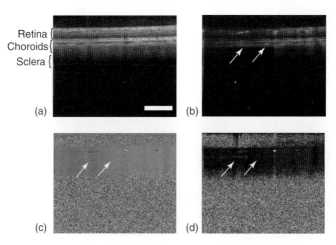

Figure 10.18 Typical *in vivo* B-scan of posterior part of the human eye. (a) Conventional OCT/OMAG structural image, where the retina and choroidal layers are demarcated, and the corresponding (b) OMAG flow image, (c) PRDOCT image with gray levels coded from $-\pi$ (black) to π (white), and (d) power Doppler OCT image. Scale bar = 500 μm. (Source: Images are reproduced from Ref. [67].)

B-scan (within 50 ms). This nonuniform subject movement can also be seen in the PRDOCT image as shown in Figure 10.18c,d.

A casual inspection of Figure 10.18 shows that the blood flow imaging is better delivered by OMAG than that by PRDOCT, because the blood flow signals as seen in the choroidal layer in Figure 10.18b are not seen in PRDOCT images (Figure 10.18c,d), as illustrated by the arrows. However, the subject movement artifacts are still present. Thus, for *in vivo* OMAG imaging of the human eye, a solution to the bulk motion artifacts is required so that the quality of OMAG blood flow image is improved. Because OMAG imaging has its origin in FDOCT, the OCT signals can be directly calculated from the captured interferograms for sequential A-scans using conventional FDOCT algorithms. It is known that the OCT signal so computed is a complex function, $\tilde{B}_{OCT}(t, z)$, which can be written as

$$\tilde{B}_{OCT}(t, z) = A(t, z) \exp[i\phi(t, z)] \tag{10.36}$$

where $A(t, z)$ and $\phi(t, z)$ are the amplitude and phase of $\tilde{B}_{OCT}(t, z)$, respectively. t is the time when the probe beam proceeds in the B-scan, and z represents the coordinate along the imaging depth. In our OMAG system, the phase term $\phi(t, z)$ can be expressed by the following equation:

$$\phi(t, z) = \phi_P(t, z) + \phi_B(t, z) + \phi_M(t, z) \tag{10.37}$$

where $\phi_P(t, z)$ is the phase term caused by the moving red blood cells, $\phi_B(t, z)$ is the phase term caused by the subject movement, and $\phi_M(t, z)$ is the phase term caused by the modulation frequency, f_M. Following PRDOCT [49, 50], the phase differences between the ith and $(i - 1)$th A-lines can be written as

$$\phi^i(t, z) = \Delta\phi_P^i(t, z) + \Delta\phi_B^i(t, z) + \Delta\phi_M^i(t, z) \tag{10.38}$$

where $\Delta\phi_P^i(t, z)$ and $\Delta\phi_B^i(t, z)$ are the phase changes caused by the moving particle and the subject movement between the ith and $(i - 1)$th A-lines, respectively. Because in OMAG system, the introduced modulation frequency, f_M, is constant during imaging, $\Delta\phi_M^i(t, z)$ is a constant value that is known *a priori*, that is

$$\Delta\phi_M^i(t, z) = 2\pi f_M T \tag{10.39}$$

where T is the time interval between adjacent A-lines. This phase term can be directly subtracted from Eq. (10.38). Thus, the phase term directly related to the movement, $\Delta\phi_m^i(t, z)$ is

$$\Delta\phi_m^i(t, z) = \Delta\phi_P^i(t, z) + \Delta\phi_B^i(t, z) \tag{10.40}$$

In Eq. (10.40), the variable t is the timing of the probe beam proceeding in a B-scan, which corresponds to the position of the probe beam, x. Thus Eq. (10.8) can be replaced by

$$\Delta\phi_m^i(x, z) = \Delta\phi_P^i(x, z) + \Delta\phi_B^i(x, z) \tag{10.41}$$

Because the OMAG system used in this study has an imaging speed of 20 000 A-scans per second, it is reasonable to assume that the subject is static within a single A-scan. Under this condition, Eq. (10.41) represents the bulk motion of subject between adjacent A-scans, plus the phase changes due to the blood flow, if presented. Usually, within a single B-scan, the regions occupied by the blood vessels are much smaller than the areas occupied by the surrounding tissue. Thus, the phase change between the ith and $(i - 1)$th A-scans caused by the bulk motion could be approximated by averaging all the phase differences along the A-scan

$$D f_m^i(x) = \frac{1}{z} \sum_z f_m^i(x, z) dz \tag{10.42}$$

to minimize the errors brought by the system noise and flow signals [13, 31]. Here $\Delta \phi_m^i(x)$ is the bulk motion corresponding to the phase difference between ith and $(i - 1)$th A-scans. Therefore, with reference to the first A-scan in the B-scan, the phases at the ith A-line caused by the bulk subject motion, $\phi_m^i(x)$, can be obtained by a recursive function

$$\phi_m^1(0) = 0, \phi_m^i(x) = \phi_m^{i-1}(x) + \Delta \phi_m^i(x), i = 2, 3, \ldots, N \tag{10.43}$$

where N is the number of A-scans that composes the B-scan. Thus far, the phase changes along the B-scan due to the bulk tissue motion, $\phi_B^i(x, z)$, have been computed. Subtracting Eq. (10.43) from Eq. (10.37) and then inserting into Eq. (10.36), we have

$$\tilde{B}'_{OCT}(x, z) = A(x, z) \exp[i(\phi_P(x, z) + \phi_M(x, z))] \tag{10.44}$$

where the frequency modulation term due to the bulk tissue motion is eliminated. Subsequently, the spectral interferograms without the tissue motion effect can be obtained via an inverse FFT to Eq. (10.44)

$$b(x, \lambda) = \text{FFT}^{-1} \left[\tilde{B}'(x, z) \right] \tag{10.45}$$

Finally, the conventional OMAG algorithm as detailed in the previous section is applied to Eq. (10.45) to obtain the OMAG flow image that would be ideally free of motion artifacts. In Eq. (10.42), the phase due to the bulk tissue motion is estimated by the averaged value of phase changes along the A-scan. However, the phases are random for the OCT signals that fall below the system noise floor. This will have a dramatic effect on the estimation of bulk tissue motion. To reduce this effect, we used the OCT structural image to segment the regions of interest, $R(x, z)$, within which the OCT signals are 15 dB above the system noise level. Only the phases within the region of interest are calculated. Below, we detail the steps to perform the segmentation to find $R(x, z)$.

First, the SD-OCT structural image was used to segment the regions of interest that represent retina and choroids. Two boundaries were determined. One corresponded to the vitreoretinal interface, that is, anterior boundary, and the other to the deepest penetration points, posterior boundary. The anterior boundary was obtained by using an algorithm that is similar to that described by Mujat *et al.* [68]. First, we used a Gaussian filter with a standard deviation of 4×4 pixels to blur the cross-sectional image (B-scan) obtained previously. Then the edge of the image was obtained by calculating the gradient of the blurred structural image. It was then converted to a binary image by setting a threshold. The first nonzero points of the binary image, represented by a curve, were detected, and the speckle noises were eliminated. The anterior boundary was then obtained by fitting and smoothing this curve.

The posterior boundary was obtained by setting a threshold to the blurred retina structural image, which was equal to the noise floor of the image obtained. The intensity was treated as the signal if it was larger than the threshold and was set to unity; on the other hand, it was treated as noise if it was smaller than the threshold and was set to zero. Using this method, the structure image was converted to a binary image. The posterior boundary was obtained by the last nonzero points after the isolated speckle noises were eliminated. The final posterior boundary was then obtained by a fitting and smoothing procedure. Finally, the region of region $R(x,z)$ was obtained by bounding the anterior and posterior boundaries as described above. The phase estimation in Eq. (10.42) is therefore performed within this region of interest

$$\Delta\phi^i_m(x) \approx \frac{1}{z} \int \Delta\phi^i_m(x,z)dz \,|z \in R(x,z) \tag{10.46}$$

To further improve the accuracy of the phase estimation, the phases in Eq. (10.46) are only calculated for the OCT signals that are stronger than a preset threshold, which is 15 dB above the system noise floor. Figure 10.19 illustrates the flow chart

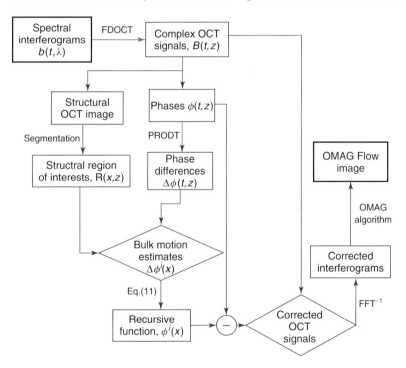

Figure 10.19 Flow chart detailing the steps to computationally compensate the bulk tissue motion artifacts in OMAG imaging of blood perfusion in retina and choroids. (Source: Image is reproduced from Ref. [67].)

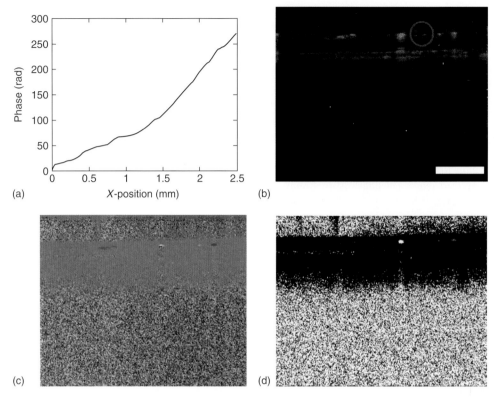

(a)

(b)

(c)

(d)

Figure 10.20 Final results after applying the motion compensation method to digitally stabilize the B-scan as detailed in Figure 10.3. (a) Accumulated changes along the B-scan from Eq. (10.42), (b) the resulting OMAG blood flow image after motion compensation. Also shown are (c) PRDOCT blood flow image and (d) Power Doppler blood flow image after motion compensation for comparison. Scale bar = 500 μm. (Source: Images are reproduced from Ref. [67].)

of the operations that are used to calculate the final OMAG flow images with the subject motion artifacts minimized.

To test the algorithm, we used the raw interferogram data for Figure 10.18. Figure 10.20 show the results after the bulk tissue motion was compensated to stabilize the B-scan image. The phase accumulation due to the bulk tissue motion amounted to ~250 rad within the single B-scan (Figure 10.20a). This phase change along the B-scan was used to compensate the spectral interferograms to obtain the final OMAG blood flow image as shown in Figure 10.20b. Compared with Figure 10.18b, the OMAG flow image after phase compensation is almost free of motion artifacts as shown in Figure 10.20b. Such results show that the algorithm described above works well. For comparison, we also applied the compensation method to compensate the phases in the OCT signals to obtain the final PRDOCT flow images. The results are given in Figure 10.20c,d for PRDOCT power DOCT images, respectively. Comparing OMAG and PRDOCT blood flow images, the former delivers superior imaging performance, as evidenced by the fact that (i) the blood signals circled in Figure 10.20b cannot be easily identified in Figure 10.20c,d and (ii) the flow signals within choroidal layer are abundant in Figure 10.20b which are, however, almost absent in PRDOCT images.

10.3.4
Doppler OMAG

The key advantage of OMAG is that only the signals backscattered by the moving blood appear in the OMAG flow output plane; this makes the blood flow imaging almost free of artifact-induced noise. However, the OMAG is incapable of providing flow velocity information like PRDOCT. This is because in the OMAG flow image, the regions that are occupied by the microstructural signals are rejected by OMAG; thus the required correlation between the adjacent A-scans within the static tissue regions are totally lost, leading to a rather noisy appearance in the output plane of flow velocity. To overcome this problem, we digitally reconstruct an ideal static background tissue that is totally optically homogeneous to replace the real hetero-geneous tissue sample in OMAG. This ideal background tissue provides a constant background signal that makes the adjacent A-scans totally correlated, leading to a dramatic increase of the phase SNR for the phase-resolved signals that represent flow velocities. This method inherits the advantages of both OMAG and PRDOCT.

The spectral interference signal captured by each pixel of the CCD camera in OMAG/SD-OCT is essentially the same, except the wavelength, λ. We assume the wave numbers of the broadband light source are from k_0 to k_0+, where $k_0 = 2\pi/\lambda_0$, and these wave numbers cover 1024 pixels of the line scan camera. Consequently, the camera records the spectral interference fringe signal formed between the reference light and the light backscattered from within sample, which can be written as a function of k_j

$$I\left(k_j\right) = S\left(k_j\right) \left\langle \left| E_R \exp\left(i2k_j r\right) + \int_{-\infty}^{\infty} a(z) \exp\left\{i2k_j[r + nz]\right\} dz \right|^2 \right\rangle$$

$$j = 1, 2, 3, \ldots, 1024 \tag{10.47}$$

where $i = -1$, $<>$ is the time average, k_j is the wave number of the light captured by the jth detector (pixel) of the CCD camera, $I(k_j)$ is the light intensity captured by the jth detector, $S(k_j)$ is the spectral density of the light source at k_j, r is the optical path length for the light traveled in the reference arm, n is the refractive index of the sample, and $a(z)$ is the magnitude of the light backscattered at depth z. In our system, each B-scan contains 1500 A-lines and covers about 2.5 mm in the lateral direction. Thus the signal captured by the jth pixel in each B-scan can be written as a function of time variable t that relates to the position of focus beam spot on the sample, steered by the x-scanning mirror. Thus

$$I\left(k_j, t\right) = S\left(k_j\right) \left\langle \left| E_R \exp\left(i2k_j r\right) + \int_{-\infty}^{\infty} a(z) \exp\{i2k_j[r + nz]\} dz \right|^2 \right\rangle$$

$$j = 1, 2, 3, \ldots, 1024 \tag{10.48}$$

Because the light backscattered from the sample is quite weak compared to the light reflected from the RM, we do not consider the self-cross-correlation between the light backscattered from different positions within the sample. We also do not consider the DC signals because they do not contribute to useful OMAG signals. Therefore, Eq. (10.48) can be written as

$$I\left(k_j, t\right) = 2S\left(k_j\right) E_R \int_{-\infty}^{\infty} a(z, t) \cos\left(2k_j n z\right) dz \tag{10.49}$$

It is clear that Eq. (10.48) is constant if the sample is totally optically homogeneous, which means that $a(z, t)$ and n do not vary within the entire sample. If this is the case, then the spatial frequency components of the sample in the lateral direction presented by Eq. (10.49) will be a delta function, shown as a red arrow in Figure 10.21a. However, in real situations, our imaging sample is often optically heterogeneous, which means that $a(z, t)$ and n are functions of time variable t. Thus, Eq. (10.49) can be expressed as

$$I\left(k_j, t\right) = 2S\left(k_j\right) E_R \int_{-\infty}^{+\infty} a\left(z_1\right) \cos\left[2k_j n(z, t) z dz\right] \tag{10.50}$$

As a consequence, Eq. (10.50) is no longer constant. The intensity captured by the CCD camera will be modulated by the heterogeneous properties of the sample along each B-scan. The spatial frequency components of a static tissue sample, which we call the heterogeneous frequencies, will exhibit as a randomly distributed function around zero frequency with a bandwidth of BW, as shown in red curve in Figure 10.21b [70].

When there is a patent blood vessel buried within motionless tissue at position (z_1, t_1), we assume that the blood cells (scattering particles) within the vessel move toward the incident beam at a velocity v. The frequency of the light backscattered from these blood cells will be modulated by its velocity. Then, Eq. (10.50) can be expressed as

$$I\left(k_j, t\right) = 2S\left(k_j\right) E_R \left[\int_{-\infty}^{\infty} a(z, t) \cos(2k_j n(t) z) dz \right.$$
$$\left. + a(z_1, t_1) \cos[2k_j n(t)(z_1 - vt)]\right] \tag{10.51}$$

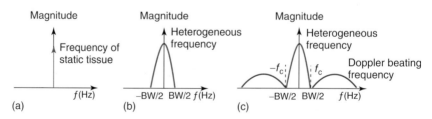

Figure 10.21 Diagram of frequency components for different tissue samples: (a) an ideal tissue sample (optically homogeneous sample) with no moving particles, (b) a real tissue sample (optically heterogeneous sample) with no moving particles, and (c) a real tissue sample (optically heterogeneous sample) with moving particles. (Source: Images are reproduced from Ref. [69].)

Here, we also do not consider the self cross-correlation signal from within the sample. The first term on the right side of Eq. (10.51) represents backscattering signals from a static sample with reflectivity of $a(z,t)$, while the second term represents backscattering from the moving particles with reflectivity of $a(z_1,t_1)$ with a velocity of v at position $a(z_1,t_1)$. Moving particles produce a frequency shift caused by the Doppler effect of the moving particles. This is illustrated in Figure 10.21c; the blue curve is the Doppler beat frequency part. Recall that the phase-resolved technique requires a correlation between adjacent A-scans to determine v of the moving particles [49], and the correlation, in conventional PRDOCT, provided by the first term on the right side of Eq. (10.51) is also required to suppress the noise signals in the nonflow regions in order to increase the flow imaging contrast. Because of the optical heterogeneity $n(z,t)$ of a tissue, $n(z,t)$ imposes a noise background onto the blood flow signals, making it difficult for PRDOCT to measure precisely the blood flow velocity, particularly in capillaries [60, 65, 67]. In contrast, OMAG eliminates the first term on the right side of Eq. (10.51) in order to image blood flow. This elimination renders the noise production due to $n(z,t)$ to a minimum, but unfortunately, results in OMAG losing its correlation condition between adjacent A-scans for the heterogeneous tissue regions. Consequently, the phase-resolved technique cannot be directly applied to OMAG blood flow signals. To solve this problem, our proposed strategy is to digitally re-construct an ideal sample background with a constant backscattering coefficient a_0 and a refractive index n_0 throughout the sample – thus creating a totally homogeneous sample that reinforces a complete correlation among OMAG A-scan signals.

$$I_0\left(k_j, t\right) = 2S\left(k_j\right) E_R \left[\int_{-\infty}^{\infty} a_0(z, t) \cos\left(2k_j n_0(z, t) z\right) dz \right] \tag{10.52}$$

where $a_0(z, t) \equiv a_0$ and $n_0(z, t) \equiv n_0$ throughout the scanned tissue sample. In condition, $a_0 = 10^{-6}$, and $n_0 = 1.35$ when we construct the homogeneous tissue background using Eq. (10.52). These values were taken according to the typical optical properties of biological tissues, that is, the average reflectivity is between 10^{-4} and 10^{-7} and the average refractive index is 1.35 [71]. The digitally reconstructed homogeneous tissue sample subsequently replaces the first term on the right side of Eq. (10.51). In doing so, OMAG blood flow signal now becomes

$$I'\left(k_j, t\right) = 2S\left(k_j\right) E_R \left[\int_{-\infty}^{\infty} a_0(z, t) \cos\left(2k_j n_0 z\right) dz \right.$$

$$\left. + E_R a\left(z_1, t_1\right) \cos\left[2k_j n\left(z_1, t_1\right)\left(z_1 - vt\right)\right] \right] \tag{10.53}$$

The construction of the ideal tissue sample does not affect OMAG signals of blood flow because it only replaces the tissue background signals with a homogeneous background without affecting the blood flow signals within the B-scan. If we treat time variable t as a constant and apply a FT on wavelength k, we can obtain

$$\tilde{I}(z, t) = \text{FT}^{-1}\left\{I\left(k_j, t\right)\right\} |k = A(z, t) \exp[i\phi(z, t)] \tag{10.54}$$

where $\varphi(z, t)$ is the phase of the analytic signal. The phase difference between adjacent A-scans, n and $n - 1$, is then evaluated

$$\Delta\phi(z, t) = \tan^{-1}\left[\frac{\mathrm{Im}\left[\tilde{I}(z, t_n) \cdot \tilde{I}(z, t_{n-1})\right]}{\mathrm{Re}\left[\tilde{I}(z, t_n) \cdot \tilde{I}(z, t_{n-1})\right]}\right] \tag{10.55}$$

On the basis of the linear relationship between phase difference between adjacent A-lines and velocity [4, 5], the velocity of flow signal imaged by OMAG can be directly written as

$$v(z, t) = \frac{\lambda\Delta\phi(z, t)}{4\pi\,\Delta t} \tag{10.56}$$

where $v(z, t)$ is the flow velocity at depth z, Δt is the time interval between adjacent A-lines. Note that there is a small constant offset induced by a_0 in Eq. (10.53), which may perturb the evaluated $\Delta\varphi(z, t)$. However, the small offset is usually at least 2 orders of magnitude smaller than the OMAG flow signals, leading to a negligible effect on the final evaluated $\Delta\varphi(z, t)$.

10.3.4.1 Signal Processing

The flow chart of the processing procedure is illustrated in Figure 10.22. It is because the image data was achieved by scanning, the variable t present in the theory section could be directly replaced by the position of the x-direction. In this case, we use x to replace t for better illustration of the cross-sectional image. The raw fringe signal, $I(k,x)$, captured by our system was first separated into two parts based on the heterodyne technique by a carefully selected frequency, f_c, along lateral direction, which depends on the characteristic of the sample and system setup.

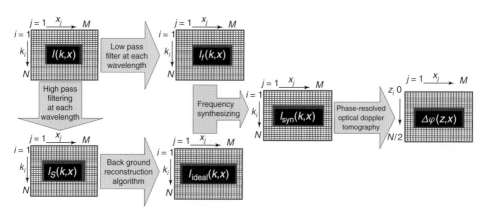

Figure 10.22 Flow chart showing the steps for DOMAG to evaluate the velocities of blood flow from a B-scan data set, $I(k,t)$. The data coordinates are indicated in the lower right corner of each data block, where t is the time variable of probe beam scanning over a sample, k is the wave number, f is the spatial frequency, and z is the imaging depth. FT$|t$ represents the Fourier transform (FT) against the time variable t in the B-scan, FT $-$ 1$|f$ indicates the inverse FT against the spatial frequency, f, and FT$|k$ is FT against the wave number k.

The static signal, $Is(k,x)$, the low frequency part, was reconstructed following the theory described above. An ideal simulation sample, Iideal(k,x), with no optical heterogeneity could be achieved by Eq. (10.49). Using a frequency synthesizing method, the flow signal, $If(k,x)$, extracted from the original fringe data by applying a high-pass filter at each wavelength, and the static signal, extracted from the ideal simulation sample by applying a low-pass filter at each wavelength, were recombined to a new synthesizing signal, $Isyn(k,x)$. After applying the PRDOCT algorithm, we could obtain the Doppler optical microangiography (DOMAG) phase difference image. Based on the following linear relationship between phase difference and velocity [34, 49], we could directly obtain the velocity information of the sample.

Because the background tissue signal was rejected previously, the DOMAG image provides two great improvements on two aspects. First, based on phase-resolved technology, the flow velocity was directly provided by DOMAG, compared to traditional OMAG. Second, the texture pattern artifacts caused by the optical heterogeneity, which could greatly reduce the performance of the PRDOCT, was successfully rejected. In consequence, the phase SNR of the DOMAG was greatly improved compared to PRDOCT.

10.3.4.2 Experimental Verification

To test the performance of our method, we first apply it on the flow phantom experiments. A phantom was made from gelatin mixed with 2% milk to simulate the background optical heterogeneity of the tissue in which a capillary tube with an inner diameter of $\sim$200 μm was submerged and $\sim$2% TiO_2 particle solution was flowing. The flow velocity of the solution was controlled by a precision syringe pump. The inclining angle of the tube toward the incident beam was set as $\sim$90°. In this experiment, each B-scan (lateral direction) contained 1000 A-lines and covered 2.5 mm. Thus, the corresponding Δx between adjacent A-lines was 2.5 μm. The resulting images are illustrated in Figure 10.23.

Figure 10.23a is the structure image obtained through the conventional FDOCT method. We use this image to get flow region in our experiment. Four points, the top, bottom, left, and right points of the inner wall, were chosen to mark the flow region. Figure 10.23b is the OMAG flow image. As we can see, the light backscattered by the fluid particles was successfully highlighted, while the background static phantom was rejected. Figure 10.23c,d are the DOMAG and PRDOCT flow images, respectively. Comparing these two images, one can see that the background character texture pattern artifacts are successfully eliminated in the DOMAG method. These artifacts are introduced by optical heterogeneity of the phantom. In consequence, the noise level of Figure 10.23c is significantly reduced compared to Figure 10.23d, PRDOCT method. These aspects could also be illustrated by Figure 10.23e. The blue curve is selected from the location marked with blue line in Figure 10.23c, while the red curve is selected from the same location marked with the red line in Figure 10.23d. The phase difference caused by the fluid particles is almost the same (the parabolic curve) using these two methods, while the noise (the flat curve) of the blue is much smaller than that of the red.

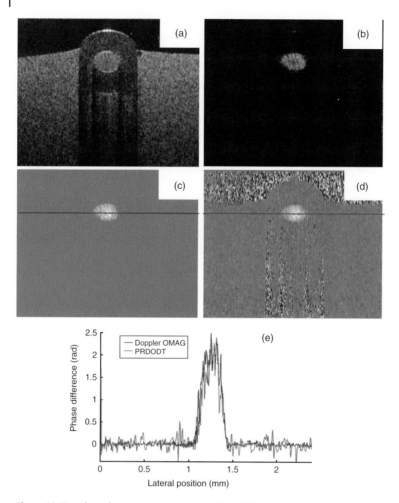

Figure 10.23 Flow phantom experiment results. (a) Structure image, (b) OMAG flow image, (c) Doppler OMAG image, (d) PRDOCT image, and (e) two lines extracted from the same depth location of DOMAG and PRDOCT. (Source: Images are reproduced from Ref. [69].)

To quantify the illustrated efficiency of the improvement demonstrated by the DOMAG method compared to PRDOCT method, we calculated N (noise, which could also be present by standard deviation of the phase differences between adjacent A-lines, $\sigma_{\Delta\phi}$), S (signal), and phase SNR of both methods. The noise in our experiment is presented by the standard deviation of the noise region. The signal, S, is evaluated through the following algorithm in the flow region:

$$S = \sum_{x=L}^{R} \sum_{z=B}^{T} (\Delta\varphi_{xz} > N) \tag{10.57}$$

Table 10.1   Evaluated noise, signal, and phase SNR of a phase difference flow image of PRDOCT and Doppler OMAG.

	$N(\Delta\phi(rad))$	S (number)	Phase SNR (dB)
DOMAG	0.036	4731	51
PRDOCT	0.405	3116	39
Improvement	92%	1.52 (unitless)	12

where $>$ returns 1 when $\Delta\phi$ is bigger than N, else it returns 0. By doing this, the signal, S, here could denote the effective detectable signal numbers and phase SNR is the ratio of these two values, S and N. The results are illustrated in Table 10.1. With our new digital background reconstruction method, the phase noise N was reduced from 0.405 to 0.036 rad, which is about 92% improvement. For the reduction of the background noise, the detectable effective signal number was also greatly improved, from 3116 to 4731, which is a 52% improvement. Based on these two aspects, the phase SNR was successfully improved by 12 dB, from 39 to 51 dB.

The phase noise we used here could also be called as the *phase sensitivity*, which could be determined by the intensity SNR of the system, X, by the following equation [55]:

$$\sigma^2_{\Delta\phi} = \left(\frac{1}{X}\right) \tag{10.58}$$

The phase sensitivity value obtained from Eq. (10.56) is the upper limit value that phase-resolved method can get in the totally correlated situation. In the above experiment, the intensity SNR of the flow region is $\sim$30 dB, which is quite common in experiments to extract a blood flow signal in *in vivo* experiment. The corresponding phase sensitivity is $\sim$0.033 rad. As we can see, the sensitivity of our method is quite close to the totally correlated situation.

10.3.4.3   *In Vivo* Imaging with DOMAG

For further testing the potential of DOMAG in noninvasive assessment of microcirculation *in vivo*, we obtained transcranial cerebrovascular images of mice. In the following experiments, the mice we used were three-month-old male C57BL/6J mice, which were purchased from commercial breeders (Charles River Laboratories), and each of them weighed 23–28 g. Twenty four hours before we performed the experiment, the hair of the mice was removed by some kind of a depilatory cream. During the experiment, the mouse was anesthetized by using 2% isoflurane ($0.2\,l\,min^{-1}$ O_2, $0.8\,l\,min^{-1}$ air). To make sure the body of the mouse was in an active condition, we used a warming blanket and a thermometer to maintain the body temperature of the mouse between 36.7 and 37.1 °C. Before the image data was acquired, a skin window of the mouse head was carefully opened using sterile technology and with skull left intact. To make the head of the animal as stable as possible, we used a custom stereotaxic imaging stage. The exposed skull of the mouse was washed with saline to maintain moisture. All animals were disposed off according to IACUC regulations. The protocol was approved by the Oregon Health and Sciences University Institutional Animal Care and Use Committee and was in compliance with the guidelines of the National Institutes of Health for care and handling of laboratory animals.

For 3D image, the amplitude of the $X-Y$ scanner was set at 2.5 mm by 2.5 mm, which contained 2000 A-lines in lateral direction and 500 B-scans in elevation direction (y-direction). Thus the distance interval between adjacent A-lines was ~1.25 μm, while the distance interval between adjacent B-scans was ~5 μm. The original raw data was first processed frame by frame, and then the flow images were recombined to provide a 3D volumetric vasculature image of the mouse head. Figure 10.24a is the conventional OCT cross-sectional structure image of the mouse head, from which the histologically important layers were clearly identified. Figure 10.24b presents the DOMAG phase difference image, $\Delta\phi(x, z)$. With the orientation of the blood vessels, which could be obtained from the volumetric vasculature image, the velocity information could be extracted from Eq. (10.57). Figure 10.24c shows the image that we got by merging Figure 10.24a,b together to present exactly where the blood flow located. The red color means the blood vessels have a forward velocity, while the green means they have a backward direction.

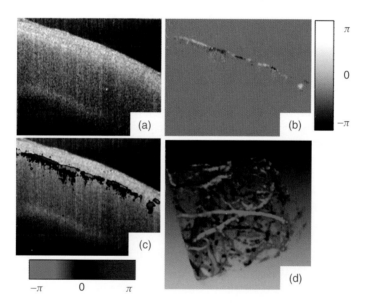

Figure 10.24 Doppler OMAG image results. (a) Conventional OCT structure image, (b) Doppler OMAG flow image, (c) OCT cross-sectional structure image showing the location of the blood flow with the forward ones coded with red color and the backward ones with green color, (d) volumetric rendering of cerebrovasculature. The red color represents the forward blood flow while the green color represents the backward blood flow.

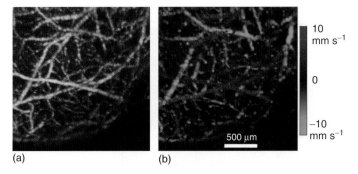

Figure 10.25 Maximum-amplitude projection view $(x-y)$ of (a) OMAG and (b) DOMAG of the cerebral blood flow in the cortical brain of the mouse shown in Figure 10.24. (Source: Images are reproduced from Ref. [69].)

To combine all two-dimensional slices, DOMAG could provide rendering 3D volumetric image of blood vessel networks, presented in Figure 10.24d. The red color denotes the flow with forward direction, while the green is the flow with backward direction.

To view in detail the blood vessel networks coded with velocity information, Figure 10.25b provides the $x-y$ projection view with the blood vessel with forward flow direction in red and backward direction in green. On the basis of the linear relationship between phase differences and velocity present in Eq. (10.57), Figure 10.25b is actually a velocity projection along the light beam. Together with the blood vessel perfusion information given by OMAG (the 2D $x-y$ projection view of blood vessel perfusion networks is presented in Figure 10.25a), DOMAG provides a tool that has the potential capability of precisely quantitatively evaluating the blood vessel.

10.3.4.4 Comparison between PRDOCT and DOMAG

In Figure 10.26, we demonstrated the differences between OMAG, conventional PRDOCT method, and DOMAG method. Figure 10.26a is a 2D conventional OCT cross-sectional structure image. The OMAG method obtained the images of microstructures via SD-OCT (Figure 10.26a), blood flow via OMAG (Figure 10.26b), and the corresponding velocities of blood flow via DOMAG (Figure 10.26c). DOMAG calculated the velocities of blood flow in functional vessels, including capillaries (white arrows, for example), and even in the vessels ~1.5 mm deep below the bone surface (red arrow). However, the PRDOCT result (Figure 10.26d) indicates that conventional DOCT fails to provide detailed velocities of blood flows in this case. The level of background phase noise is an important metric when quantifying blood flow, particularly in capillaries, because this metric affects our ability to extract useful flow signals from the noisy background. Using the method described in Section 10.3.4.2, the noise level for PRDOCT was typically 0.5 rad, largely due to the heterogeneous property of the tissue sample as seen in Figure 10.26d and as discussed in Section 10.3.4, suggesting that PRDOCT might

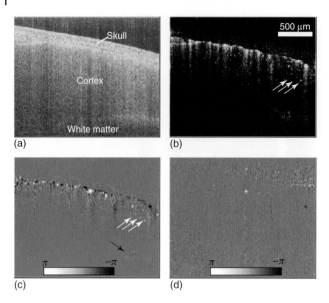

Figure 10.26 Comparison between OMAG and PRDOCT B-scan imaging of the cortical brain in mice *in vivo*. (a) OMAG structural image (i.e., SD-OCT) and the corresponding (b) OMAG flow image, (c) DOMAG flow velocity image, and (d) PRDOCT flow velocity image. See the text for explanation of the arrows. (Source: Images are reproduced from Ref. [69].)

not be able to measure blood flow velocities $<1.1\,\text{mm s}^{-1}$ when the A-scan rate is at $\sim 20\,\text{kHz}$. However, DOMAG was able to reduce this noise level to 0.034 rad, which is comparable to the phantom experiments shown in Section 10.4.1, suggesting an approximate 15-fold improvement in imaging blood flow velocities over conventional PRDOCT in this *in vivo* imaging case. Thus, we expect that DOMAG will be a good candidate tool to quantify blood flow within perfused tissue.

To further show the advantages of DOMAG in imaging the blood flow velocities over PRDOCT, we compared 3D DOMAG and PRDOCT images evaluated from a scanned tissue volume from the mouse brain cortex with the skull left intact. Figure 10.27 (shown as projection images to x–y) illustrates the difference between OMAG, DOMAG, and PRDOCT imaging of cerebral blood flow (CBF) in mice under the same experimental conditions. To obtain the PRDOCT flow image, we had to use algorithms established in [67, 68] to reduce the noise artifacts, where algorithms for minimization of the sample motion artifacts, segmentation of regions of interest, and correction of phase-wrapping errors were implemented. Note that it did not require performing the segmentations in DOMAG in order to render the 3D image as the phase noise level was low in the entire 3D space. These results indicate that DOMAG (Figure 10.27b) could reliably determine the velocities of blood flows within almost all vessels in the scanned tissue. Not surprisingly, PRDOCT (Figure 10.27c) can be erroneous in quantifying blood flows within the scanned tissue due to noise produced in PRDOCT, which masks slow flows ($<1.1\,\text{mm s}^{-1}$) in small vessels. Furthermore, blood vessel diameters seen in

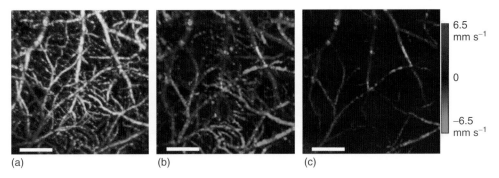

(a) (b) (c)

Figure 10.27 Comparison between *in vivo* 3D OMAG and PRDOCT imaging of the cortical brain in mice with the intact skull. Shown are the maximum *x–y* projection views of (a) OMAG cerebral blood flow image, (b) DOMAG flow velocity image, and (c) PRDOCT flow velocity image. The physical size of scanned tissue volume was 2.5 × 2.5 × 2.0 mm³. White bar = 500 μm. (Source: Images are reproduced from Ref. [69].)

the DOMAG and OMAG images were significantly larger than those in the DOCT images, suggesting a clear advantage of DOMAG over DOCT in quantifying blood flow in the scanned tissue.

The reason for these differences is that the performance of conventional PRDOCT is limited by the background texture noise pattern caused by the optical hetero-geneity, that is, microstructures, of the tissue sample [21]. On the other hand, DOMAG uses an ideal reconstructed sample as the tissue background, which makes the adjacent OMAG A-scans totally correlated, maximally satisfying the cor-relation requirement for the phase-resolved technique. As a consequence, DOMAG reduces the background phase noise to a minimum. This improves the capability of DOMAG to detect low blood velocity near the wall of the blood vessel, and as a result, the diameter of blood vessel detected by DOMAG is larger than that by PRDOCT, as seen in Figure 10.27.

An alternative way to better illustrate the phase noise levels is to use 3D plots of cross-sectional images (B-scans). Shown in Figure 10.28 is such an illustration for a typical B-scan of the cortical brain in mice. Figure 10.27a is the conventional PRDOCT flow velocity plot, without applying the segmentation approach to eliminate the random phases in low-signal regions. The flow signals are pointed by the black arrows and the noise in the useful signal region is pointed with red arrow. In the low-OCT-signal regions, for example, the region above tissue surface where there is no light reflectivity and the region deep in the tissue where the detected optical signal is low due to the light attenuation, the evaluated phases will exhibit random phase noise signals in PRDOCT. From Figure 10.28a, it is clear that the noise in the low-signal region overwhelmed the useful flow signals, thus segmentation is often needed in PRDOCT to exclude this random noise. After segmentation of the tissue regions of interest using the methods in [67, 68], a better view is given in Figure 10.28b to show the effects of background noise in the tissue region. In Figure 10.28b, the noise pointed with

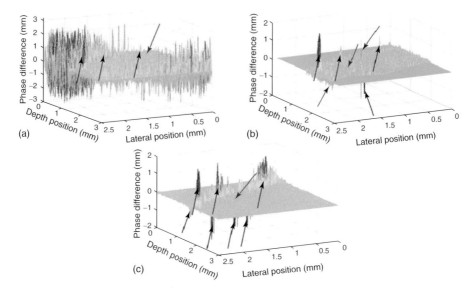

Figure 10.28 3D flow images. (a) Conventional PRDOCT flow image without segmentation, (b) conventional PRDOCT flow image with segmentation, and (c) Doppler OMAG flow image. (Source: Images are reproduced from Ref. [69].)

a red arrow is so high that it prevents the small blood vessel signals from being detected. We should pay special attention to those pointed by blue arrows, where it is difficult to distinguish between blood signals and noise. For DOMAG, shown in Figure 10.28c, the background noise is very small compared to the blood vessel signals, which improves significantly the imaging performance for DOMAG. It should be noted that Ren *et al.* previously proposed a moving-scatterer-sensitive optical Doppler optical coherence tomography (MSS-DOCT) technique for *in vivo* blood flow imaging using SD-OCT [72, 73]. In their method, a delayed-line filter was used to suppress the influence of stationary scatterers by subtracting adjacent complex axial scans before applying the phase-resolved method to calculate the Doppler frequency shift. There are distinct differences between DOMAG and MSS-DOCT in that (i) the former operates on the wave number domain signals, that is, interferograms, while MSS-DOCT operates on the time domain signals, that is, complex OCT images and (ii) DOMAG filters out the signals caused by the static scattering components from the entire B-scan signals, while the latter uses delay-line filters applied to the neighborhood A-scans to suppress the static signals.

10.4
Applications of OMAG

Because of its exceptionally high spatial resolution and velocity sensitivity, several basic research and clinical applications of OMAG have been demonstrated, which includes monitoring cortical hemodynamics and cerebral vascular perfusion mapping in rodent models for brain research, cerebral blood perfusion, and vascular plasticity following TBI in rodent models, screening vasoactive drugs, monitoring changes in tissue morphology, and hemodynamics following pharmacological intervention and mapping, and imaging ocular blood flow.

10.4.1
In Vivo Imaging of Mouse Cerebral Blood Perfusion and Vascular Plasticity Following Traumatic Brain Injury Using OMAG

TBI often causes alterations in CBF that are thought to influence secondary pathophysiology and neurologic outcome in human brain. Inadequate CBF is an important contributor to mortality and morbidity after TBI [74]. Despite the importance of cerebral vascular dysfunction in TBI pathophysiology, the effect of trauma on CBF has been less well studied than the effect of trauma on the brain [75]. Similarly, our understanding of the rehabilitation and autoregulation of cerebrovascular blood circulation after TBI also remains incomplete. In this regard, a noninvasive technique for imaging *in vivo* blood flow, down to capillary level resolution, would be of great value.

Three-month-old C57 BL/6 mice (20–30 g) were used in the study to show the potential of OMAG for monitoring changes in dynamic CBF following TBI *in vivo*. The experimental protocol was in compliance with the Federal guidelines for care and handling of small rodents and approved by the Institutional Animal Care and Use Committee. Before OMAG imaging, the mouse head was shaved and depilated. During the imaging, the animal was immobilized in a custom-made stereotaxic stage and was lightly anesthetized with isoflurane (0.21 min^{-1} O$_2$, 0.81 min^{-1} air). The body temperature was kept between 35.5 and 36.5 °C by use of a warming blanket and monitored by a rectal thermal probe throughout the experiment. An incision of ∼1 cm was made along the sagittal suture, and the frontal, parietal, and interparietal bones were exposed by pulling the skin to the sides. The animal was then positioned under the OMAG scanning probe. In order to acquire the CBF images over a large area of the cortex, the scan was performed clockwise, which resulted in six OMAG images covering areas between anterior coronal suture (Bregma) and posterior coronal suture (Lambda). The total image acquisition time for the six OMAG scans was ∼8 min. For each 3D OMAG image, a volumetric segmentation algorithm [60] was applied to isolate the blood flow signals within the cortex, and a maximum projection method was then used to project the blood flow signals onto the *x–y* plane in order to reduce the image size. The final image, representing the CBF over the mouse cortex, was obtained by stitching six resulting images together and cropping, covering an area of ∼4.2 × 7.2 mm^2 over the mouse head.

Before inducing TBI, a control OMAG image was acquired as the baseline for later comparison. Then the mouse was subjected to TBI. In order to induce a traumatic lesion in the cortex, a 30-gauge needle was disinfected and used to puncture a round and vertical hole with a depth of 1.5 mm measured from the upper surface of the skull. The bleeding was washed out using medical-grade saline. About 30 min after the onset of TBI, OMAG imaging was initiated at the same region as the control. After imaging, the animal was sutured, disinfected, and injected with antibiotics, and then returned to the cage for rehabilitation. A series of OMAG images were taken on the same animal on days 1 (24 h after TBI),

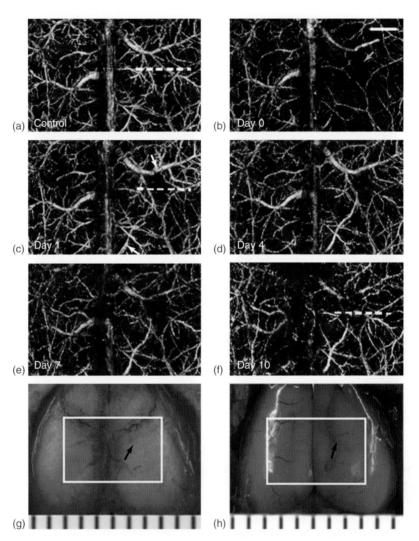

Figure 10.29 3D OMAG imaging of the cortex during TBI in mice. Compared to baseline (a), progressive vessel regulation (vessels are pointed by white arrows) and neovascularization at traumatic area develop during TBI rehabilitation. The site of injury is pointed by green arrow. (g,h) The photographs of the brain cortex with and without skull on the same mouse. The area in (a–f) corresponds to the area marked with dashed white box in (g) and (h). The scale bar represents 1.0 mm. (Source: Images are reproduced from Ref. [77].)

4, 7, and 10. Finally, the animal was euthanized by cervical dislocation, and digital images of the head were taken (cf. Roper Scientific PhotometricsCoolsnap). Next the skin and skull on the head were carefully removed to expose the dorsal blood vessels of the brain, which were then photographed to be compared with images from the OMAG system.

A typical series of OMAG CBF images is shown in Figure 10.29 and the cross-sectional structure and perfusion images corresponding to the dashed line positions in Figure 10.29 are shown in Figure 10.30. Figure 10.29a is the OMAG image from baseline, that is, the control, where it shows the capability of OMAG to delineate the dynamic CBF, down to capillary-level resolution, within the cortex while the skull was left intact. At 30 min after TBI, a reduction of CBF (cerebral ischemia) over the entire cortex was seen in the OMAG image (Figure 10.29b). The reduction of CBF might be due to the posttraumatic hemorrhage caused by the external injury that leaves the blood in the space between the meninges and cortex, near the TBI site (pointed by the green arrow). However, the CBF reduction was not even across the cortex as seen in Figure 10.29b, with the ipsilateral reduction more severe than the reduction in the contralateral region. Another possible reason for the reduction of CBF seen in the OMAG image might be the possible bleeding that partially blocks the light penetration into the deeper tissues (i.e., light absorption due to the clotted blood); however, the clotted blood will be most likely localized near the TBI site. At the TBI site, the blood flow was totally ceased, due to hemostasis. Furthermore, the vessel constriction was apparent in the ipsilateral region, which might be caused by acute cerebrovascular regulation to prevent the occurrence of hypoxic–ischemic reaction [76].

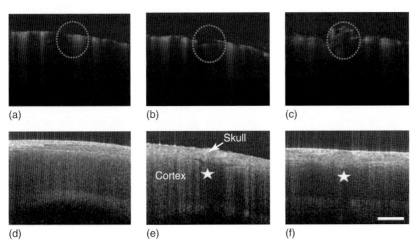

(a)   (b)   (c)

(d)   (e)   (f)

Figure 10.30 Cross sections (slices) of microstructure (d–f) and blood perfusion (a–c) of the mouse brain during pretraumatic (a,d) and posttraumatic (b,e, c,f) phases. They correspond to the dashed white line position in Figure 10.29. The areas in dashed circle show the evolution of neovascularization, and the trauma zone in the cortex is marked by a white star. (Source: Images are reproduced from Ref. [77].)

During the progress of rehabilitation, OMAG is able to visualize the changes of CBF in the same injured animal over time. At day 1, vasoconstriction disappeared and the blood perfusion almost returned to the baseline, apart from the site of injury (Figure 10.29c). However, the vessel dilation seemed to occur near the TBI site, particularly for the vessels pointed by the white arrows and their associated branches. The needle-induced lesion area is still absent from the blood circulation (Figures 10.29c and 10.30b). From days 4 to 7, the new blood vessels started to appear in the traumatic region, indicating that the neovascularization was taking place (Figure 10.29d,e). The neovascularization was more evident at day 10 (Figures 10.29f and 10.30c); however, the blood flows over the cortex seen in the previous OMAG images was increasingly difficult to detect by the OMAG system at day 10. The reason for this difficulty is that the thickness of cranium doubled (Figure 10.30f) when compared with the control (Figure 10.30d) and this reduced the amount of light to reach the cortex because of the well-known light scattering phenomenon [71]. The increased thickness of cranium was most probably due to the infection caused by the experimental procedures, although the antibiotics were applied to the animal daily. This can be eliminated for future systematic studies on TBI through careful and skilled surgical procedures. Despite this infection in the current study that doubled the cranium thickness, OMAG still offers the opportunity to visualize the changes of global CBF that may aid our understanding of the cerebral vascular plasticity on TBI.

For comparison, the direct photographs of the brain cortex with and without skull just after the OMAG imaging at day 10 are shown in Figure 10.29g,h, respectively, where the TBI site is identified by the black arrow. Seeing the blood vessels through the cranium is almost impossible (Figure 10.29g). Comparing between Figure 10.29h and OMAG images, the agreement on the major vascular network over the brain cortex is achieved. More importantly, the microvessels unobserved in Figure 10.29h are seen in OMAG images, suggesting the OMAG's capability to monitor the cerebral vascular circulation after TBI at capillary level resolution.

The ability to noninvasively record and map the variations of CBF would greatly contribute to our understanding of the complex nature involved following TBI. Because the moving red blood cells in patent vessels, including capillaries can be precisely localized in OMAG, any functional vessel up to the depth of 2.00 mm is able to be imaged under OMAG. Our current experimental results have shown the capability of OMAG to monitor the response of the cerebral circulation to TBI and to visualize the neovascularization following TBI. The noted increases in newly formed vessels after TBI may serve to alleviate secondary neuronal damage by improving local blood flow and metabolite delivery to the nutrient-deprived neurons. Our understanding of the mechanism of new vessel formation still remains incomplete. On the basis of the volumetric imaging of OMAG with improved resolution, OMAG may provide a powerful tool to investigate and visualize neovascularization following TBI on the same animal over a long period. Specifically, if combined with immunocytochemistry, OMAG may aid the investigations on elucidating whether both angiogenesis and vasculogenesis or either of them participates in promoting neovascularization [78]. However, due to the coagulation of red blood cells from broken vessels on the site of injury in the current study, observation of the generation of precursor microvessels will possibly be inhibited, if this beginning event happens before the blood clot is partially absorbed. Currently, our group is developing algorithms to quantitatively assess the CBF from the OMAG measurements so that the accurate angiodynamics following TBI can be provided.

In summary, we have studied the dynamic CBF over the mouse brain on TBI by use of the OMAG imaging *in vivo*. The CBF before and after trauma were mapped at the resolution level of capillary flow in real time without interfering with the mouse brain in a significant way, because the cranium was left intact for the OMAG procedure. We have shown the potential of OMAG to image neovascularization by monitoring the 3D vasculature around the traumatic region during the rehabilitation process. These results indicate that OMAG may provide a powerful tool to investigate and understand the TBI mechanism, which could aid the development of novel therapeutic strategies in the treatment of TBI.

10.4.2
Retinal and Choroidal Microvascular Perfusion Mapping with OMAG

Accurate 3D imaging of microvascular blood perfusion has great significance in ophthalmology. There is a growing body of evidence which suggests that vascular abnormalities and dysregulation may contribute to the development of several major ocular diseases as different as glaucoma, diabetic retinopathy, or age-related macular degeneration, and so on. Much effort has been made to investigate the ocular microvascular perfusion in detail. However, direct 3D visualization and investigation of the ocular microcirculation is complicated by the fact that the posterior pole of the eye is nourished mainly by two different vascular beds, the retina and the choroid, in which the retina have several layers and sublayers. In terms of physiological and pathological conditions, the retinal and choroidal microvascular systems exhibit significant differences, which are reviewed elsewhere [79]. High-resolution noninvasive techniques for depth-resolved *in vivo* imaging of ocular microvascular perfusion are not currently available as a diagnostic tool in ophthalmology. Such a technique could have a significant impact on better understanding of retinal pathogenesis and early diagnosis and facilitate preventive retinal treatment.

To demonstrate the performance of OMAG imaging of the posterior chamber of the eye *in vivo*, we performed experiments using the system described in Section 10.3.1 on the volunteers in our laboratory. The whole experiment was done in a darkroom. To reduce the eye and head movement, the volunteer was asked to stare at a fixed position during the experiment, and at the same time, the head of the volunteer was placed on a custom-made stage, which helped the volunteer to relax during the experiment. Every 3D spectral interferogram data set captured by the OMAG system was composed of 1000 A-scans on a frame (B-scan) and 200 frames in the elevation direction (C-scan), from which the volumetric structural

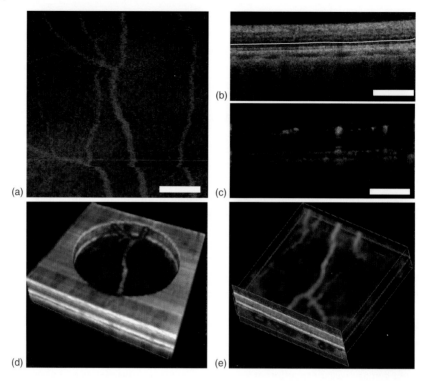

Figure 10.31 *In vivo* volumetric imaging of the posterior chamber of an eye from a volunteer. (a) OCT fundus image of the scanned volume as described in [33]. (b) OCT cross-sectional image at the position marked yellow in (a), in which four lines as shown result from the segmentation method that is used to separate the blood flows in retina and choroids. (c) Fly-through movie that represents the 2D OMAG flow images within the scanned volume. (d) Volumetric rendering of the merged structural and flow images with a cut through in the center of structural image. (e) Volumetric rending of the blood flow image where flows in retina are coded with green and those in choroids with red. Scale bar = 500 μm. (Source: Images are reproduced from Ref. [67].)

and blood flow images were obtained. This data volume was acquired over an area ∼2.5 mm × 2.5 mm in approximately 10 s.

Figure 10.31 shows the *in vivo* imaging results produced by one volume data set captured at a position near the optic disk. Figure 10.31a gives the OCT fundus projection image obtained by integrating signals along the depth direction from the volumetric OCT structural images using the method proposed by Jiao *et al.* [80], where the major blood vessels over the retina can be seen, but not in the choroid. Figure 10.31b represents one cross-sectional image within the volumetric OCT image at the position marked by the yellow line in Figure 10.31a. Figure 10.31c and the associated movie show the fly-through 2D OMAG flow images of the cross sections after the bulk motion was corrected as described in the section titled "Motion Compensation OMAG", where it can be seen that the blood flows within the retina and that the choroidal layers are clearly delineated. The results also demonstrate that the motion compensation method as described in the section titled "Motion Compensation OMAG" Section 10.3.3.1.6 worked well for the volumetric OMAG imaging. In addition, we should pay attention to the dilation and contraction of the area of flow cross section in the movie, which are most likely caused by the heartbeat of the volunteer. In the retinal region, not only some big vessels but also the capillary vessels are presented. Although the blood flow in the vessels in the choroid region are slow, which is difficult to be detected by PRDOCT, it can be captured by OMAG imaging method. Because OMAG gives the volumetric structural and flow images simultaneously, the 3D vasculatures can be merged into the 3D structural image. Such merged volumetric image is illustrated in Figure 10.31d, where a cut-through view in the center of volumetric structural image is used to better appreciate how the blood vessels innervate the tissue. To separately view the blood vessels within the retinal and choroidal layers, we used a segmentation method to produce two masks, from the three-dimensional OMAG structural image, that represent the retina and choroids. In a cross-sectional view, the mask that represents the retina is shown as the red and yellow lines in Figure 10.31b, and that which represents the choroid as the green and blue lines. To render the volumetric flow image, the blood flow signals within the boundaries of two masks are coded with green color (retina) and red color (choroid). The result is shown in Figure 10.31e, where the flow image shows us two vessel networks with good connection between vessels.

Currently, the OMAG imaging system has a limited field of view. One typical 3D image covers a volume of $2 \times 2 \times 2 \, mm^3$ in the posterior segment of the eye. Figure 10.32 shows one example of 3D perfusion maps from a healthy volunteer. Figure 10.32a,b demonstrates the 3D volumetric blood vessel networks in the retina and choroid. In Figure 10.32c, the retinal blood vessels (coded in green) and choroidal blood vessels (coded in red) are merged together to present their relative positions. Together with a cross-sectional B-scan structure image, Figure 10.32c also demonstrates the positions of blood vessels relative to the structure.

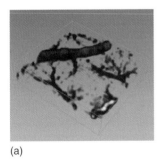 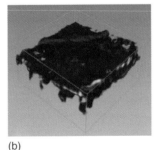 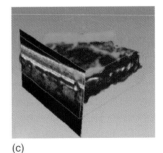

(a) (b) (c)

Figure 10.32 Volumetric image of blood vessel networks in (a) retina and (b) choroid. (c) Combined volumetric image, together with a cross-sectional structure image. (Source: Images are reproduced from Ref. [81].)

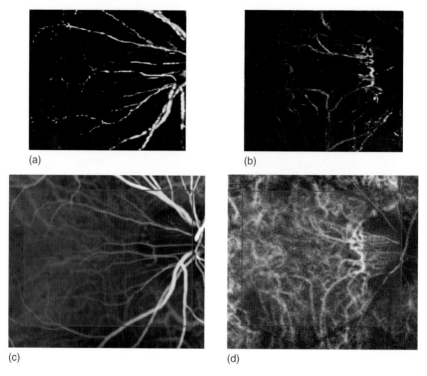

(a)

(b)

(c)

(d)

Figure 10.33 Wide-field of view blood perfusion maps for (a) retina and (b) choroids, compared with (c) fluorescein angiography and (d) indocyanine green angiography. (Source: Images are reproduced from Ref. [81].)

To achieve wide-field imaging of fundus vasculature (7.4 mm × 7.4 mm) with this technique, we sequentially scanned different areas of the posterior part of human eye with multiple 3D data sets. Each of these small 3D data sets covered around 2 mm × 2 mm × 2 mm area. In both lateral and elevation directions, we introduced a ~0.2 mm overlap between every two small data set, in order to make no blank space during the whole image stitching process. The images in Figure 10.33 were created from 16 3D datasets captured using a predesigned scan pattern. Figure 10.33a,b shows blood flow maps from the retina and choroid, respectively, using OMAG. These results compare favorably with clinical fluorescein angiography (FA) – see Figure 10.33c – and indocyanine green angiography (ICGA) – see Figure 10.33d – from the same volunteer. Furthermore, OMAG sees more microblood vessels in the foveal region than FA (marked by the white ellipse).

By comparison, the OMAG results demonstrated very good agreement with the clinical FA and ICGA results. By scrutinizing the appearances of the blood vessels, almost all noticeable vessels presented by FA and ICGA images are demonstrated by OMAG imaging. Furthermore, in the retinal perfusion map in Figure 10.33a, the OMAG results demonstrated more microcirculation information in the fovea region than that of the FA image. The main advantages of OMAG compared to FA and ICGA are that the images are obtained without injected contrast agents and the vessels can be correlated with the depth of location in the retina or choroid. These two advantages of OMAG wide field of view perfusion maps indicate that this imaging modality will potentially be a very powerful tool for *in vivo* clinical application in the future.

10.4.3
Volumetric Imaging of Cochlear Blood Perfusion in Rodent with OMAG

The motivation behind the study of cochlear microcirculation is the hypothesis that it plays an important role in maintaining the normal homeostatic environment in the inner ear and also the assumption that some cochlear diseases are vascular in nature. It is hypothesized that these disorders can be treated by increasing blood flow to the inner ear. It is known that there is high metabolic demand of cochlear tissues such as stria vascularis [82, 83], and that ischemia may have potential role in cochlear injury following noxious insults such as sound [84–86] or ototoxic drugs [87]. It is also possible that vascular change scan be part of the etiology of sudden deafness syndrome [88, 89] and Meniere's disease [90, 91]. Imaging to measure cochlear blood flow could be accomplished for the vascular network of the osseous spiral lamina that can be visualized via the round window membrane, a natural opening into the cochlea. There is a clear need for understanding the mechanisms controlling the cochlear blood flow. The study of blood flow in cochlea has interested auditory investigators for centuries. There have been many research activities, with applications of various techniques to measure cochlear blood flow. Intravital microscopy [92, 93] was used for the first direct observation of cochlear blood flow. Intravital microscopy allowed visualization of the major vascular beds of the lateral wall and the basilar membrane in the living animal [87]. With this technique, vessel lumen diameter, changes in blood flow pattern, and flow rate can be assessed under resting conditions and with experimental manipulations. However, the technique requires the removal of otic capsule over the lateral wall vessels to permit direct visualization. Under the best of conditions, it is a very invasive procedure.

In order to demonstrate the potential for using OMAG for studying *in vivo* cochlear blood flow and imaging the cochlear microstructures for small animal models, we obtained detailed cochlea blood perfusion images of gerbils. The gerbil was chosen as our animal model for its relatively thin bony otic capsule. The experimental protocol was in compliance with the Federal Guidelines for care and handling of small rodent and was approved by the Oregon Health and Science University Institutional Animal Care and Use Committee. The middle ears of two deeply anesthetized gerbils were surgically exposed to provide a window for OMAG imaging. The surface of the cochlea was wiped with a cotton pledget to remove the periosteum vessels. The animals were wrapped in a heating pad that was thermoregulated to 38.5 °C. The animals were then placed under the OMAG

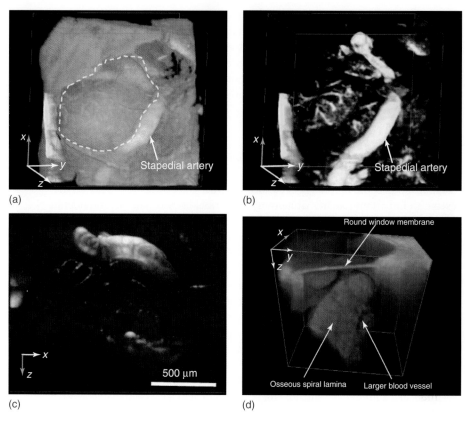

(a)

(b)

(c)

(d)

Figure 10.34 OMAG image of the gerbil cochlea in three dimension. Image volume is 2.0 × 2.0 × 2.0 mm³. (a) Image of microstructures within the scanned tissue, where the location of the cochlea is indicated by the dashed outline. (b) Corresponding volumetric image of the blood perfusion within the cochlea. (c) 2D projection view (x–z view) of blood flow (b) in the cochlea; the image shows the blood vessel network, including capillaries, in the first turn of the cochlea. (d) OMAG imaging of cochlea in gerbils through the round window *in vivo*. The imaged tissue volume = 2.0 × 2.0 × 2.0 mm³ (x-y-z). The OMAG probe beam was directed from the top. (Source: Images are reproduced from Ref. [94].)

scanning probe, as described earlier, and full 3D scans of the cochlea of the prepared animals were then taken. The animal preparation provided us with a wide optical view for the OMAG to image. Figure 10.34a shows *in vivo* 3D OMAG image of gerbil cochlea. The imaging volume was 2 × 2 × 2 mm³. The final images are scaled to the physical dimensions using a refractive index of 1.35 for typical biological tissues. Figure 10.34a shows the image of the microstructures within the imaged tissue volume. In Figure 10.34b, 3D OMAG image of the blood vessels in the bone and in the tissue just inside the bony otic capsule is shown. Figure 10.34c is the 2D projection of the 3D image in Figure 10.34b. In the projection image, one can see the blood vessel network, including the capillaries, in the first turn of the cochlea.

Figure 10.34d illustrates the visualization of the osseous spiral lamina in the base of the cochlea. This structure can easily be seen via the thin round window membrane, avoiding attenuation of the signal by otic capsule bone. The osseous spiral lamina contains arterioles, venules, and capillaries. Deeper spiral modiolar artery and vein might be accessible for measurement. This lamina possibly represents the easiest location to obtain an estimate of the quality of cochlear blood flow.

10.5
Summary

OMAG is an emerging imaging modality with clear potential in many basic research and medical imaging applications. Because of its exceptionally high spatial resolution and velocity sensitivity, it may provide useful information regarding microcirculation in a number of applications, both in clinical and basic research. For example, OMAG may one day be used to screen for vasoactive drugs, monitor changes in tissue morphology and hemodynamics following pharmacological intervention and photodynamic therapy, evaluate the efficacy of laser treatment in patients with a vascular birthmark (port wine stain), assess the depth of burn wounds, map cortical hemodynamics for brain research, and image blood flow around the eye. Quantification of the local metabolic rate of oxygen consumption would be an exciting extension for OMAG. Another interesting direction would be to combine OMAG with other high-resolution imaging tools, such as laser speckle imaging, confocal microscopy, and two-photon microscopy. The fruitful cellular and molecular information provided by these modalities, based on scattering or fluorescence contrast, will be highly complementary.

Acknowledgments

We thank many of our colleagues who have contributed to the OMAG project at the Biophotonics and Imaging Laboratory and Department of Biomedical Engineering at the Oregon Health and Science University, particularly the graduate students and postdoctoral fellows. Dr. Wang also acknowledges grant supports from the National Heart, Lung, and Blood Institute (**1R01 HL093140-01**), National Institutes of Health (**R01 HL093140-01, R01EB009682-01**, and the American Heart Association Grant-in-Aid (**0855733G**).

References

1. Hertzman, A.B. and Spealman, C.R. (1937) Observation on the finger volume pulse recorded photoelectrically. *Am. J. Physiol.*, **119**, 334.

2. Challoner, A.V.J. (1979) in *Non-Invasive Physiological Measurements*, vol. 1 (ed. P. Rolfe), Academic Press, London, p. 125.

3. Holti, G. and Mitchell, K.W. (1979) in *Non-Invasive Physiological Measurements*, vol. 1 (ed. P. Rolfe), Academic Press, London, p. 113.

4. Kety, S.S. (1949) Measurement of regional circulation by the local clearance of radioactive sodium. *Am. Heart J.*, **38**, 321.

5. Sejrsen, P. (1971) Measurement of cutaneous blood flow by freely diffusible radioactive isotopes. Methodological studies on the washout of krypton-85 and xenon-13 from the cutaneous tissue in man. *Dan. Med. Bull.*, **18** (Suppl. 3), 9.

6. Groner, W., Winkelman, J.W., Harris, A.G., Ince, C., Bouma, G.J., Messmer, K., and Nadeau, R.G. (1999) Orthogonal polarization spectral imaging: a new method for study of the microcirculation. *Nat. Med.*, **5** (10), 1209.

7. Nadeau, R.G. and Groner, W. (2001) The role of a new noninvasive imaging technology in the diagnosis of anemia. *J. Nutr.*, **131** (5), 1610S.

8. Wayland, H. and Johnson, P.C. (1967) Erythrocyte velocity measurements in microvessels by a two-slit photometric method. *Am. J. Physiol.*, **22**, 333.

9. Bollinger, A., Butti, P., Barras, J.P., Trachsler, H., and Siegenthaler, W. (1974) Red blood cell velocity in nailfold capillaries of man measured by a television microscopy technique. *Microvasc. Res.*, **7**, 61.

10. Stevenson, J.G., Brandestini, M.A., Weiler, T., Howard, E.A., and Eyer, M. (1979) Digital multigate Doppler with color echo and Doppler display – diagnosis of atrial and ventricular septal defects. *Circulation*, **205**, 60–62.

11. Iga, A.M., Sarkar, S., Sales, K.M., Winslet, M.C., and Seifalian, A.M. (2006) Quantitating therapeutic disruption of tumor blood flow with intravital video microscopy. *Cancer Res.*, **66**, 11517–11519.

12. Jain, R.K., Munn, L.L., and Fukumura, D. (2002) Dissecting tumour pathophysiology using intravital microscopy. *Nat. Rev. Cancer*, **2**, 266–276.

13. Goertz, D.E., Christopher, D.A., Yu, J.L., Kerbel, R.S., Burns, P.N., and Foster, F.S. (2000) High-frequency color flow imaging of the microcirculation. *Ultrasound Med. Biol.*, **26**, 63–71.

14. Briers, J.D. (2001) Laser Doppler, speckle and related techniques for blood perfusion mapping and imaging. *Physiol. Meas.*, **22**, 35–66.

15. Caselli, A., Bedi, D.S., O'Connor, C., Shah, C., and Veves, A. (2002) Assessment of laser Doppler perfusion imager's in vivo reliability: can it be used for a prospective analysis. *J. Laser Appl.*, **14**, 198–202.

16. Hassan, M., Little, R.F., Vogel, A., Aleman, K., Wyvill, K., Yarchoan, R., and Gandjbakhche, A.H. (2004) Quantitative assessment of tumor vasculature and response to therapy in kaposi's sarcoma using functional noninvasive imaging. *Technol. Cancer Res. Treat.*, **3**, 451–457.

17. Sorensen, J., Bengtsson, M., Malmqvist, E.L., Nilsson, G., and Sjoberg, F. (1996) Laser Doppler perfusion imager (LDPI)--for the assessment of skin blood flow changes following sympathetic blocks. *Acta Anaesthesiol. Scand.*, **40**, 1145–1148.

18. Grinvald, A., Lieke, E., Frostig, R.D., Gilbert, C.D., and Wiesel, T.N. (1986) Functional architecture of cortex revealed by optical imaging of intrinsic signals. *Nature*, **324**, 361–364.

19. Wang, X.D., Pang, Y., Ku, G., Xie, X., Stoica, G., and Wang, L.-H. (2003) Non-invasive laser-induced photoacoustic tomography for structural and functional imaging of the brain in vivo. *Nat. Biotechnol.*, **21**, 803–806.

20. Zhang, H.F., Maslov, K., Stoica, G., and Wang, L.H.V. (2006) Functional photoacoustic microscopy for high resolution and noninvasive in vivo imaging. *Nat. Biotechnol.*, **24**, 848–851.

21. Wang, R.K. and Ma, Z.H. (2006) Real-time flow imaging by removing texture pattern artifacts in spectral-domain optical Doppler tomography. *Opt. Lett.*, **31** (20), 3001–3003.

22. Yun, S.H., Tearney, G.J., de Boer, J.F., and Bouma, B.E. (2004) Motion artifacts in optical coherence tomography with frequency-domain ranging. *Opt. Express*, **12** (13), 2977–2998.

23. Wang, R.K., Jacques, S.L., Ma, Z., Hurst, S., Hanson, S., and Gruber, A.

(2007) Three dimensional optical angiography. *Opt. Express*, **15**, 4083–4097.

24. Hausler, G. and Lindner, M.W. (1998) Coherence radar and spectral radar – new tools for dermatological diagnosis. *J. Biomed. Opt.*, **3**, 21–31.

25. Fercher, A.F., Mengedoht, K., and Werner, W. (1988) Eye-length measurement by interferometry with partially coherent light. *Opt. Lett.*, **13**, 1867–1869.

26. Hitzenberger, C.K., Drexler, W., and Fercher, A.F. (1992) Measurement of corneal thickness by laser doppler interferometry. *Invest. Ophthalmol. Vis. Sci.*, **33**, 98–103.

27. Izatt, J.A., Hee, M.R., Swanson, E.A., Lin, C.P., Huang, D., Schuman, J.S., Puliafito, C.A., and Fujimoto, J.G. (1994) Micrometer-scale resolution imaging of the anterior eye with optical coherence tomography. *Arch. Ophthalmol.*, **112**, 1584–1589.

28. Clivaz, W., Marquis-Weible, F., Salathe, R.P., Novak, R.P., and Gilgen, H.H. (1992) High-resolution reflectometry in biological tissue. *Opt. Lett.*, **17**, 4–6.

29. Schmitt, J.M., Knüttel, A., and Bonner, R.F. (1993) Measurement of optical properties of biological tissues by low-coherence reflectometry. *Appl. Opt.*, **32**, 6032–6042.

30. Clivaz, X., Marquis-Weible, F., Salathé, R.P., Novak, R.P., and Gilgen, H.H. (1992) High resolution relfectometry in biological tissues. *Opt. Lett.*, **17**, 4–6.

31. Swanson, E.A., Izatt, J.A., Hee, M.R., Huang, D., Lin, C.P., Schuman, J.S., Puliafito, C.A., and Fujimoto, J.G. (1993) In vivo retinal imaging by optical coherence tomography. *Opt. Lett.*, **18**, 1864–1866.

32. Choma, M., Sarunic, M., Yang, C., and Izatt, J. (2003) Sensitivity advantage of swept source and Fourier domain optical coherence tomography. *Opt. Express*, **11**, 2183–2189.

33. Chen, Z.P., Milner, T.E., Dave, D., and Nelson, J.S. (1997) Optical Doppler tomographic imaging of fluid flow velocity in highly scattering media. *Opt. Lett.*, **22**, 64–66.

34. Chen, Z.P., Milner, T.E., Srinivas, S., Wang, X.J., Malekafzali, A., van Gemert, M.J.C., and Nelson, J.S. (1997) Non-invasive imaging of in vivo blood flow velocity using optical Doppler tomography. *Opt. Lett.*, **22**, 1–3.

35. Izatt, J.A., Kulkarni, M.D., Yazdanfar, S., Barton, J.K., and Welsh, A.J. (1997) In vivo color Doppler imaging of picoliter blood volumes using optical coherence tomography. *Opt. Lett.*, **22**, 1439–1441.

36. Yazdanfar, S., Kulkarni, M.D., and Izatt, J.A. (1997) High-resolution of in-vivo cardiac dynamics using color Doppler optical coherence tomography. *Opt. Express*, **1**, 424–431.

37. Kulkarni, M.D., van Leeuwen, T.G., Yazdanfar, S., and Izatt, J.A. (1997) Velocity-estimation accuracy and frame-rate limitations in color Doppler optical coherence tomography. *Opt. Lett.*, **23**, 1057–1059.

38. Ding, Z., Zhao, Y., Ren, H., Nelson, J., and Chen, Z. (2002) Real-time phase-resolved optical coherence tomography and optical Doppler tomography. *Opt. Express*, **10**, 236–245.

39. White, B.R., Pierce, M.C., Nassif, N., Cense, B., Park, B.H., Tearney, G.J., Bouma, B.E., Chen, T.C., and de Boer, J.F. (2003) In vivo dynamic human retinal blood flow imaging using ultra-high-speed spectral domain optical Doppler tomography. *Opt. Express*, **11**, 3490–3497.

40. Leitgeb, R.A., Schmetterer, L., Drexler, W., Fercher, A.F., Zawadzki, R.J., and Bajraszewski, T. (2003) Real-time assessment of retinal blood flow with ultrafast acquisition by color Doppler Fourier domain optical coherence tomography. *Opt. Express*, **11**, 3116–3121.

41. Leitgeb, R.A., Schmetterer, L., Hitzenberger, C.K., Fercher, A.F., Berisha, F., Wojtkowski, M., and Bajraszewski, T. (2004) Real-time measurement of in vitro flow by Fourier-domain color Doppler optical coherence tomography. *Opt. Lett.*, **29**, 171–173.

42. Chen, Z., Zhao, Y., Srinivas, S.M., Nelson, J.S., Prakash, N., and Frostig, R.D. (1999) Optical Doppler tomography. *IEEE J. Sel. Top. Quantum Electron.*, **5**, 1134–1141.

43. Makita, S., Hong, Y., Yamanari, M., Yatagai, T., and Yasuno, Y. (2006) Optical coherence angiography. *Opt. Express*, **14**, 7821–7840.

44. Choma, M.A., Ellerbee, A.K., Yazdanfar, S., and Izatt, J.A. (2006) Doppler flow imaging of cytoplasmic streaming using spectral domain phase microscopy. *J. Biomed. Opt.*, **11**, 024014.

45. Mariampillai, A., Standish, B.A., Munce, N.R., Randall, C., Liu, G., Jiang, J.Y., Cable, A.E., Vitkin, I.A., and Yang, V.X.D. (2007) Doppler optical cardiogram gated 2D color flow imaging at 1000 fps and 4D in vivo visualization of embryonic heart at 45 fps on a swept source OCT system. *Opt. Express*, **15**, 1627–1638.

46. Wehbe, H., Ruggeri, M., Jiao, S., Gregori, G., Puliafito, C.A., and Zhao, W. (2007) Automatic retinal blood flow calculation using spectral domain optical coherence tomography. *Opt. Express*, **15**, 15193–15206.

47. Zhao, Y., Chen, Z., Saxer, C., Xiang, S., de Boer, J.F., and Nelson, J.S. (2000) Phase-resolved optical coherence tomography and optical Doppler tomography for imaging blood flow in human skin with fast scanning speed and high velocity sensitivity. *Opt. Lett.*, **25**, 114–116.

48. Wang, R.K. (2004) High resolution visualisation of fluid dynamics with Doppler optical coherence tomography. *Meas. Sci. Technol.*, **15**, 725–733.

49. Zhao, Y.H., Chen, Z.P., Ding, Z.H., Ren, H., and Nelson, J.S. (2002) Real-time phase-resolved functional optical coherence tomography by use of optical Hilbert transformation. *Opt. Lett.*, **25**, 98–100.

50. Ren, H.W., Ding, Z.H., Zhao, Y.H., Miao, J., Nelson, J.S., and Chen, Z.P. (2002) Phase-resolved functional optical coherence tomography: simultaneous imaging of in situ tissue structure, blood flow velocity, standard deviation, birefringence, and Stokes vectors in human skin. *Opt. Lett.*, **27**, 1702.

51. Evans, D.H. and McDicken, W.N. (2000) *Doppler Ultrasound: Physics. Instrumentation and Signal Processing*, John Wiley & Sons, Ltd, Chichester.

52. Leitgeb, R., Hitzenberger, C.K., and Fercher, A.F. (2003) Performance of Fourier domain vs. time domain optical coherence tomography. *Opt. Express*, **11**, 889–894.

53. de Boer, J.F., Cense, B., Park, B.H., Pierce, M.C., Tearney, G.J., and Bouma, B.E. (2003) Improved signal-to-noise ratio in spectral-domain compared with time-domain optical coherence tomography. *Opt. Lett.*, **28**, 2067–2069.

54. Zhang, J. and Chen, Z.P. (2005) In vivo blood flow imaging by a swept laser source based Fourier domain optical Doppler tomography. *Opt. Express*, **13**, 7449–7459.

55. Vakoc, B.J., Yun, S.H., de Boer, J.F., Tearney, G.J., and Bouma, B.E. (2005) Phase-resolved optical frequency domain imaging. *Opt. Express*, **13**, 5483–5492.

56. Yun, S.H., Tearney, G.J., de Boer, J.F., and Bouma, B.E. (2004) Motion artifacts in optical coherence tomography with frequency-domain ranging. *Opt. Express*, **12**, 2977–2998.

57. Park, B.H., Pierce, M.C., Cense, B., Yun, S.H., Mujat, M., Tearney, G., Bouma, B., and de Boer, J. (2005) Real-time fiber-based multi-functional spectral-domain optical coherence tomography at 1.3 μm. *Opt. Express*, **13**, 3931–3944.

58. Szkulmowski, M., Szkulmowska, A., Bajraszewski, T., Kowalczyk, A., and Wojtkowski, M. (2008) Flow velocity estimation using joint spectral and time domain optical coherence tomography. *Opt. Express*, **16**, 6008–6025.

59. Bachmann, A.H., Villiger, M.L., Blatter, C., Lasser, T., and Leitgeb, R.A. (2007) Resonant Doppler flow imaging and optical vivisection of retinal blood vessels. *Opt. Express*, **15**, 408–422.

60. Wang, R.K. and Hurst, S. (2007) Mapping of cerebro-vascular blood perfusion in mice with skin and skull intact by Optical Micro-AngioGraphy at 1.3 μm wavelength. *Opt. Express*, **15**, 11402.

61. Wang, R.K. and Subhash, H.M. (2009) Optical Microangiography: high-resolution 3-D imaging of blood flow. *Opt. Photonics News*, **20**, 40–46.

62. Wang, R.K. (2007) In vivo full range complex Fourier domain optical coherence tomography. *Appl. Phys. Lett.*, **90**, 054103.

63. Bedrosian, E.A. (1963) Product theorem for Hilbert transforms. *Proc. IEEE*, **51**, 868–869.

64. Hahn, S.L. (1996) in *The Transforms and Applications Handbook* (ed. A.D. Poularikas), CRC, p. 463.

65. Wang, R.K. (2007) Three-dimensional optical micro-angiography maps directional blood perfusion deep within microcirculation tissue beds in vivo. *Phys. Med. Biol.*, **52**, N531.

66. Wang, R.K. (2008) Directional blood flow imaging in volumetric optical microangiography achieved by digital frequency modulation. *Opt. Lett.*, **33**, 1878–1880.

67. An, L. and Wang, R.K. (2008) In vivo volumetric imaging of vascular perfusion within human retina and choroids with optical micro-angiography. *Opt. Express*, **16**, 11438–11452.

68. Mujat, M., Chan, R.C., Cense, B., Park, B.H., Joo, C., Akkin, T., Chen, T.C., and de Boer, J.F. (2005) Retinal nervefiber layer thickness map determined from optical coherence tomography images. *Opt. Express*, **13**, 9480–9491.

69. Wang, R.K. and An, Lin. (2009) Doppler optical micro-angiography for volumetric imaging of vascular perfusion in vivo. *Opt. Express*, **17**, 8926–8940.

70. Wang, R.K. (2007) Fourier domain optical coherence tomography achieves full range complex imaging in vivo by introducing a carrier frequency during scanning. *Phys. Med. Biol.*, **52** (19), 5897–5907.

71. Tuchin, V. (2007) *Tissue Optics: Light Scattering Methods and Instruments for Medical Diagnosis*, SPIE, ISBN-0819464333.

72. Ren, H.W., Sun, T., MacDonald, D.J., Cobb, M.J., and Li, X.D. (2006) Real-time in vivo blood-flow imaging by moving-scatterer-sensitive spectral-domain optical Doppler tomography. *Opt. Lett.*, **31** (7), 927–929.

73. Ren, H. and Li, X. (2006) Clutter rejection filters for optical Doppler tomography. *Opt. Express*, **14** (13), 6103–6112.

74. Werner, C. and Engelhard, K. (2007) Pathophysiology of traumatic brain injury. *Br. J. Anaesth.*, **99** (1), 4–9.

75. Bouma, G.J. and Muizelaar, J.P. (1992) Cerebral blood flow, cerebral blood volume, and cerebrovascular reactivity after severe head injury. *J. Neurotrauma.*, **9**, S333–S348.

76. Guyton, C.A. (2006) *Textbook of Medical Physiology*, W.B. Saunders, Philadelphia, pp. 195–202.

77. Jia, Y., Alkayed, N., and Wang, R.K. (2009) Potential of optical microangiography to monitor cerebral blood perfusion and vascular plasticity following traumatic brain injury in mice in vivo. *J. Biomed. Opt.*, **14**, 040505.

78. Morgan, R., Kreipke, C.W., Roberts, G., Bagchi, M., and Rafols, J.A. (2007) Neovascularization following traumatic brain injury: possible evidence for both angiogenesis and vasculogenesis. *Neurol. Res.*, **29** (4), 375–381.

79. Bill, A. (1990) Sperber GO: control of retinal and choroidal blood flow. *Eye*, **4**, 319–325.

80. Jiao, S., Knighton, R., Huang, X., Gregori, G., and Puliafito, C.A. (2005) Simultaneous acquisition of sectional and fundus ophthalmic images with spectral-domain optical coherence tomography. *Opt. Express*, **13**, 444–452.

81. An, L., Subhush, H.M., Wilson, D.J., and Wang, R.K. (2010) High-resolution wide-field imaging of retinal and choroidal blood perfusion with optical microangiography. *J. Biomed. Opt.*, **15**, 026011.

82. Chou, J.T.Y. and Rodgers, K. (1962) Respiration of tissues lining the mammalian membranous labyrinth. *J. Laryngol. Otol.*, **76**, 341–351.

83. Thalmann, R., Miyoshi, T., and Thalmann, I. (1972) The influence of ischemia upon the energy reserves of inner ear tissues. *Laryngoscope*, **82**, 2249–2272.

84. Axelsson, A., Vertes, D., and Miller, J. (1981) Immediate noise effects on cochlear vasculature in the guinea pig. *Acta Otolaryngol.*, **91**, 237–246.

85. Hawkins, J. Jr. (1971) The role of vaso-constriction in noise-induced hearing loss. *Ann. Otol. Rhinol. Laryngol.*, **80**, 903–913.

86. Quirk, W.S. and Seidman, M.D. (1995) Cochlear vascular changes in response to loud noise. *Otol. Neurotol.*, **16**, 322–325.

87. Lawrence, M. (1970) Circulation in the capillaries of the basilar membrane. *Laryngoscope*, **80**, 1364–1375.

88. Millen, S., Toohill, R., and Lehman, R. (1982) Sudden sensorineural hearing loss: operative complication in non-otologic surgery. *Laryngoscope*, **92**, 613–617.

89. Plasse, H., Spencer, F., Mittleman, M., and Frost, J. (1980) Unilateral sudden loss of hearing: an unusual complication of cardiac operation. *J. Thorac. Cardiovasc. Surg.*, **79**, 822–826.

90. Prazma, J., Rodgers, G.K., and Pillsbury, H.C. (1983) Cochlear blood flow: effect of noise. *Arch. Otolaryngol.*, **109**, 611–615.

91. Selmani, Z., Pyykkö, I., Ishizaki, H., and Marttila, T.I. (2001) Cochlear blood flow measurement in patients with Meniere's disease and other inner ear disorders. *Acta Otolaryngol.*, **121**, 10–13.

92. Weille, F.L., Gargano, S.R., Pfister, R., Martinez, D., and Irwin, J.W. (1954) Circulation of the spiral ligament and stria vascularis of living guinea pig: experimental study. *AMA Arch. Otolaryngol.*, **59**, 731–738.

93. Perlman, H.B. and Kimura, R.S. (1955) Observations of the living blood vessels of the cochlea. *Ann. Otol. Rhinol. Laryngol.*, **64**, 1176–1192.

94. Choudhury, N., Chen, F., Shi, X., Nuttall, A.L., and Wang, R.K. (2009) Volumetric imaging of blood flow within cochlea in gerbil in vivo. *IEEE J. Sel. Top. Quantum Electron.*, **16**, 524–529.

11
Photoacoustic Tomography of Microcirculation

Song Hu and Lihong V. Wang

11.1
Introduction

Microcirculation, the periphery of the cardiovascular system, is responsible for supplying gases and nutrients to biological tissues. Disorders in microcirculation break the homeostasis of metabolism and may ultimately lead to organ morbidity. Thus, *in vivo* imaging of microcirculation is of physiological, pathophysiological, and clinical significance.

While optical microscopy [1–5] has been widely used to dissect the delicate features of the microvasculature, label-free microvascular imaging beyond the soft penetration limit (ballistic or quasiballistic regime) of biological tissues [6] has proved to be challenging. Photoacoustic tomography (PAT), by detecting endogenous or exogenous optical absorption contrasts acoustically, extends the penetration limit of high-resolution microvascular imaging to the optical diffusive regime [7]. In label-free PAT, red blood cells (RBCs) are usually irradiated by a short-pulsed laser beam. The resulting transient thermoelastic expansion induces high-frequency ultrasonic waves (photoacoustic waves), which encode the spatial distribution of RBCs and thus can be used to reconstruct a three-dimensional (3D) image of the microvascular structure and hemoglobin concentration [8]. With multiwavelength measurements, PAT can further differentiate oxyhemoglobin (HbO_2 or O_2Hb) and deoxyhemoglobin (HbR or Hb) to quantify hemoglobin oxygen saturation (sO_2) [9]. With improved temporal resolution, blood flow rate can also be assessed by analyzing RBC dynamics [10].

This chapter provides a comprehensive review of microvascular aspects of PAT, including system designs, imaging methods, and recent progress in biomedical applications. Photoacoustic theories, technical details of other embodiments of PAT, and more biomedical applications can be found in the literature [6, 11–13]. For this chapter, all the microvascular images were produced with a 7 ns wavelength-tunable laser system unless otherwise specified.

Microcirculation Imaging, First Edition. Edited by Martin J. Leahy.
© 2012 Wiley-VCH Verlag GmbH & Co. KGaA. Published 2012 by Wiley-VCH Verlag GmbH & Co. KGaA.

11.2
PAT Systems

PAT has two major embodiments: photoacoustic microscopy (PAM) and photoacoustic computed tomography (PACT). PAM is based on two-dimensional (2D) raster scanning of the overlapping dual foci of optical illumination and acoustic detection. According to the different mechanisms used to achieve lateral resolution, PAM can be further classified into two forms: optical-resolution photoacoustic microscopy (OR-PAM) [14] and acoustic-resolution photoacoustic microscopy (AR-PAM) [15, 16]. Instead of using time-intensive raster scanning, PACT uses a linear or curved ultrasound array to achieve dynamic acoustic focusing over the entire region of interest (ROI), with the aid of a reconstruction algorithm. Such array-based PACT systems enable real-time imaging of hemodynamics [17]; however, the image quality needs to be improved [17, 18].

11.2.1
High-Resolution PAM

In PAM, the dual foci of optical illumination and ultrasonic detection are usually configured coaxially and confocally to maximize the detection sensitivity. A smaller overlapped focal area provides higher lateral resolution. In OR-PAM [14, 19], a diffraction-limited optical focus, which is much smaller than the ultrasonic focus, provides micrometer lateral resolution within the optical quasiballistic regime ($\sim$1 mm) or submicrometer lateral resolution within the optical ballistic regime ($\sim$0.1 mm) [6, 20]. In AR-PAM, by contrast, the acoustic focus – smaller than the optical focus [16] – affords 50 μm resolution in the optical diffusive regime (>3 mm). The penetration depth and spatial resolution of PAM can be scaled simultaneously, while the ratio of the penetration depth to the axial resolution (referred to as *relative spatial resolution*) remains as high as 200, which is adequate for high-resolution imaging [7].

An OR-PAM system is shown in Figure 11.1 [21]. To ensure laser safety, the pulsed laser beam is first attenuated by a tunable neutral density filter. Then, a fraction of the pulse energy (10–100 nJ) is spatially filtered by a pinhole and focused by a microscope objective into a diffraction-limited spot (5 μm in diameter) for photoacoustic excitation. To monitor the fluctuation in laser energy, 5% of the incident light is reflected by an optical beam sampler to a photodiode. The remaining light passes to an acoustic-optical beam splitter, which is positioned under the objective to separate the optical illumination in the vertical direction and the acoustic detection in the horizontal direction. The acoustic-optical beam splitter consists of two right-angle prisms and a thin layer of silicone oil. The prism glass and silicone oil have similar optical refractive indices but very dissimilar acoustic impedances, which makes the layer optically transmissive but acoustically reflective [22]. Through time-resolved ultrasonic detection and 2D raster scanning of the acoustic-optical dual foci or the experimental object along the transverse plane, a complete volumetric view of the biological tissue is recorded [8].

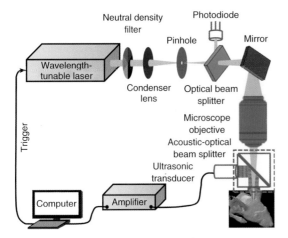

Figure 11.1 Schematic of an optical-resolution photoacoustic microscopy system.

OR-PAM, similar to other ballistic imaging modalities (confocal microscopy, two-photon microscopy, and optical coherence tomography), is strongly subject to optical scattering, which degrades the optical focusing and thereby limits the maximum penetration to ~1 mm in biological tissues. However, this limitation can be overcome by taking advantage of the "weak" acoustic scattering in tissues (1000 times smaller than the optical scattering). Maslov *et al.* [15] have developed AR-PAM, which maintains a relatively high lateral resolution (~50 μm) beyond the quasiballistic regime.

An AR-PAM system is shown in Figure 11.2 [16]. The light from a tunable dye laser, pumped by an Nd:YAG laser, is delivered through a multimode optical fiber, expanded by a conical lens, and then weakly focused into the biological

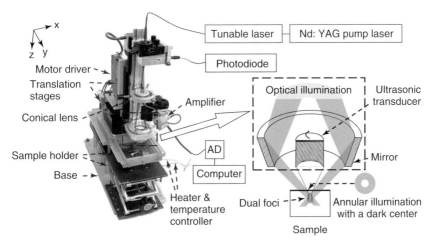

Figure 11.2 The dark-field acoustic-resolution photoacoustic microscopy system.

sample by an optical condenser. A ring-shaped optical illumination was formed on the sample surface with a dark center. The use of an optically dark zone greatly reduces surface signals and provides an ideal location for transducer placement. A high-frequency ultrasonic transducer with a custom-made spherical focusing lens is placed coaxially with the optical lenses. The ultrasonic and optical foci overlap each other to produce a confocal configuration. Note that although the lateral resolution of AR-PAM is achieved by acoustic focusing, optical illumination is still weakly focused here to enhance regional photon deposition.

11.2.2
Real-Time PACT

Although PAM offers label-free microvascular imaging with high resolution and sensitivity, its current implementation is subject to a time-intensive image acquisition process caused by the limited rates of raster scanning and laser repetition. To enable real-time monitoring of acute hemodynamics, array-based PACT has been actively studied [17, 23–25]. Raster scanning can be eliminated by numerically focusing the photoacoustic signals detected by the ultrasound array to essentially everywhere within the optical illumination. The limitation in laser repetition rate can be partially overcome by using a full-field optical illumination of the entire ROI, where a complete tomographic image can be acquired with a single laser shot.

A 512 element ring-shaped array-based PACT system is shown in Figure 11.3 [17, 24]. A pulsed laser beam is expanded by a concave lens and then homogenized by a diffuser to provide uniform incident fluence over the entire ROI. The ring-shaped array encircles the ROI to detect photoacoustic signals within the plane perpendicular to the optical axis. The universal back-projection algorithm [26] is applied to reconstruct tomographic views of the biological tissues in the detection plane. This array-based PACT system can achieve a maximum imaging

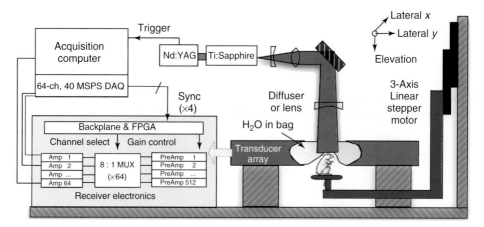

Figure 11.3 Schematic of the 512 element ring-shaped array-based photoacoustic computed tomography system.

rate of 1 fps. Improvements in the data acquisition system can further increase the temporal resolution [24].

11.3
Microcirculation Parameters Quantified by PAT

Taking advantage of the endogenous optical absorption contrast of hemoglobin– the major constituent of RBCs and the primary oxygen carrier in the blood stream – PAT can quantify important multiple functional parameters, such as the concentration of total hemoglobin ([HbT]), sO_2, and blood flow, within individual microvessels. These quantification methods form the technical core of the microvascular aspects of PAT and have been used in neurovascular and metabolic studies [9, 27, 28]. Note that PAT can also visualize the metastasis of tumor cells in the microcirculation by capitalizing on other endogenous chromophores (such as melanin) or exogenous contrast agents [29, 30].

11.3.1
Total Hemoglobin Concentration and Microvascular Structure

In the visible spectral range, hemoglobin is the predominant optical absorber in the blood stream. The photoacoustic signal generated within a blood vessel is proportional to hemoglobin absorption. However, the two major forms of hemoglobin (HbO_2 and HbR) have distinct absorption spectra, and thus the measured photoacoustic signal usually depends on hemoglobin concentration as well as oxygenation. Fortunately, in the visible and near-infrared regions of the hemoglobin absorption spectra, there are many isosbestic points (390, 422, 452, 500, 530, 545, 570, 584, and 797 nm), where the molar extinction coefficients of HbO_2 and HbR are equal [11]. Thus, photoacoustic signals acquired at such wavelengths reflect [HbT] only, regardless of sO_2. These isosbestic wavelengths are also preferred for imaging of microvascular structure because both oxygenated arteries and deoxygenated veins can be imaged simultaneously without any oxygenation-induced bias in signal strength.

The [HbT] mapping of an entire mouse ear was acquired by OR-PAM at the isosbestic wavelength of 570 nm (Figure 11.4). The signal strength, represented by the pixel brightness in grayscale, indicates [HbT]. The lower brightness in small capillaries indicates a lower [HbT] compared with that in the large arterial and venous trunks. From the microvascular structure delineated by OR-PAM, we can clearly distinguish the artery (open arrow) and the vein (diamond arrow) that form an arterial–venous pair. We can further trace the venous branching down to the capillary network through as many as 11 bifurcations (closed arrows).

11.3.2
Hemoglobin Oxygen Saturation

While an isosbestic wavelength is used to sense the [HbT], the dependence of light absorption on hemoglobin oxygen saturation is used to measure sO_2.

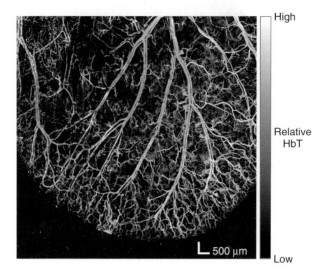

High

Relative
HbT

500 μm

Low

Figure 11.4 Optical-resolution photoacoustic microscopy
of the total hemoglobin concentration and microvascular
branching in a living mouse ear.

Multiwavelength PAT can image the relative concentrations of both HbO_2 and
HbR and consequently measure sO_2 within single microvessels.

In the visible spectral range, HbO_2 and HbR are the two dominant absorbers in
blood. Thus, the blood absorption coefficient can be expressed as [31]

$$\mu_a\left(\lambda_i, x, y, z\right) = \varepsilon_{HbR}\left(\lambda_i\right) \cdot [HbR] + \varepsilon_{HbO_2}\left(\lambda_i\right) \cdot [HbO_2] \tag{11.1}$$

where $\mu_a\left(\lambda_i, x, y, z\right)$ is the blood absorption coefficient at wavelength λ_i and position
(x, y, z); $\varepsilon_{HbR}\left(\lambda_i\right)$ and $\varepsilon_{HbO_2}\left(\lambda_i\right)$ are the molar extinction coefficients of HbR
and HbO_2, respectively; and [HbR] and [HbO_2] are their relative concentrations.
Assuming that the optical fluence is wavelength independent, we can use the
detected photoacoustic signal amplitude $\Phi\left(\lambda_i, x, y, z\right)$ to represent $\mu_a\left(\lambda_i, x, y, z\right)$ in
Eq. (11.1) and calculate [HbR] and [HbO_2] as relative values. Afterward, the sO_2 can
be computed as

$$sO_2 = \frac{[HbO_2]}{[HbR] + [HbO_2]} \tag{11.2}$$

Note that [HbT] = [HbR] + [HbO_2].

The sO_2 of a $1 \times 1\ mm^2$ region in a living nude mouse ear was mapped by
OR-PAM with dual wavelengths (570 and 578 nm) as shown in Figure 11.5. We
can clearly distinguish paired arteries and veins by their sO_2 values ($\sim$0.95 vs
$\sim$0.75). Note that the sO_2 values varied in the same blood vessel by $\sim$10% in
some specific regions (arrows in Figure 11.5), and the shapes of these regions look
like sebaceous glands. The inaccuracy in the sO_2 calculation is likely due to the
wavelength-dependent optical scattering of the glands.

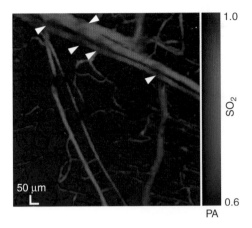

Figure 11.5 Optical-resolution photoacoustic microscopy of the hemoglobin oxygen saturation in a living mouse ear.

11.3.3
Blood Flow and Cell Counting

Blood flow is closely associated with neuronal activity and tissue metabolism. More importantly, combining the measurements of blood flow, [HbT], sO$_2$, and vessel morphology has the potential to quantify tissue oxygen metabolism with high spatial resolution. Recently, Fang *et al.* [32] reported the photoacoustic Doppler effect, where the relative motion between the photoacoustic source and acoustic detector induces a Doppler shift in the detected photoacoustic signal with respect to the source modulation frequency. They measured flow in tissue-mimicking phantoms using photoacoustics based on intensity-modulated continuous-wave laser excitation [33].

A schematic of the photoacoustic Doppler flowmetry (PADF) system is shown in Figure 11.6a [33]. Optically absorbing particles with a flow speed of v are excited with an intensity-modulated laser beam to induce photoacoustic waves. The detected photoacoustic waves undergo a Doppler shift expressed as [32]

$$f_{PAD} = f_0 \frac{v}{v_s} \cos \theta \tag{11.3}$$

where f_0 is the frequency of the intensity modulation, v_s is the speed of sound, and θ is the angle subtended by the propagating direction of the detected photoacoustic wave and the traveling direction of the particles. As shown in Figure 11.6b, f_{PAD} is linearly proportional to v. A flow speed as low as 27 µm s^{-1} can be measured through f_{PAD}.

Although the PADF described in Figure 11.6 can detect blood flows as slow as the average capillary flow, it can detect the flow only along the ultrasonic axis. Recently, Fang and Wang [34] modified OR-PAM for M-mode photoacoustic particle flow imaging, which is able to detect capillary flow perpendicular to the ultrasonic axis. M-mode means "motion mode," where the dual optical and ultrasonic foci

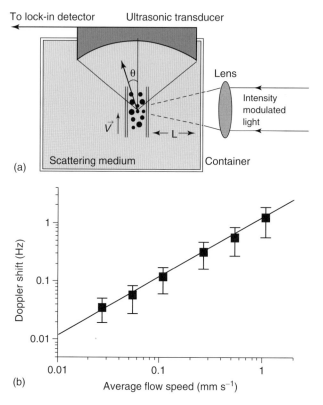

(a)

(b)

Figure 11.6 (a) Schematic of photoacoustic Doppler flowmetry. (b) Photoacoustic Doppler shift versus particle flow speed.

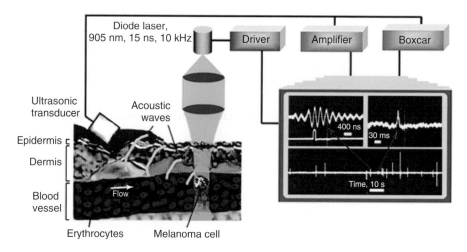

Figure 11.7 Schematic of photoacoustic flow cytometry.

are kept stationary to record the motion of absorbing particles along the acoustic axis. Yao *et al.* further extended this technology to all types of blood vessels with a concept called *photoacoustic* Doppler bandwidth broadening and applied it to measure the microvascular blood flow in small animals *in vivo* [10, 35].

The M-mode photoacoustic flowmetry that Fang *et al.* used for transverse flow measurements can also be applied to monitoring cell trafficking in the microcirculation. In photoacoustic flow cytometry (Figure 11.7), a pulsed laser beam is focused and kept stationary within a targeted blood vessel or lymph vessel, and individual cells passing through this detection point are excited and detected with an ultrasonic transducer [36, 37]. On the basis of the spectral features of endogenous chromophores (such as melanin) or exogenous contrast agents (such as nanoparticles), single metastatic cells or circulating bacteria can be detected, identified, and destroyed *in vivo* in real time [29, 30, 37, 38].

11.4
Biomedical Applications

Since PAT can image and characterize multiple important microcirculation parameters, including [HbT], sO_2, blood flow, and vascular morphology, it holds broad applications in microcirculation-related physiological, pathophysiological, and clinical studies. A few recent applications are covered here, and more applications can be found in the literature [11].

11.4.1
Longitudinal Monitoring of Tumorlike Angiogenesis

A major obstacle in tumor or ischemic angiogenesis research is the lack of imaging tools for studying the temporal features of angiogenesis in intact animals. *Ex vivo* histology requires animal termination and thus disables chronic monitoring. *In vivo* optical microscopy, such as intravital microscopy, confocal microscopy, or multiphoton microscopy, allows repetitive imaging; however, the required angiographic contrast agents may alter the behavior of the intrinsic microcirculation. OR-PAM, enabling *in vivo* label-free imaging of the intact microvasculature down to single capillaries, is ideal for longitudinal studies of tumor or ischemic angiogenesis.

Recently, we applied OR-PAM to study the kinetics of hypoxia-inducible factor (HIF)-mediated angiogenesis in a transgenic mouse model [39]. Continuous induction of doxycycline caused the overexpression of HIF-1α, a master regulatory factor of angiogenesis. Throughout 30 day HIF activation, OR-PAM clearly observed a progressive and ultimately remarkable increase in microvascular density and tortuosity in transgenic mice (Figure 11.8). By contrast, control experiments on a nontransgenic mouse evidenced no noticeable changes in microvascular morphology (Figure 11.9).

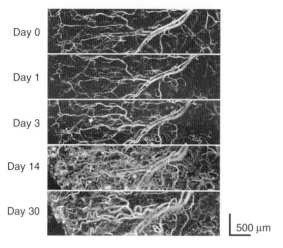

Figure 11.8 Longitudinal monitoring of HIF-mediated angiogenesis in a transgenic mouse using optical-resolution photoacoustic microscopy. Optical wavelength: 570 nm.

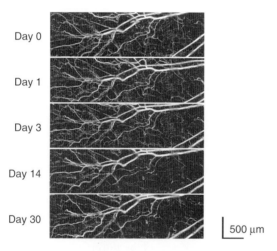

Figure 11.9 Longitudinal monitoring of a nontransgenic mouse using optical-resolution photoacoustic microscopy. Optical wavelength: 570 nm.

11.4.2
Transcranial Imaging of Cortical Microvasculature

Advances in cortical microvascular imaging of small animal models greatly facilitate the understanding of neurovascular coupling, the relationship between local neural activity and subsequent changes in cerebral hemodynamics. However, high-resolution cortical imaging through intact mouse skulls remains challenging for pure optical modalities because the optical scattering and absorption of the skull significantly degrade the spatial resolution and signal-to-noise ratio (SNR). Moreover, the invasive procedure and the required injection of angiographic agents discourage longitudinal monitoring of brain plasticity, the changing of brain function to compensate for injury or disease and to adapt to new environments. Label-free PAT provides a solution by breaking through the optical diffusion limit. AR-PAM has successfully demonstrated mouse brain imaging through both intact scalp and skull [27]. This noninvasive feature is highly desirable for chronic studies of cortical plasticity. However, its current spatial resolution (70 μm laterally) is not adequate to resolve capillary networks that are directly coupled with neuronal metabolism. By moderately sacrificing the penetration depth, OR-PAM has enabled *in vivo* capillary imaging through intact mouse skulls [9], which is favorable for chronic studies.

The label-free OR-PAM imaged oxygen gradients in the mouse cortical microcirculation (Figure 11.10). Two optical wavelengths were used for sO_2 mapping. Figure 11.10a,b shows the maximum amplitude projection (MAP) images of a 2×2 mm^2 ROI acquired at 570 and 578 nm, respectively. Figure 11.10c shows the corresponding 3D microvascular morphology, and Figure 11.10d shows the sO_2 mapping. In Figure 11.10a, the microvessels labeled with CL appear to be single capillaries. In Figure 11.10d, the red vessels (sO_2 values >90%) are believed to be arteries, whereas the green ones (sO_2 values as low as 60–70%) are likely to be veins. However, there is no clear cutoff between arteries and veins in sO_2 values; instead, the blood oxygenation of microvasculature is closely associated with its branching order and the local tissue metabolic rate [40, 41]. To demonstrate the oxygen gradients in the cortical microcirculation, we selectively analyzed a postcapillary venular tree (Figure 11.10e) and a precapillary arteriolar tree (Figure 11.10f) extracted from Figure 11.10d. A negative linear correlation between the branching order and the mean sO_2 value was observed in both the arteriolar and venular trees (arteriolar tree: $R^2 = 0.98$, $p = 0.01$; venular tree: $R^2 = 0.75$, $p = 0.14$), as shown in Figure 11.10g. The oxygen gradient in the arteriolar tree (~12% from order 1 to 4) implies that, besides capillaries, precapillary arterioles may also participate in blood–tissue oxygen exchange, while the oxygen gradient in the venular tree (~9% from order 1 to 4) suggests that a diffusional shunt is present between arterioles and venules.

11.4.3
Label-Free Ophthalmic Microangiography

Visual impairment due to pathological ocular microcirculation is highly prevalent worldwide. Fluorescence angiography, the current gold standard for ocular microvascular imaging, requires the injection of contrast agents that can cause pain, complications, or even death [42]. Moreover, the angiographic agents may fail to perfuse if there is conspicuous leakage in the pathological vasculature.

Recently, OR-PAM has demonstrated label-free microvascular imaging in both the anterior and posterior ocular segments [21, 43]. Figure 11.11a shows a projected angiogram of the iris microcirculation obtained by label-free OR-PAM at 570 nm

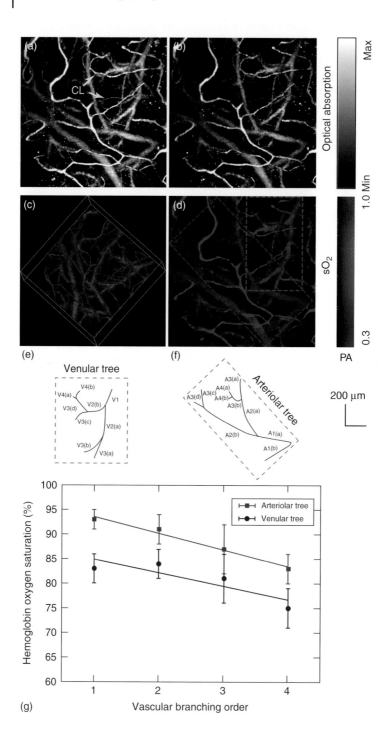

Figure 11.10 Label-free optical-resolution photoacoustic microscopy of oxygen gradients in a living mouse cortex through the intact skull. Maximum amplitude projection images acquired at (a) 570 and (b) 578 nm. (c) Volumetric mapping of the total hemoglobin concentration acquired at 570 nm. (d) Vessel-by-vessel mapping of the hemoglobin oxygen saturation (sO_2). (e) A venular tree with branching orders (boxed by blue dashed lines in (d)). (f) An arteriolar tree with branching orders (boxed by red dashed lines in (d)). (g) The sO_2 value versus the vascular branching order in the precapillary arteriolar tree and the postcapillary venular tree. The square and round markers represent the mean sO_2 values in each branching order, and the error bars stand for the standard deviations of the mean sO_2 values. The calculated sO_2 values are shown in the color bar. PA: photoacoustic signal amplitude. The scale bar applies to (a), (b), and (d).

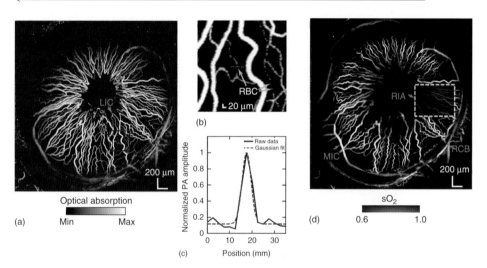

Figure 11.11 Label-free optical-resolution photoacoustic microscopy of the iris microvasculature in a living mouse. (a) Maximum amplitude projection (MAP) image acquired at 570 nm. (b) Close-up of the boxed area in (a). The arrows indicate individual red blood cells (RBCs) in iris capillaries. (c) Photoacoustic amplitude profile of a RBC crossed by the red dashed line in (b). (d) MAP image of the same region in (a) overlaid by the hemoglobin–oxygen saturation mapping of the boxed region of interest. CP, ciliary process; LIC, lesser iris circle; MIC, major iris circle; PA, photoacoustic signal; RCB, recurrent choroidal branch; and RIA, radial iris artery.

[21]. The tight optical focusing and the high detection sensitivity enabled OR-PAM to visualize individual RBCs traveling along iris capillaries (Figure 11.11b, a close-up of the boxed region in Figure 11.11a). According to the Gaussian fit of the cross-sectional photoacoustic signal profile (Figure 11.11c), an imaged RBC (crossed by the red dashed line in Figure 11.11b) was estimated to be 6 µm in diameter. Note that the laser exposure applied here was 30 times below the American National Standards Institute (ANSI) safety limit. The low-level exposure, in combination with the label-free feature, enables repetitive imaging. As a simple demonstration, the region in Figure 11.11a was reimaged in Figure 11.11d. With the focal plane lowered toward the posterior segment, Figure 11.11d better visualized the peripheral vascular structures such as the ciliary process (CP), the

recurrent choroidal branch (RCB), and the major iris circle (MIC) that bifurcates into multiple radial iris arteries (RIAs), except that the lesser iris circles (LICs) were slightly blurred. Besides the out-of-focus issue, Figures 11.11a,d show essentially no difference in the microvascular morphology, which implies that this laser exposure level did not cause any visible destruction to the ocular vasculature. In addition to vascular morphology, we further obtained a vessel-by-vessel sO_2 map of a smaller ROI with dual wavelengths (570 and 578 nm) (the dashed line box in Figure 11.11d), where we could clearly identify the RIAs, and we also could observe the transition in blood oxygenation from arteries to veins.

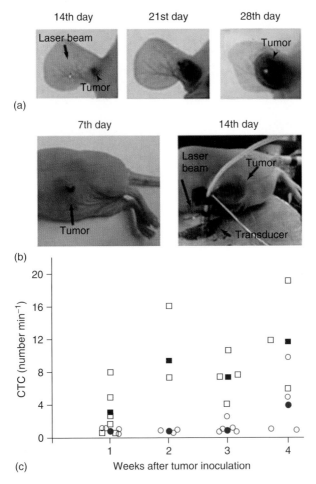

Figure 11.12 Melanoma tumor growth in mouse ear (a) and (b) abdomen. (c) The time courses of the circulating rate of melanoma cells in a 150 μm abdomen vessel after tumor inoculation in the ear (open circle) and abdomen (open square). Filled circles and filled squares are the corresponding mean values.

11.4.4
Real-Time Monitoring and Destruction of Circulating Cancer Cells

The circulation of tumor cells in the blood stream is prognostic of cancer metastasis. However, due to the limited sensitivity, conventional methods have difficulty in detecting sparse circulating tumor cells before malignant metastasis. Photoacoustic flow cytometry introduced in Section 11.3.3 provides a promising solution.

Photoacoustic counting of circulating melanoma cells has been shown in the mouse ear (Figure 11.12a) and the abdomen (Figure 11.12b) with melanoma tumor inoculation [30]. A 150 μm diameter vessel that is ~1.5 mm from the primary tumor margin in the abdomen was subject to a four-week monitoring by photoacoustic flow cytometry. One week after the abdomen tumor inoculation, ~3 melanoma cells were detected in the abdomen vessel per minute, which was likely due to migration and intravasation. Starting from the second week, more melanoma cells (>7 cells min^{-1}) were detected in the abdominal vessel, which likely indicated the starting of the metastatic process in the vicinity of the primary tumor. By contrast, there were very few melanoma cells detected in the abdominal vessel even three weeks after tumor inoculation in the mouse ear, which suggests that prominent metastasis did not occur until three to four weeks after tumor inoculation (Figure 11.12c).

Note that with increased laser energy photoacoustic flow cytometry can further destroy tumor cells. For example, after 1 h exposure to the abdominal skin vessels with a laser pulse energy of 450 mJ cm^{-2} (the photodamage threshold of the circulating tumor cells), Zharov et al. observed a significant decrease in the tumor cell detection rate, from 12 cells min^{-1} down to 0.5–1 cells min^{-1}. However, in the few days following this procedure, the circulating tumor cell count recovered back to the initial levels as new tumor cells entered into the microcirculation.

11.5
Discussion and Perspectives

PAT, capable of detecting endogenous hemoglobin contrast with highly scalable spatial resolution and penetration depth, holds great potential for fundamental physiological research and clinical care. Its primary advantages include the following:

1) Relying on the endogenous hemoglobin contrast guarantees that OR-PAM images only RBC-perfused microvasculature, the functional vascular subset responsible for tissue oxygen supply.
2) The high nonradiative quantum yield of hemoglobin enables high imaging sensitivity, down to the single RBC level (contrast-to-noise ratio is ~20 dB with 570 nm laser excitation).
3) The label-free feature and low laser exposure level enable repetitive imaging for disease monitoring and treatment evaluation.

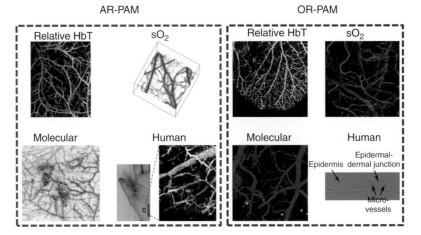

Figure 11.13 Current status of acoustic- and optical-resolution photoacoustic microscopy for microcirculation imaging.

4) Spectroscopic measurements enable functional imaging of sO$_2$ on a single vascular basis.
5) Multiparameter imaging of the microcirculation (including [HbT], sO$_2$, blood flow, and vascular morphology) holds the potential for quantification of the oxygen metabolism rate within a single modality, guaranteeing the same sample time and volume.

Currently, the two microscopy implementations of PAT – AR-PAM and OR-PAM – have achieved *in vivo* high-resolution functional [8, 9, 16, 22, 44] and molecular [45, 46] imaging of the microcirculation in small animal models. With a laser exposure level well within the ANSI safety standards, AR-PAM has further demonstrated human subcutaneous imaging [16] and OR-PAM also has shown its potential in human cutaneous imaging (Figure 11.13).

Although promising, PAT still requires further refinements in the following aspects.

11.5.1
Fluence Compensation for Accurate sO$_2$ Measurements

As mentioned in Section 11.3.2, the optical fluence is assumed to be wavelength independent during sO$_2$ quantification, which is an approximation. However, to recover more accurate sO$_2$ values, fluence compensation becomes necessary. The inaccuracy in sO$_2$ calculation due to the wavelength-dependent optical scattering of the sebaceous gland shown in Figure 11.5 is a good example.

Substantial efforts have been undertaken on this topic [31, 47–50]. However, the existing numerical models require further refinements to take into account the strong heterogeneity in the structure and composition of biological tissues, and the experimental approaches are still quite invasive and represent tentative measures. Recently, Rajian *et al.* employed a known-spectrum optical contrast agent for fluence compensation in tissue-mimicking phantoms [51]. This noninvasive method holds the potential for *in vivo* fluence compensation.

11.5.2
High-Speed Imaging for Clinical Applications

As shown in Figure 11.13, OR-PAM has demonstrated cross-sectional imaging of human cutaneous microcirculation with high spatial resolution and adequate penetration depth (up to 1 mm in the cuticle region, data not shown). However, the pronounced motion artifact during the data acquisition prevented us from getting good volumetric images. The rates of raster scanning, laser repetition, and data acquisition must be improved to facilitate an effective clinical translation.

In conclusion, PAT has potentially broad applications in microcirculation imaging, yet much effort still needs to be invested to mature this technology. We are looking forward to seeing PAT fully ensconced among mainstream microcirculation imaging technologies.

Animal Ethics

All experimental animal procedures were carried out in conformance with the laboratory animal protocol approved by the School of Medicine Animal Studies Committee of Washington University in St. Louis.

Acknowledgments

The authors appreciate Prof James Ballard's close reading of the manuscript. This work was sponsored by National Institutes of Health Grants **R01 EB000712, EB000712A2S1, R01 EB00071207S2, R01 EB008085, R01 CA113453901, U54 CA136398, and 5P60 DK02057933**. Prof Wang has financial interests in Microphotoacoustics, Inc. and Endra, Inc. However, neither supported this work.

References

1. Groner, W., Winkelman, J.W., Harris, A.G., Ince, C. *et al.* (1999) Orthogonal polarization spectral imaging: a new method for study of the microcirculation. *Nat. Med.*, **5**, 1209–1212.

2. Iga, A.M., Sarkar, S., Sales, K.M., Winslet, M.C., and Seifalian, A.M. (2006) Quantitating therapeutic disruption of tumor blood flow with intravital video microscopy. *Cancer Res.*, **66**, 11517–11519.

3. Kleinfeld, D., Mitra, P.P., Helmchen, F., and Denk, W. (1998) Fluctuations and stimulus-induced changes in blood flow observed in individual capillaries in layers 2 through 4 of rat neocortex. *Proc. Natl. Acad. Sci. U.S.A.*, **95**, 15741–15746.

4. Laemmel, E., Genet, M., Le Goualher, G., Perchant, A. *et al.* (2004) Fibered confocal fluorescence microscopy (Cell-viZio) facilitates extended imaging in the field of microcirculation. A comparison with intravital microscopy. *J. Vasc. Res.*, **41**, 400–411.

5. Wang, R.K., Jacques, S.L., Ma, Z., Hurst, S. *et al.* (2007) Three dimensional optical angiography. *Opt. Express*, **15**, 4083–4097.

6. Wang, L.V. and Wu, H. (2007) *Biomedical Optics: Principles and Imaging*, John Wiley & Sons, Inc., Hoboken, NJ.

7. Wang, L.V. (2009) Multiscale photoacoustic microscopy and computed tomography. *Nat. Photon.*, **3**, 503–509.

8. Hu, S., Maslov, K., and Wang, L.V. (2009) Noninvasive label-free imaging of microhemodynamics by optical-resolution photoacoustic microscopy. *Opt. Express*, **17**, 7688–7693.

9. Hu, S., Maslov, K., Tsytsarev, V., and Wang, L.V. (2009) Functional transcranial brain imaging by optical-resolution photoacoustic microscopy. *J. Biomed. Opt.*, **14**, 040503.

10. Yao, J., Maslov, K., and Wang, L.V. (2010) Transverse flow measurement using photoacoustic Doppler bandwidth broadening: phantom and in vivo studies. *Proc. SPIE*, **7564**, 756402.

11. Hu, S. and Wang, L.V. (2010) Photoacoustic imaging and characterization of the microvasculature. *J. Biomed. Opt.*, **15**, 011101.

12. Wang, L.V. (2008) Tutorial on photoacoustic microscopy and computed tomography. *IEEE J. Sel. Top. Quantum Electron.*, **14**, 171–179.

13. Wang, L.V. (2009) *Photoacoustic Imaging and Spectroscopy*, CRC Press, Boca Raton, FL.

14. Maslov, K., Zhang, H.F., Hu, S., and Wang, L.V. (2008) Optical-resolution photoacoustic microscopy for in vivo imaging of single capillaries. *Opt. Lett.*, **33**, 929–931.

15. Maslov, K., Stoica, G., and Wang, L.V. (2005) In vivo dark-field reflection-mode photoacoustic microscopy. *Opt. Lett.*, **30**, 625–627.

16. Zhang, H.F., Maslov, K., Stoica, G., and Wang, L.V. (2006) Functional photoacoustic microscopy for high-resolution and noninvasive in vivo imaging. *Nat. Biotechnol.*, **24**, 848–851.

17. Li, C., Aguirre, A., Gamelin, J., Maurudis, A. *et al.* (2010) Real-time photoacoustic tomography of cortical hemodynamics in small animals. *J. Biomed. Opt.*, **15**, 010509.

18. Xu, M. and Wang, L.V. (2006) Photoacoustic imaging in biomedicine. *Rev. Sci. Instrum.*, **77**, 041101.

19. Maslov, K., Ku, G., and Wang, L.V. (2010) Photoacoustic microscopy with submicron resolution. *Proc. SPIE*, **7564**, 75640W.

20. Garcia-Uribe, A., Balareddy, K.C., Zou, J., and Wang, L.V. (2008) Micromachined fiber optical sensor for in vivo measurement of optical properties of human skin. *IEEE Sens. J.*, **8**, 1698–1703.

21. Hu, S., Rao, B., Maslov, K., and Wang, L.V. (2010) Label-free photoacoustic ophthalmic angiography. *Opt. Lett.*, **35**, 1–3.

22. Hu, S., Maslov, K., and Wang, L.V. (2009) In vivo functional chronic imaging of a small animal model using optical-resolution photoacoustic microscopy. *Med. Phys.*, **36**, 2320–2323.

23. Gamelin, J., Aguirre, A., Maurudis, A., Huang, F. *et al.* (2008) Curved array photoacoustic tomographic system for small animal imaging. *J. Biomed. Opt.*, **13**, 024007.

24. Gamelin, J., Maurudis, A., Aguirre, A., Huang, F. *et al.* (2009) A real-time photoacoustic tomography system for small animals. *Opt. Express*, **17**, 10489–10498.

25. Yang, X., Maurudis, A., Gamelin, J., Aguirre, A. *et al.* (2009) Photoacoustic tomography of small animal brain with a curved array transducer. *J. Biomed. Opt.*, **14**, 054007.

26. Xu, M. and Wang, L.V. (2005) Universal back-projection algorithm for photoacoustic computed tomography. *Phys. Rev. E*, **71**, 016706.

27. Stein, E.W., Maslov, K., and Wang, L.V. (2009) Noninvasive, in vivo imaging of blood-oxygenation dynamics within

the mouse brain using photoacoustic microscopy. *J. Biomed. Opt.*, **14**, 020502.

28. Wang, X., Pang, Y., Ku, G., Xie, X. *et al.* (2003) Noninvasive laser-induced photoacoustic tomography for structural and functional in vivo imaging of the brain. *Nat. Biotechnol.*, **21**, 803–806.

29. Galanzha, E.I., Shashkov, E.V., Kelly, T., Kim, J.W. *et al.* (2009) In vivo magnetic enrichment and multiplex photoacoustic detection of circulating tumour cells. *Nat. Nanotechnol.*, **4**, 855–860.

30. Galanzha, E.I., Shashkov, E.V., Spring, P.M., Suen, J.Y., and Zharov, V.P. (2009) In vivo, noninvasive, label-free detection and eradication of circulating metastatic melanoma cells using two-color photoacoustic flow cytometry with a diode laser. *Cancer Res.*, **69**, 7926–7934.

31. Zhang, H.F., Maslov, K., Sivaramakrishnan, M., Stoica, G., and Wang, L.H.V. (2007) Imaging of hemoglobin oxygen saturation variations in single vessels in vivo using photoacoustic microscopy. *Appl. Phys. Lett.*, **90**, 3.

32. Fang, H., Maslov, K., and Wang, L.V. (2007) Photoacoustic Doppler effect from flowing small light-absorbing particles. *Phys. Rev. Lett.*, **99**, 184501.

33. Fang, H., Maslov, K., and Wang, L.V. (2007) Photoacoustic Doppler flow measurement in optically scattering media. *Appl. Phys. Lett.*, **91**, 3.

34. Fang, H. and Wang, L.V. (2009) M-mode photoacoustic particle flow imaging. *Opt. Lett.*, **34**, 671–673.

35. Yao, J., and Wang, L.V. (2010) Transverse flow imaging based on photoacoustic Doppler bandwidth broadening. *J. Biomed. Opt.*, **15**, 021303.

36. Zharov, V.P., Galanzha, E.I., Shashkov, E.V., Khlebtsov, N.G., and Tuchin, V.V. (2006) In vivo photoacoustic flow cytometry for monitoring of circulating single cancer cells and contrast agents. *Opt. Lett.*, **31**, 3623–3625.

37. Zharov, V.P., Galanzha, E.I., Shashkov, E.V., Kim, J.W. *et al.* (2007) Photoacoustic flow cytometry: principle and application for real-time detection of circulating single nanoparticles, pathogens,

and contrast dyes in vivo. *J. Biomed. Opt.*, **12**, 051503.

38. Galanzha, E.I., Shashkov, E.V., Tuchin, V.V., and Zharov, V.P. (2008) In vivo multispectral, multiparameter, photoacoustic lymph flow cytometry with natural cell focusing, label-free detection and multicolor nanoparticle probes. *Cytometry A*, **73**, 884–894.

39. Hu, S., Oladipupo, S., Yao, J., Santeford, A.C. *et al.* (2010) Optical-resolution photoacoustic microscopy of angiogenesis in a transgenic mouse model. *Proc. SPIE*, **7564**, 756406.

40. Kobayashi, H. and Takizawa, N. (1996) Oxygen saturation and pH changes in cremaster microvessels of the rat. *Am. J. Physiol.*, **270**, H1453–H1461.

41. Tsai, A.G., Johnson, P.C., and Intaglietta, M. (2003) Oxygen gradients in the microcirculation. *Physiol. Rev.*, **83**, 933–963.

42. Hurley, B.R. and Regillo, C.D. (2009) in *Fluorescein Angiography: General Principles and Interpretation in Retinal Angiography and Optical Coherence Tomography* (ed. J. Fernando Arevalo), Springer, New York, 27–42.

43. Jiao, S.L., Jiang, M.S., Hu, J.M., Fawzi, A., *et al.* (2010) Photoacoustic ophthalmoscopy for in vivo retinal imaging. *Opt. Express*, **18**, 3967–3972.

44. Zhang, H.F., Maslov, K., Li, M.L., Stoica, G., and Wang, L.H.V. (2006) In vivo volumetric imaging of subcutaneous microvasculature by photoacoustic microscopy. *Opt. Express*, **14**, 9317–9323.

45. Hu, S., Yan, P., Maslov, K., Lee, J.-M., and Wang, L.V. (2009) Intravital imaging of amyloid plaques in a transgenic mouse model using optical-resolution photoacoustic microscopy. *Opt. Lett.*, **34**, 3899–3901.

46. Li, L., Zemp, R.J., Lungu, G., Stoica, G., and Wang, L.V. (2007) Photoacoustic imaging of lacZ gene expression in vivo. *J. Biomed. Opt.*, **12**, 020504.

47. Laufer, J., Elwell, C., Delpy, D., and Beard, P. (2005) In vitro measurements of absolute blood oxygen saturation using pulsed near-infrared photoacoustic spectroscopy: accuracy and resolution. *Phys. Med. Biol.*, **50**, 4409–4428.

48. Laufer, J., Delpy, D., Elwell, C., and Beard, P. (2007) Quantitative spatially resolved measurement of tissue chromophore concentrations using photoacoustic spectroscopy: application to the measurement of blood oxygenation and haemoglobin concentration. *Phys. Med. Biol.*, **52**, 141–168.

49. Maslov, K., Zhang, H.F., and Wang, L.V. (2007) Effects of wavelength-dependent fluence attenuation on the noninvasive photoacoustic imaging of hemoglobin oxygen saturation in subcutaneous vasculature in vivo. *Inverse Probl.*, **23**, S113–S122.

50. Wang, X., Xie, X., Ku, G., Wang, L.V., and Stoica, G. (2006) Noninvasive imaging of hemoglobin concentration and oxygenation in the rat brain using high-resolution photoacoustic tomography. *J. Biomed. Opt.*, **11**, 024015.

51. Rajian, J.R., Carson, P.L., and Wang, X. (2009) Quantitative photoacoustic measurement of tissue optical absorption spectrum aided by an optical contrast agent. *Opt. Express*, **17**, 4879–4889.

12
Fluorescence and OCT Imaging of Microcirculation in Early Mammalian Embryos

Irina V. Larina, Mary E. Dickinson, and Kirill V. Larin

Proper formation of the heart and vasculature relies on a complex balance between genetic signaling events and mechanical stimuli [1–3]. Primary genetic defects that affect cell differentiation or tissue patterning can lead to alterations in cardiac function and blood flow, producing complicated secondary defects. On the other hand, defective blood flow can secondarily affect signaling pathways within cells that are required for normal development. Therefore, to characterize cardiovascular development and to understand the nature of cardiovascular congenital abnormalities, it is important to take into account both genetic and mechanical factors, such as blood flow and heart contractions.

Since mammalian embryos develop *in utero*, currently available imaging techniques do not allow embryonic imaging and hemodynamic analysis *in vivo* with high spatial and temporal resolution. To overcome this limitation, live static mouse embryo culture protocols have been developed to allow live imaging at the embryonic stages from the 6.5 to about 10.5 dpc [4]. The embryos can be maintained in culture for over 24 h to provide an access for optical imaging while the heart is beginning to beat and remodeling into a chambered pump, blood circulation is establishing, and vasculature is forming and remodeling.

This chapter describes how two optical approaches, confocal microscopy of vital fluorescent reporters and optical coherence tomography (OCT), can be used for live imaging of microcirculation during development in cultured mouse embryos. Confocal microscopy combined with fluorescent protein reporter lines gives the advantage of performing live imaging with subcellular resolution. We describe mouse transgenic lines, which can be used for hemodynamic analysis by tracking individual blood cells as well as for visualization of the developing vasculature. While confocal microscopy allows for exceptional spatial resolution, its imaging depth is limited to about 200–300 μm. This limitation can be addressed by using OCT (as described in Chapter 10), which allows 3D imaging millimeters into tissue, although at the expense of lower spatial resolution (2–10 μm). Here we describe how OCT can be applied for hemodynamic analysis in deep embryonic vessels during development.

Microcirculation Imaging, First Edition. Edited by Martin J. Leahy.
© 2012 Wiley-VCH Verlag GmbH & Co. KGaA. Published 2012 by Wiley-VCH Verlag GmbH & Co. KGaA.

12.1
Mouse Embryo Manipulations for Live Imaging

In mice, blood cells and endothelial cells are first detected in blood islands of the embryonic yolk sac at 7.5 dpc. Formation of the embryonic heart starts at about the same time. By about 8.5 dpc, the embryonic heart tube starts to beat thereby circulating plasma through the vascular system. It takes a few hours for the heartbeat to become strong enough to pick up blood cells from the blood islands into the circulation. Within the next 24 h, shear stress generated by the circulating blood cells facilitates remodeling of the vascular plexus into more mature hierarchical circulatory system. At the same time, the heart tube expands, loops, forms chambers and valves, and by about 14.5 dpc, it remodels into a four-chambered functional pump with appropriate inflow and outflow. Mouse embryo manipulation and static embryo culture protocols described below allow live imaging for over 24 h and were optimized for 7.5–10.5 dpc stages. Since these stages correspond to the most structural rearrangements of the yolk sac vasculature and the heart, the described methodology provides an opportunity for hemodynamic analysis and time-lapse imaging during critical stages of development to understand dynamic aspects of cardiovascular formation.

For timed pregnancies, mating pairs are set overnight and checked for the presence of a vaginal plug every morning (a presence of the plug is taken as 0.5 dpc). At the desired stage, the female is sacrificed and the embryos are dissected out of the uterus with the yolk sac intact. The dissection medium consists of DMEM/F-12 (Invitrogen), 10% fetal bovine serum (FBS) (Invitrogen), and 10 mM penicillin/streptomycin (Invitrogen). The medium should be freshly prepared ($\sim$50 ml per pregnant female) and preheated to 37 °C. The dissection station is also preheated and maintained at 37 °C using a custom-made heater box and a conventional heater. Freshly dissected embryos are transferred to the 37 °C 5% CO_2 incubator for recovery for at least 30 min.

It is critically important to maintain the temperature of the imaging stage at 37 °C throughout the duration of the imaging session. For fluorescence imaging, this can be achieved with a custom-built incubation system fitted around the scope, although it was found that the embryo culture technique is more robust if a commercial incubation system is used (such as from Carl Zeiss, Inc.) since it provides precise control of the temperature and CO_2 and is equipped with a humidifier. For OCT imaging, we position the whole scanning head of the OCT system inside the commercial 37 °C, 5% CO_2 incubator.

For fluorescence imaging, mouse embryos can be cultured in glass bottom culture dishes (MatTek), which have a glass cover slip attached to the microwell in the bottom of the dish. Alternatively, Lab-Tek 2-well chambers with glass cover slip bottoms (Nunc) can be used. The glass bottom culture dishes use about 3 ml of the culture medium, while the Lab-Tek chambers use about 2 ml. The glass cover slip in the bottom of the chambers allows for imaging with inverted microscopes. For the OCT imaging, the embryos are cultured in 30 mm culture dishes with about 5 ml of medium.

If embryo culture experiments are limited to a few hours, embryos can be imaged in the DMEM/F-12 (Invitrogen) medium prepared for embryo dissection as described above. However, for longer imaging sessions (such as visualization of vascular plexus formation, remodeling, and endothelial cell tracking), the culture medium should be supplemented with rat serum as follows: two parts of the DMEM/F12, one part of the rat serum, supplemented with penicillin/streptomycin (Invitrogen). Even though the rat serum is commercially available through different sources, we prefer extracting the rat serum in the laboratory. Using the commercially available serum resulted in very inconsistent results, probably caused by the traces of anesthetics used during blood extraction as well as variations in serum extraction and handling. On the other hand, home-made rat serum consistently allowed us to maintain embryos in static culture for over 24 h.

For rat serum preparation, adult male Sprague Dawley rats are used. Usually, 30 rats provide about 50–100 ml of serum. It is critically important to use ether for rat anesthesia, because it evaporates easily from the serum, while other anesthetic agents remain in the serum and can affect embryonic growth and survival. Blood is collected from an anesthetized rat through the dorsal aorta exposed by abdominal incision into a Vacutainer blood collection tube (BD Biosciences) using Vacutainer blood collection set (BD Biosciences). After the extraction, the tube is placed on ice for up to 40 min during blood extraction from other rats. The tubes with blood are centrifuged at 1300 g for 20 min, and the supernatant (blood serum) is collected by pooling. If the supernatant looks pink in some tubes, it is because of lysis of the red blood cells; discarding those tubes is recommended. The serum is centrifuged again at 1300 g for 10 min to get rid of the remaining blood cells, and the remaining supernatant serum is collected by pooling. The serum should be heat-inactivated at 56 °C for 30 min with the lid unscrewed to allow ether evaporation. For further ether evaporation, the tubes are left overnight at 4 °C with lids unscrewed, then filtered using 0.45 μm filter (Nalgene®), and stored in 1 ml aliquots at −80 °C for up to one year.

One of the major limitations for successful experiments is a sample drift over time caused by the embryo growth as well as possible floating and rotation. To prevent excessive movement and floating of the embryo, a part of decidua can be left attached to the embryo during the dissection or, alternatively, a piece of a hair can be placed over the embryo to keep it in the same position.

The described mouse embryo manipulation and static culture protocols have been successfully used for live imaging and hemodynamic analysis using confocal microscopy of transgenic embryos with vital fluorescent reporters [2, 5, 6] as well as OCT [7, 8].

12.2
Imaging Vascular Development and Microcirculation Using Confocal Microscopy of Vital Fluorescent Markers

Time-lapse confocal imaging of vital fluorescent reporter in transgenic animals is a powerful tool to analyze early development and research cellular consequences of genetic manipulations [9–12]. Several transgenic mouse lines have been generated that express fluorescent proteins in specific tissues of the embryo, for example, ε-globin-GFP expressing green fluorescent protein (GFP) in primitive erythroblasts, Flk1-H2B::EYFP expressing nuclear yellow fluorescent protein (YFP) in the endothelial cells, and Oct4-GFP expressing GFP in primordial germ cells. Live imaging of transgenic embryos carrying fluorescent markers crossed to different mutant lines expands the possibilities in studying molecular mechanisms and signaling events regulating embryonic development.

A transgenic fluorescent reporter mouse model useful for hemodynamic analysis in early embryos was generated by Dyer *et al.* [13]. These animals carry GFP under control of ε-globin promoter, which drives GFP expression in primitive erythroblasts. Blood cells brightly labeled with the GFP are first detected in the blood islands of the embryonic yolk sac before the beginning of the heartbeat. A few hours after the beginning of the heartbeat (about 8.5 dpc), when the plasma flow is stronger, the blood cells leave the blood islands and join the circulation. These events can be directly studied using this reporter in live embryo culture. Using ε-globin-EGFP transgenic mouse line, expressing GFP in embryonic blood cells it is possible to visualize the initiation of blood formation, to quantify early circulation events, and to characterize mutants with circulation defects [2, 5].

Classical point-scanning confocal microscopy is too slow to record the motion of the rapidly moving blood cells. To overcome this limitation, several groups have used a line-scanning approach where, instead of the full-frame imaging, the scanning is performed along a designated line, either along or perpendicular to the vessel [5, 14, 15]. If the scanning line is set perpendicular to the vessel, the circulating blood cells are crossing the line, the number of scans and time it takes for each cell to go across the line can be recorded. The length of the cell trace divided by time reveals the velocity. If the scanning line is set parallel to the flow, the blood cells are moving along the line and their velocity can also be measured. These techniques provide valuable hemodynamic measurements in live vessels and are still widely used, although they are time consuming since only a single line recording can be performed at a time.

The recent development of fast-scanning, line-based confocal microscopes provide the opportunity for full-frame real-time imaging of rapid dynamic events. If the brightness of the fluorescent marker permits, the Zeiss LSM 5 LIVE confocal microscope allows one to acquire 512×512 pixel images at the rate of up to 120fps. This is about 100 times faster than using regular standard confocal microscope. Since the blood flow in early embryos is in the range of millimeters per second, the dynamics of all blood cells in the field of view can be followed with superior temporal and spatial resolution for detailed hemodynamic analysis.

To visualize and analyze microcirculation in the embryonic yolk sac, image processing software Imaris (Imaris 5.0.3, Bitplane) can be used. Figure 12.1 shows an example of blood flow imaging in cultured ε-globin-GFP embryos using a Zeiss LSM 5 LIVE fast-scanning confocal microscope and Imaris processing. The imaging is performed at 10.5 dpc when the yolk sac vasculature is remodeled into a network of large vessels with high flow and branching from them are smaller

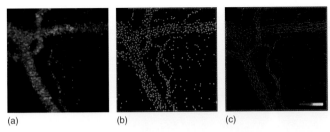

(a)   (b)   (c)

Figure 12.1 Live imaging of microcirculation in the embryonic yolk sac of Tg(ε-globin-GFP) mice at 10.5 dpc with fast-scanning confocal microscopy. (a) A frame from a time lapse acquired at 60 fps. Green dots represent individual circulating blood cells labeled by the GFP. (b) Spots corresponding to the individual blood cells. (c) Tracks formed by the moving blood cells over 50 frames. Different colors correspond to different time points according to the scale.

vessels with lower flow. An image sequence (512 × 512 pixels) was acquired at 60 fps using 10 × magnification. Figure 12.1a shows a representative frame from the time lapse with green dots correspond to individual blood cells circulating through the yolk sac vasculature. To visualize and analyze the microcirculation in the embryonic yolk sac, each distinguishable GFP-labeled cell in the focal plane was automatically associated with a spot, as shown in Figure 12.1b. This procedure was performed in Surpass mode of the Imaris software using the "Add new spots" function in the Objects window (we usually set minimal diameter of the detected spots to 7 μm). The number of nuclei-associated spots can be adjusted by changing the threshold for spot identification to include or exclude the cells that are partially out of focus. Once the spots are generated, they can be automatically tracked via the "Tracking" function in the Spots menu (it is best to use the "Autoregressive Motion" algorithm and set the "maximum distance" traveled between the neighboring images as 10 μm). Figure 12.2c shows tracks representing the dynamics of the GFP-labeled blood cells over the course of 50 frames. The color of the tracks changes from blue to white according to the timescale as shown on the bar. Quantitative statistics of the spot movements can be extracted for further analysis to reveal the heart rate and blood flow profiles in a variety of vessels at different phases of the cardiac cycle.

To visualize the developing embryonic vasculature, two transgenic mouse lines are particularly useful, namely, Tg(Flk1-myr::mCherry) and Tg(Flk1-H2B::EYFP). In both transgenic lines, the fluorescent proteins are expressed in the embryonic endothelium and endocardium [6, 16]. In the Tg(Flk1::myr-mCherry) line, the fluorescent protein mCherry is fused to a myristoylation motif (myr), which allows for membrane localization of the fluorescent protein and, therefore, outlines the structure of the vasculature and reveals cellular morphology and cell–cell boundaries between the endothelial cells. In the Tg(Flk1-H2B::EYFP) line, the expression of the YFP is localized to the nuclei of the endothelial cell to allow analysis of endothelial cell migration, division, and apoptosis. Intercrossing these markers allows identifying each endothelial cell within a vessel to reveal the distribution of individual cells within each vessel segment.

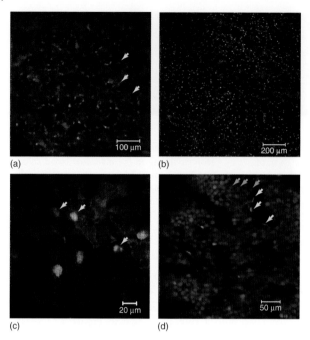

Figure 12.2 Live imaging of the developing vasculature in Tg(Flk1-myr::mCherry) X Tg(Flk1-H2B::EYFP) mice using confocal microscopy. (a) Premature vascular plexus of the embryonic yolk sac labeled by mCherry (red) and EYFP (yellow) at 8.5 dpc. (b) Remodeled yolk sac vasculature at 10.5 dpc. (c) Vascular plexus of the 8.5 dpc yolk sac at 63 × magnification in homozygous Tg(Flk1::myr-mCherry) × Tg(Flk1::H2B-EYFP) embryos. The boundaries between the endothelial cells are clearly outlined by the mCherry. (d) The vasculature is labeled by mCherry and EYFP while the blood cells are labeled with GFP (green) in Tg(Flk1-myr::mCherry) × Tg(Flk1-H2B::EYFP) × Tg(ε-globin-GFP) mice at 8.5 dpc. Yellow arrows indicate some of the EYFP-labeled nuclei of the endothelial cells; green arrows indicate GFP-labeled blood cells.

The fluorescence of mCherry and EYFP is first detectable at 7.5 dpc (also known as the *early headfold stage*) in the blood islands of the yolk sac. At this stage, the fluorescence is relatively dim and is only detectable in homozygous embryos. At 8.0 dpc, the markers label the vascular plexus as it develops in the embryonic yolk sac. By 8.5 dpc, the vascular plexus is brightly outlined by the mCherry with clearly distinguishable YFP-labeled nuclei (Figure 12.2a). Both markers remain in the endothelial cells as the vascular plexus of the embryonic yolk sac undergoes remodeling into a more mature circulatory system consisting of larger vessels that branch into progressively smaller vessels. Figure 12.2b shows the remodeling yolk sac vasculature at 10.5 dpc, labeled by the mCherry and the EYFP. Membrane boundaries between endothelial cells are distinguishable in some cells at high magnification; for example, Figure 12.2c shows a fragment of an 8.5 dpc yolk sac homozygous for both fluorescent markers at 63 × magnification. In the embryo proper, the markers are coexpressed from 8.5 dpc until late gestation throughout the vasculature of different embryonic tissues, such as the trunk, skin, brain, and eye. During late gestation, expression of myr::mCherry and H2B::EYFP decreases in major blood vessels but remains in some smaller vessels throughout postnatal life.

Endothelial markers mCherry and EYFP can be combined with the blood-specific GFP marker. Figure 12.2d shows an image acquired with fast-scanning confocal microscopy from an embryonic yolk sac at 8.5 dpc where the Flk1-driven myr::mCherry and the H2B::EYFP are combined with the GFP expressed in the embryonic blood cells. Although the imaging was performed at 30 fps, the vasculature and the blood cells are clearly outlined. While the excitation and emission spectra of the GFP and the EYFP spectra overlap significantly, they can be distinguished. In the example shown, the EYFP and the EGFP were excited at 488 nm, while the mCherry was excited at 532 nm simultaneously. The emission was detected using only two channels: BP 500–525 and 560–675. The EGFP fluorescence is detected entirely by the first channel, and the EYFP fluorescence is mostly detected by the first channel. However, since its emission spectrum is shifted toward longer wavelengths relative to the EGFP, there is some signal detected in the second channel as well. The mCherry is only detected by the second channel. This difference can be used to distinguish between the fluorophores. Because the ε-globin-EGFP transgene allows one to track individual blood cells and perform detailed hemodynamic analysis, this combination of labels provides an opportunity to study the correlation between hemodynamic and structural changes during vascular remodeling, thereby allowing a better understanding of the roles that blood flow and shear stress play in vascular formation and how disturbing these processes contributes to cardiovascular birth defects and diseases.

12.3
Live Imaging of Mammalian Embryonic Development and Circulation with OCT

While fluorescence microscopy allows visualizing microcirculation and endothelial morphology with subcellular resolution, its imaging depth is limited to about 200 μm. In the cultured mouse embryo, this imaging depth restricts the imaging to the yolk sac and very superficial layers of the embryo immediately underneath the yolk sac, while deeper vessels remain inaccessible for this methodology. Also, the imaging plane of the confocal microscope is always perpendicular to the scanning beam: as a result, if a blood vessel is not lying within the imaging plane, the blood cells cannot be tracked even with fast-scanning microscopy, since it would require changing of the focal plane position and would not be fast enough to follow the cells. For the yolk sac vasculature, it is not a problem since it is relatively flat and is parallel to the imaging plane; however, for other vascular structures, which do not meet this requirement, fluorescence microcirculation imaging is challenging. These limitations can be addressed by using OCT. OCT is 3D imaging modality with the capability to image 2–3 mm into soft tissue with a resolution of 2–20 μm [17, 18]. OCT has significant advantages over other methods such as laser scanning microscopy, which has limited imaging depth, or ultrasound biomicroscopy and micro-MRI, which allow deep tissue imaging but with lower spatial resolution, which makes OCT an ideal imaging technique for studying early embryonic mouse development.

In the experiments described here, we used modified swept source optical coherence tomography (SS-OCT) based on the Thorlabs SL1325-P16 system with output power $P = 12$ mW at central wavelength $\lambda_0 = 1325$ nm and spectral width $\Delta\lambda = 110$ nm. The scanning rate over the full operating wavelength

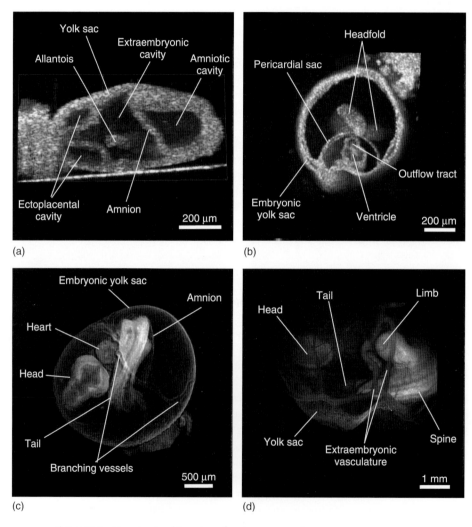

Figure 12.3 Live structural imaging of early mouse embryos with SS-OCT. 3D reconstructions of live cultured embryos at (a) 7.5 dpc, (b) 8.5 dpc, (c) 9.5 dpc, and (d) 10.5 dpc. (Adapted from Ref. [19].)

range is 16 kHz, resulting in the A-scan acquisition and processing rate of 16 kHz. The scanning head of the OCT system was positioned inside the commercial cell culture incubator set at 37 °C, 5% CO_2. The dissection station was heated and maintained at 37 °C using custom-made heater box and conventional heater.

The embryos were handled as described earlier in this chapter. Figure 12.3a–d shows examples of 3D reconstructions of live mouse embryos at different developmental stages acquired with SS-OCT. The reconstructions provided sufficient details about embryonic structures, as labeled on the panels.

Implementation of Doppler processing in OCT facilitates the acquisition of both structural and velocity information with the same spatial and temporal resolution [20]. If the direction of the blood flow is known, blood flow at each pixel can be reconstructed according to the formula [21]

$$v = \frac{\Delta\varphi}{2n\dfrac{2\pi}{\lambda}\tau\cos\beta} \tag{12.1}$$

where $\Delta\varphi$ is a Doppler phase shift calculated between successive A-scans, n is a refractive index, τ is time between A-scans, and β is an angle between the flow direction and the laser beam. An angle β can be calculated from structural 2D and 3D data sets acquired from the embryos. In the experiments presented here, refractive index was taken as $n = 1.4$.

Figure 12.4 shows an example of hemodynamic analysis in a yolk sac vessel and the dorsal aorta deep within the 9.5 dpc mouse embryo [7], when the blood flow is well established. Structural (Figure 12.4a) and Doppler (Figure 12.4b) images of part of the yolk sac and the embryonic trunk were taken at 256 A-scans per frame. Strong Doppler signals were detected from two regions. Different colors indicate opposite directions of the flow in these structures. The Doppler phase shift was measured and blood flow velocity profiles were reconstructed along the lines shown in Figure 12.4a corresponding to the yolk sac vessel and the dorsal aorta (Figure 12.4c,e). The angle between the direction of the flow and the scanning beam required for the velocity calculation was determined from the structural data sets acquired from the embryo. As expected, the velocity profiles across the vessel have a parabolic shape. The peak flow velocity across the vessels was plotted versus time (Figure 12.4d,e) and reveals the periodicity of the cardiac cycle, which can be used to calculate the heart rate of the embryo as well as to study hemodynamic changes during the heartbeat. The results of yolk sac measurements made with this system were similar to values previously measured by fast-scanning confocal microscopy [5], while the dorsal aorta flow profiles are unique for this imaging technique and demonstrate the advantage of the Doppler SS-OCT over the confocal microscopy to detect blood flow in deep tissues, suggesting that Doppler SS-OCT is an effective way to make blood flow measurements in early embryos.

Hemodynamic analysis with Doppler OCT can also be performed at early stages of circulation while blood flow is being established[8]. Figure 12.5a shows a structural image of the dorsal aorta within the 8.5 dpc embryo and corresponding

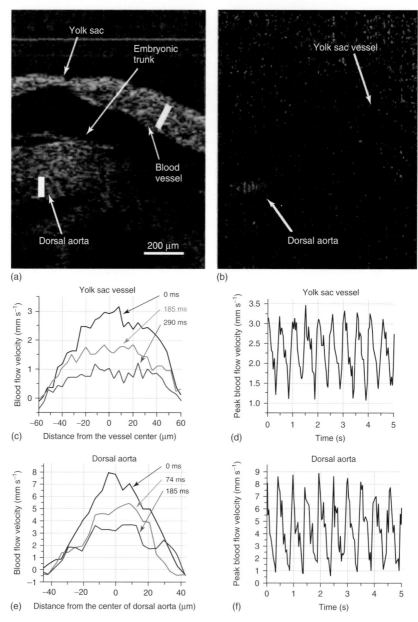

Figure 12.4 Live hemodynamic analysis with Doppler SS-OCT in cultured mouse embryo at 9.5 dpc. (a) Structural image of 9.5 dpc embryo showing fragments of a yolk sac and an embryonic trunk. (b) Corresponding color-coded Doppler SS-OCT image showing strong signals produced by blood flow in the yolk sac vessel and a dorsal aorta. (c,e) Blood flow velocity profiles and (d,f) dynamics of the peak blood flow velocity in a vessel of the yolk sac and the dorsal aorta, respectively, measured along the lines shown in (a) at different phases of the heartbeat cycle. (Adapted from Ref. [7].)

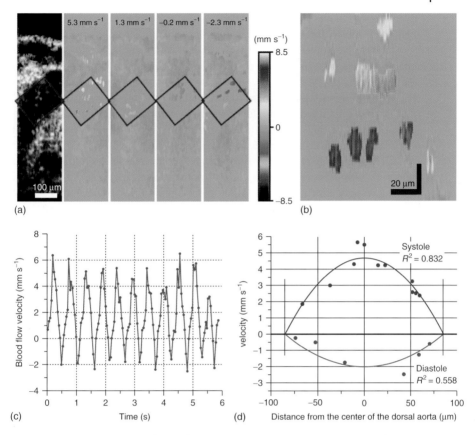

Figure 12.5 Hemodynamic analysis with SS-OCT in 8.5 dpc cultured mouse embryos from individual circulating blood cells. (a) Structural and corresponding color-coded Doppler velocity images acquired at different phases of the heartbeat cycle. Green corresponds to an absence of cells or zero velocity. Individual blood cells are distinguishable in the dorsal aorta. (b) Magnified view of the same area showing the Doppler signal from single cells as well as a small group of cells. (c) Average blood flow velocity as a function of time in the corresponding area of the dorsal aorta. Each data point corresponds to the Doppler OCT velocity measurement from an individual cell. The data points were regressed using parabolic fit. (d) Blood flow velocity profiles. Each data point corresponds to the Doppler OCT velocity measurement from an individual cell. The data points were regressed using parabolic fit. (Adapted from Ref. [8].)

Doppler velocity maps acquired at different phases of the heartbeat cycle from the same area of the embryo just a few hours after the beginning of heartbeat when blood circulation first begins. At this stage, the majority of blood cells are still found in the blood islands with limited numbers of circulating erythroblasts [2]. The Doppler velocity images were taken at 512 A-scans per frame at 25 fps. Doppler shift signal from a small group of cells as well as individual circulating blood cells is clearly distinguishable in the images (Figure 12.5a,b). Doppler velocities from all individual detectable blood cells in Figure 12.5a were measured for each acquired Doppler time frame in the time lapse. Figure 12.5c shows an average blood flow velocity plotted versus time. Dynamics of the blood flow velocity in time reveal the pulsatile nature of the flow and allow analyzing hemodynamic changes during the heartbeat. The heart rate (about 2 beats per second) correlates well with previously reported measurements at this embryonic stage, and the flow velocity values acquired in the dorsal aorta are similar to published blood flow measurements in the yolk sac at the same embryonic stage [5], supporting the physiological relevance of these data.

Blood blow velocity profiles across the vessel at different phases of the heartbeat cycle were reconstructed by analyzing individual time frames and measuring the Doppler velocity shift from each visible blood cell and the distance of the blood cell to the vessel wall. The data points for each time frame were regressed using parabolic fit. Figure 12.5d shows the data points and the corresponding fits for different phases of the cardiac cycle. Even though the profiles were reconstructed from very limited number of cells, it is clear that cell velocity is greater in the center of the vessel than near the vessel wall, and the measurements fit well with the parabolic profile suggesting that laminar flow is present. These measurements demonstrate that SS-OCT can provide sensitive spatially resolved hemodynamic measurements at the earliest stages of blood circulation.

12.4
Summary

Since the major function of the heart is to pump blood, the pattern of blood flow is an essential parameter for characterization of cardiodynamics. In addition, mechanical stimuli from the blood flow and heart contraction are as important for proper formation of the cardiovascular system as are molecular signaling events. For these reasons, live hemodynamic analysis in early mammalian embryos is a critically important tool in studying cardiovascular birth defects. In this chapter, we described mouse embryo manipulation and static culture protocols, which allow live optical imaging and hemodynamic analysis during early stages of development. We discussed two optical approaches for microcirculation analysis in early mouse embryos, namely, fast-scanning confocal microscopy of vital fluorescent reporters and Doppler OCT. These approaches provide complementary analyses: while confocal microscopy in combination with vital fluorescent reporters can be used for subcellular analysis of vascular development and hemodynamics in the embryonic yolk sac and superficial embryonic tissues right underneath the yolk sac with subcellular resolution, OCT can be used for dynamic 3D structural embryonic imaging and blood flow analysis deep within the embryonic circulatory system with resolution of single cells. These complementary approaches can be applied in a wide range of embryonic studies and can potentially answer many interesting questions about the formation of the cardiovascular system and the nature of congenital abnormalities.

References

1. Hove, J.R., Koster, R.W., Forouhar, A.S., Acevedo-Bolton, G., Fraser, S.E., and Gharib, M. (2003) Intracardiac fluid forces are an essential epigenetic factor for embryonic cardiogenesis. *Nature*, **421**, 172–177.

2. Lucitti, J.L., Jones, E.A.V., Huang, C., Chen, J., Fraser, S.E., and Dickinson, M.E. (2007) Vascular remodeling of the mouse yolk sac requires hemodynamic force. *Development*, **134**, 3317–3326.

3. Yashiro, K., Shiratori, H., and Hamada, H. (2007) Haemodynamics determined by a genetic programme govern asymmetric development of the aortic arch. *Nature*, **450**, 285–288.

4. Jones, E.A.V., Crotty, D., Kulesa, P.M., Waters, C.W., Baron, M.H., Fraser, S.E., and Dickinson, M.E. (2002) Dynamic in vivo imaging of postimplantation mammalian embryos using whole embryo culture. *Genesis*, **34**, 228–235.

5. Jones, E.A.V., Baron, M.H., Fraser, S.E., and Dickinson, M.E. (2004) Measuring hemodynamic changes during mammalian development. *Am. J. Physiol. Heart Circ. Physiol.*, **287**, H1561–H1569.

6. Larina, I., Shen, W., Kelly, O., Hadjantonakis, A., Baron, M., and Dickinson, M. (2009) A membrane associated mCherry fluorescent reporter line for studying vascular remodeling and cardiac function during murine embryonic development. *Anat. Rec.*, **292**, 333–341.

7. Larina, I.V., Sudheendran, N., Ghosn, M., Jiang, J., Cable, A., Larin, K.V., and Dickinson, M.E. (2008) Live imaging of blood flow in mammalian embryos using Doppler swept source optical coherence tomography. *J. Biomed. Opt.*, **13**, 0605061–0605063.

8. Larina, I.V., Ivers, S., Syed, S., Dickinson, M.E., and Larin, K.V. (2009) Hemodynamic measurements from individual blood cells in early mammalian embryos with Doppler swept source OCT. *Opt. Lett.*, **34**, 986–988.

9. Hadjantonakis, A.K., Dickinson, M.E., Fraser, S.E., and Papaioannou, V.E. (2003) Technicolour transgenics: imaging tools for functional genomics in the mouse. *Nat. Rev. Genet.*, **4**, 613–625.

10. Megason, S.G., and Fraser, S.E. (2003) Digitizing life at the level of the cell: high-performance laser-scanning microscopy and image analysis for in toto imaging of development. *Mech. Dev.*, **120**, 1407–1420.

11. Lichtman, J.W. and Fraser, S.E. (2001), The neuronal naturalist: watching neurons in their native habitat *Nat. Neurosci.*, **4** (Suppl. 4), 1215–1220.

12. Kulesa, P.M. (2004) Developmental imaging: insights into the avian embryo. *Birth Defects Res. C Embryo Today*, **72**, 260–266.

13. Dyer, M.A., Farrington, S.M., Mohn, D., Munday, J.R., and Baron, M.H. (2001) Indian hedgehog activates hematopoiesis and vasculogenesis and can respecify prospective neurectodermal cell fate in the mouse embryo. *Development*, **128**, 1717–1730.

14. Dirnagl, U., Villringer, A., and Einhaupl, K.M. (1992) In vivo confocal scanning laser microscopy of the cerebral microcirculation. *J. Microsc. (Oxford)*, **165**, 147–157.

15. Kleinfeld, D., Mitra, P.P., Helmchen, F., and Denk, W. (1998) Fluctuations and stimulus-induced changes in blood flow observed in individual capillaries in layers 2 through 4 of rat neocortex. *Proc. Natl. Acad. Sci. U.S.A.*, **95**, 15741–15746.

16. Fraser, S.T., Hadjantonakis, A.-K., Sahr, K.E., Willey, S., Kelly, O.G., Jones, E.A.V., Dickinson, M.E., and Baron, M.H. (2005) Using a histone yellow fluorescent protein fusion for tagging and tracking endothelial cells in ES cells and mice. *Genesis*, **42**, 162–171.

17. Huang, D., Swanson, E.A., Lin, C.P., Schuman, J.S., Stinson, W.G., Chang, W., Hee, M.R., Flotte, T., Gregory, K., Puliafito, C.A. *et al.* (1991) Optical coherence tomography. *Science*, **254**, 1178–1181.

18. Tomlins, P.H. and Wang, R.K. (2005) Theory, developments and applications of optical coherence tomography. *J. Phys. D: Appl. Phys.*, **38**, 2519–2535.

19. Larin, K.V., Larina, I.V., Liebling, M., and Dickinson, M.E. (2009) Live imaging of early developmental processes in mammalian embryos with optical coherence tomography. *J. Innovative Opt. Health Sci.*, **2**, 253–259.

20. Chen, Z., Milner, T., Srinivas, S., Wang, X., Malekafzali, A., van Gemert, M., and Nelson, J. (1997) Noninvasive imaging of in vivo blood flow velocity using optical Doppler tomography. *Opt. Lett.*, **22**, 1119–1121.

21. Vakoc, B., Yun, S., de Boer, J., Tearney, G., and Bouma, B. (2005) Phase-resolved optical frequency domain imaging. *Opt. Express*, **13**, 5483–5493.

13
High Frequency Ultrasound for the Visualization and Quantification of the Microcirculation

F. Stuart Foster

13.1
Introduction

Aberrant microcirculatory morphology and hemodynamics are signatures of many human diseases such as cancer, macular degeneration, diabetes, psoriasis, and many others. The need for noninvasive means to visualize these processes in biomedical research and clinical practice is compelling. In preclinical research, detailed knowledge of microvascular patterning and hemodynamics in mouse models of disease contribute to the quantification of both the normal physiology and that of disease progression. The systematic investigation of new therapies and combinations of therapies can be conducted to inform the development of strategies suitable for clinical investigation. From the clinical point of view, imaging tools for the microcirculation offer the potential to characterize disease progression and determine response to therapy enabling timely modifications to the therapeutic strategy. Imaging findings may also carry prognostic information that is important for patient management. In this chapter, microcirculation imaging is explored in the context of cancer, although the concepts are equally applicable in other microvascular disease areas.

For many years, the importance of angiogenesis in cancer has been clear and the rationale for the development of targeted antiangiogenic and antivascular therapeutics well articulated. In the past decade, targeting of the vascular endothelial growth factor (VEGF) pathway has shown clinical benefit in patients with metastatic colorectal cancer, advanced nonsmall cell lung cancer, hepatocellular carcinoma, metastatic breast cancer, and renal cell carcinoma. However, the results of antiangiogenic therapies have been modest in terms of survival benefit, and the cracks in our understanding of how these drugs work – and sometimes fail to work – are now evident. Most prominent is the lack of understanding of the mechanisms of action of the drugs, the inability to identify which patients might ultimately benefit from treatment, the lack of effective biomarkers to predict and track treatment response, and the development of resistance to therapy. There is an urgent need to better understand the biological underpinnings of targeted therapeutics and to design better approaches to combine therapies in such a way as to minimize resistance effects. Few studies have been carried out which take advantage of a noninvasive biomarker of vascular response both in preclinical models of targeted therapy and in patients: this chapter focuses on the development of micro-ultrasound for this role.

Ultrasound imaging systems are found in every radiology and cardiology department in the world and are the basis of hundreds of millions of clinical imaging studies each year [1]. The maximum imaging frequencies of clinical systems are typically 12–15 MHz, and they can provide resolution on the order of 300 μm at the higher end of this spectrum. In preclinical imaging, where the imaging target is often a mouse or rat, this is a serious limitation because the structures under investigation are often so small that they cannot be adequately resolved. Examples of mouse structures that fall into this category include cardiac, cancer, and neuromicrocirculations. To address this deficiency, a new ultrasound technology referred to as *micro-ultrasound* has been developed in the 15–80 MHz range. In this chapter, relevant background on the physics of ultrasound are summarized and the implementation of mechanical and linear array-based micro-ultrasound systems are described with examples of applications in the assessment of the microcirculation in mice.

13.2
Ultrasound Fundamentals

The general theory of ultrasound imaging has been well explored by many authors [2, 3]. In general, design factors are determined by three principle considerations: resolution, maximum imaging depth, and imaging frame rate. Not surprisingly, these factors cannot be considered independently but must be approached through a series of compromises. All ultrasound imaging systems rely on the propagation of mechanical (ultrasonic) waves from a transducer into tissue and the subsequent interactions of these waves with mechanical discontinuities in the tissue. At each discontinuity, a small reflected wave (scatter) called an *echo* is created and its energy is detected by the transmitting transducer. The range, z, of the scattering structure is determined by the time of flight of the ultrasound to and from the target via the simple equation

$$z = \frac{c\,t}{2} \tag{13.1}$$

where c is the speed of sound. The propagation of ultrasound in a medium implies a traveling wave for which the wavelength, frequency, and speed of sound are governed by the wave equation

$$\frac{\partial^2 p}{\partial t^2} = c^2 \nabla^2 p \tag{13.2}$$

where p represents acoustic pressure and c is the speed of sound and represents the second-order spatial derivative (Laplacian) operating on pressure. On the basis of this equation, it can be shown that

$$\lambda = \frac{c}{f} \qquad (13.3)$$

Assuming linearity, Eq. (13.2) has harmonic solutions of the form

$$p(\bar{r}, t) = \mathrm{Re}\left\{P(\bar{r}) \cdot e^{j\omega t}\right\} \qquad (13.4)$$

in which P represents a complex spatially dependent solution to the diffraction integral for specific aperture boundary conditions. A complete examination of diffraction is beyond the scope of this chapter, but $P(r)$ can be thought of as the spatial distribution of pressure arising from the transmission of ultrasound from a particular transducer aperture. It therefore takes into account the effects of focusing and propagation. Equation (13.4) is further complicated by the fact that ultrasound scanners use short pulses with significant bandwidth necessitating an integral over frequency to determine the spatial and temporal distribution of ultrasound. Figure 13.1 shows a typical low-pressure ultrasound pulse that is suitable for imaging. Note that the pulse is confined to a few cycles (Figure 13.1a) centered at a frequency of 30 MHz with bandwidth extending from <20 MHz to >40 MHz as shown in Figure 13.1b. Equations (13.2) and (13.3) assume linearity as discussed above, but when beams with high peak pressures are transmitted into tissue nonlinear effects can become important and can, in fact, be exploited to improve image quality. Nonlinearity arises from the fact that the speed of sound expressed in Eq. (13.2) is itself a function of pressure and acoustic velocity. Acoustic velocity, v, in this case is distinct from speed of sound in that it represents the actual velocity of the molecules arising from the acoustic pressure. A more accurate nonlinear representation of speed of sound in Eq. (13.2) is given by

$$c = (c_0 + \beta v)^2 \qquad (13.5)$$

where

$$\beta = 1 + \frac{B}{2A} \qquad (13.6)$$

and B/A represents the ratio of the second- and first-order terms in the expansion of the expression for pressure. B/A is often referred to as the *nonlinear parameter* in ultrasound and ranges in value from about 5 for water to about 12 for fatty tissues. Nonlinear propagation has a significant and cumulative effect on the propagation of ultrasound at relevant power levels. Essentially, the regions of compression travel slightly faster than the regions of rarefaction causing the wave to sharpen up, ultimately leading to a shock front. This leads to the generation of harmonics in the pulse spectrum. Modern ultrasound instruments routinely exploit nonlinear propagation to perform "tissue harmonic imaging" to improve the quality of ultrasound images.

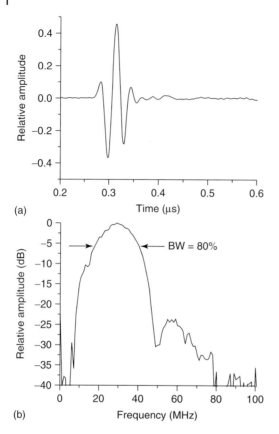

(a)

(b)

Figure 13.1 Transmitted waveform from a 30 MHz array probe measured at the elevation focus of the transducer (VisualSonics MS400). The temporal length of the pulse is confined to a few cycles of 30 MHz ultrasound, while the spectrum shows a very wide bandwidth of ~80% leading to high axial resolution.

13.2.1
Resolution

The ultimate imaging performance of any ultrasound scanner is determined by the frequency, geometry of its transducer, and tissue properties in accordance with the laws of diffraction. These issues are reviewed by Foster *et al.* [4] who described the trade-offs between resolution, penetration, and system dynamic range. The resolution of the image is determined by the beam distribution (lateral direction) and the pulse bandwidth (axial direction). Simple expressions for lateral resolution (R_{lat}), axial resolution (R_{ax}), and depth of field (DOF) for a spherical radiator at the focus are

$$R_{lat} = \bar{\lambda} \frac{\text{focal length}}{\text{diameter}} = \bar{\lambda}(f\text{-number}) \tag{13.7}$$

$$R_{ax} = \frac{1}{2}\frac{c}{BW} \tag{13.8}$$

$$DOF = 7\bar{\lambda}(f-number)^2 \tag{13.9}$$

where $\bar{\lambda}$ is the average wavelength, c is the speed of sound (1.5 mm µs^{-1}), and BW is the bandwidth of the transducer (megahertz). The ratio of the focal length to the diameter is often referred to as the *f-number*. Equation (13.7) is valid only for a focused transducer in the focal zone or for an unfocused transducer at axial distances beyond the far-field transition. Depending on the choice of frequency and f-number, the resolution can vary over several orders of magnitude. Thus, a typical clinical system with a center frequency of 5 MHz, an f-number of 2, and bandwidth of 2.5 MHz will have lateral resolution of 0.6 mm and axial resolution of 300 µm. By comparison, a micro-ultrasound scanner with similar geometry but with a center frequency of 50 MHz will have lateral and axial resolutions of 60 and 25 µm, respectively.

The frequency-dependent attenuation of ultrasound limits the total ultrasound path in tissue to about 600 wavelengths round trip or a maximum depth of 300 wavelengths. On the basis of this criterion, imaging 10–30 mm of mouse or human tissue suggests minimum wavelengths of 33 µm (45 MHz) to 100 µm (15 MHz), respectively. This range is ideal for imaging of mice and rats. Note that fixing the bandwidth at 50% results in axial resolution approximately twice that of lateral resolution but that this is only true over a comparatively narrow DOF. This leads to one of the central issues in ultrasound, which is how to sweep the focus over the entire field of view in an effective manner. Generally, this problem is solved by the use of a linear array of transducers in which the delay patterns of transmit and receive are manipulated to achieve a focus that dynamically sweeps from near to far. Dynamic focusing and phased linear arrays are firmly entrenched as the dominant technology for ultrasound imaging.

13.2.2
Reflectivity and Signal Strength

Signal strength or brightness in ultrasound images is determined by the reflectivity of the tissues being imaged. From a theoretical point of view, prediction of the reflected signal requires solution of the inhomogeneous wave equation and detailed knowledge of the mechanical properties of tissue. In particular, the acoustic impedance, Z, defined as the product of density and speed of sound

$$Z = \rho_0 c \tag{13.10}$$

is critical in determining reflectivity. In general, two regimes are important: (i) reflection at surfaces with dimensions $\gg \lambda$ and (ii) situations where the reflector dimension is $\ll \lambda$. The latter situation is referred to as *Rayleigh scatter*. In regime 1, ultrasound waves are reflected from large interfaces such as that between the liver and kidney and are governed by a reflection coefficient defined by

$$R = \frac{(Z_2 - Z_1)}{(Z_2 + Z_1)} \tag{13.11}$$

where Z_2 and Z_1 are the acoustic impedances of the tissues forming the interface. In soft tissues, values of the reflection coefficient are in the range of ~ 0.0001–0.1 but can become very significant in the presence of bone or air. In the scatter regime, reflectivity is more complex. In the simplest situation (Rayleigh scatter), the scattered pressure from a solid sphere of radius a is given by

$$D_{(\varphi)} = \frac{k^2 a^3}{3} \left(\frac{\kappa - \kappa_0}{\kappa_0} + \frac{3\rho - 3\rho_0}{2\rho + \rho_0} \mathrm{Cos}\varphi \right) \tag{13.12}$$

where k is the wave number in the medium, κ is the compressibility of the particle, and φ is the scattering angle. Not surprisingly, the amplitude of the pressure scattered by a small sphere is strongly dependent on size, frequency (via k), compressibility, density, and scattering angle. Red blood cells are generally considered to be Rayleigh scatterers, but this assumption begins to break down at some of the higher frequencies discussed here.

13.2.3
Doppler Quantification of Blood Flow

Ultrasound is well established as a means of measuring blood flow or, more precisely, blood velocity using the Doppler principle. Scattering of ultrasound from moving red blood cells leads to a shift in the frequency of scattered ultrasound in comparison to the frequency of the insonifying pulse. The expression for velocity of blood flow, v, is given by

$$v = \frac{f_{\mathrm{d}}\, c}{(2 f_0\, \mathrm{Cos}(\theta))} \tag{13.13}$$

where f_{d} is the Doppler frequency shift, f_0 is the insonifying frequency, c is the local speed of sound, and θ is the angle between the axis of beam propagation and the flow velocity vector. Doppler information may be displayed in a variety of ways to contribute functional information on the flow of blood in the vascular system. Pulsed Doppler is used to display blood velocity as a function of time (the Doppler waveform) at a particular location in space. This is very useful for the detailed evaluation of local hemodynamics but is not helpful for mapping the vasculature. To perform this function, the display of the average velocity calculated on a pixel-by-pixel basis using Doppler estimators is performed. The latter mapping is referred to as *color flow* imaging. Since velocity is a vector, color flow images are encoded with flow toward the transducer represented in shades of red and flow away from the transducer in shades of blue. Another important display method involves integrating the power in the Doppler spectrum for each pixel and displaying this information as a "Power Doppler" image. Such displays are linearly proportional to blood volume and are displayed on an orange to yellow scale superimposed on the grayscale ultrasound image.

Early work demonstrating Doppler detection of blood flow changes with breast tumors began 20 years ago. Since then, attempts have been made to correlate conventional ultrasound Doppler findings with tumor stage and/or patient prognosis. It is, however, clear that these methods are sensitive only to large vessel flow, that is, arterioles and venules larger than about 50 μm. This situation has recently changed with the introduction of three important innovations in the field of ultrasound imaging: (i) the development of a generation of new microbubble (MB) contrast agents, (ii) the development of new nonlinear signal processing tools to permit effective separation and display of the echo from the microvascular pool, and (iii) the development of micro-ultrasound and high-frequency Doppler, which enable noninvasive imaging of microscopic structure and blood flow with unprecedented spatial resolution.

13.3
Instrumentation

The growing demand for imaging tools in the biological community led to successful commercialization of micro-ultrasound in the early 2000s [5] (Figure 13.2a). These systems were based on mechanically scanned single-element transducers operating in the 15–80 MHz range and provided resolution in the

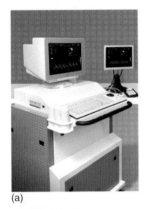

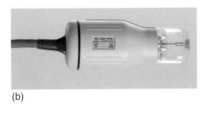

(b)

(a)

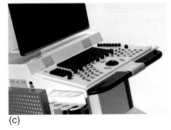

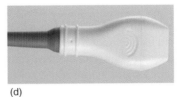

(c)   (d)

Figure 13.2 High frequency micro-ultrasound imaging systems developed over the past 10 years have enabled effiecient, high resolution, quantitative analysis of animal models of disease. Earlier systems (a) relied on mechanically steered single element scanheads (b). More recently, fully beamformed scanners (c) have been developed using novel high frequency arrays (d). The latter devices use no mechanical actuation and improve the depth of field of the imaging system.

40–200 µm range depending on frequency and aperture configuration according to Eqs. (13.7–13.9). Photographs of the scanner and scanhead of the mechanical scanner are given in Figure 13.2a and b, respectively. The scanhead contains the high-frequency transducer in a sealed liquid-filled compartment that is coupled to the mouse skin using an ultrasound gel. Remarkably, these probes were capable of reaching frame rates in excess of 100 Hz. Several hundred peer-reviewed papers using the single-element-scanned micro-ultrasound platform have now been published. Overviews related to applications of micro-ultrasound in developmental biology in mice are available [6–10] in the area of cardiovascular research [11–14] and in the area of cancer [15–19]. While single-element systems have fared well in the market, they suffer from serious limitations in DOF. This is due to the fact that the single transducer has a fixed focus in space analogous to a camera with a fixed focus lens. In addition, single elements are limited in their ability to provide functional maps of Doppler blood flow in real time and in their ability to image contrast agents. In 2009, systems based on linear transducer array technology were finally introduced to solve these problems [20]. Arrays offer the flexibility to change the point of focus electronically as the ultrasound propagates back to the sensor thus extending the DOF. The new imaging technology was commercialized by VisualSonics and enables the frequency of systems based on linear transducer arrays to be extended from 15 MHz to above 50 MHz. Photographs of the linear array instrument and scanhead that currently defines the field of micro-ultrasound imaging are shown in Figure 13.2c and d, respectively.

13.3.1
Imaging Protocols

Animals studied under approved protocols are positioned on an imaging platform that presents the region to be imaged to a scanhead rigidly attached to a mechanical positioning system as shown in Figure 13.3a. This allows hands-free positioning and capture of the images. The animal is first anesthetized using a 2% isoflurane mixture in oxygen or air, and hair (if present) is removed using a depilatory cream. The mouse is then restrained on the heated imaging platform with surgical tape to maintain normal body temperature of the animal during imaging. A warmed ultrasonic gel is applied to the mouse's skin to couple the scanhead and imaging commences. Key physiological parameters are captured from the platform including heart rate, temperature, respiration, and ECG. These signals are gathered through paw and temperature probes and integrated with the real-time micro-ultrasound images. A typical imaging configuration is illustrated in Figure 13.3a in which the system operator has a mouse on the imaging platform with required instrumentation. A flexible but lockable arm holds the transducer adjacent to the tissue to be imaged. In the background, the anesthesia delivery, induction chamber, and monitoring equipment are shown on the right. Images such as the one shown in Figure 13.3b show the results of an upper abdominal image of an adult mouse. The depiction of organs and other vascular structures is remarkably similar to human images made at much lower frequencies. Visible are

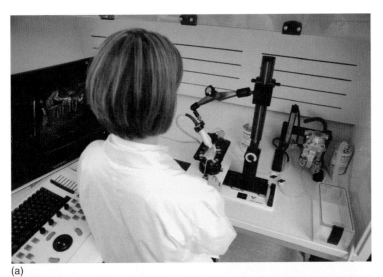

(a)

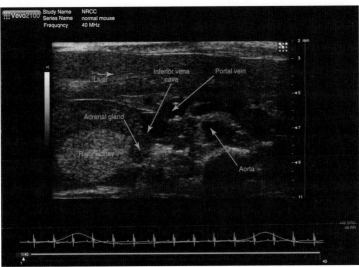

(b)

Figure 13.3 (a) The imaging system of Figure 13.2c being used to image a mouse. The mouse is anesthetized and lying on a heated stage and is monitored for heart rate, breathing, and, in some cases, blood pressure. Scanning is preformed after removal of hair (if necessary) and after the application of a heated gel to the region of interest. The Ultrasound scanhead is mounted on a "Rail System" inside a biosafety cabinet to reduce jitter in the image due to hand motion. (b) Example of a still frame from a real-time sequence of images of the abdominal region of the mouse. This "B-scan" image shows, from left to right, a section through the kidney, adrenal gland, the vena cava, portal vein, and the aorta.

the overlying liver, the right kidney, adrenal gland, vena cava, aorta, and portal vein. An additional accessory to the imaging platform is an injection mount that allows for the guidance of precise injections or biopsies *in vivo* through the real-time imaging guidance of the micro-ultrasound system. For ultrasound contrast and targeted imaging studies (described in detail in Section 13.3.2), MB agents such as MicroMarker (VisualSonics, Toronto) or Definity (Lantheus, Montreal) can be reconstituted according to manufacturer's specifications and injected via tail vein in volumes that typically do not exceed 100 μl.

13.3.2
Microbubble Contrast Agents

The introduction of ultrasound MB contrast agents has created a significant opportunity for visualization of the microcirculation [21, 22]. Recent reviews of the physics and imaging modes for contrast ultrasound are given by Ferrara *et al.* [23] and Borden *et al.* [24]. Current generations of these agents consist of MBs, which range in diameter from <1 to 5 μm, rendering them suitable for intravenous injection. A typical contrast agent consists of a thin flexible or rigid shell composed of albumin, lipid, or polymer confining a gas such as nitrogen, or a perfluorocarbon. The choice of shell and gas has an important influence on the properties of the agent. While Eq. (13.5) indicates that nonlinear propagation of ultrasound results in the creation of harmonics, scatter from MBs is governed by somewhat more complex interactions that result in the creation of other spectral features unique to MBs. The radial motion of the wall of an MB under insonation is most often described by the Rayleigh–Plesset or Keller–Miksis equations as described in [23]. It is a fortunate coincidence of nature that insonation in the MHz frequency range excites bubble resonance due to the compressible nature of the gas inside the bubble. The frequency of this resonance is a function of the gas properties and the shear modulus of the MB shell given by

$$f_0 = \frac{1}{2\pi a_e} \sqrt{\frac{3\kappa p_0 + 12 G_s \dfrac{d_{Se}}{a_e}}{\rho_L}} \tag{13.14}$$

where f_0 is the resonant frequency, a_e is the equilibrium bubble radius, κ is the polytropic exponent of the gas, p_0 is the atmospheric pressure, G_s and d_S are the shear modulus and thickness of the shell, respectively, and ρ_L is the density of the surrounding liquid [25]. With increased incident amplitudes, the bubbles can be driven to oscillate asymmetrically resulting in the scattering of energy to harmonic multiples of the transmit frequency (f_0) and to noninteger multiples of the fundamental such as $1/2f_0$, $3/2f_0$, $5/2f_0$, and so on. The component at $1/2$ the fundamental is referred to as the *subharmonic*, while the other noninteger harmonics are referred to as *ultraharmonics*.

The challenge of MB contrast imaging has been to develop specific pulse sequences and signal processing that maximize detection efficiency for signals arising from MBs while suppressing signals arising from tissue or nonlinear propagation. This has generally required the development of pulse sequences in which the phase difference and amplitude of the insonifying pulse is manipulated to suppress or enhance particular linear and nonlinear components. For example, one conceptually simple approach to separate linear from nonlinear signals is to send an ultrasound pulse like the one in Figure 13.1a followed by a second identical pulse shifted in phase by 180°. When the echoes from these experiments are subtracted, the result is zero for linear scatter and nonzero for nonlinear scatter. This technique, known as *pulse inversion imaging*, was developed by Hope-Simpson and colleagues [26] and is now a standard approach on clinical instruments. Techniques such as harmonic imaging [27] and pulse inversion [26] exploit the second harmonic ($2f_0$) to provide greater contrast with respect to the surrounding tissue. Burns and Hope-Simpson [28] patented the concept of combining phase and amplitude processing for optimized nonlinear contrast imaging and Doppler. This idea was further refined by Haider and Chiao [29] and evolved into commercially available contrast pulse sequences (CPSs). Eckersley *et al.* [30] showed that phase and amplitude modulation (PIAM) provided 14–18 dB enhancement of contrast signals over linear scatterers for insonifying pulses having a center frequency of 2.5 MHz. The detection of energy in the subharmonic and ultraharmonic frequency range has also been explored by a number of investigators [31–35] and is of particular interest because these signals arise only from MB interactions. At diagnostic frequencies, PIAM processing retains an advantage over subharmonic imaging in that resolution is not compromised. In the micro-ultrasound frequency range, Needles *et al.* have shown optimal contrast imaging with amplitude modulation approaches [36]. Figure 13.4 shows vials of commercially available MicroMarker contrast available from VisualSonics (Figure 13.4a) and a dark field micrograph of Definity (Lantheus Medical Imaging) showing MB sizes from 1 to ~5 μm.

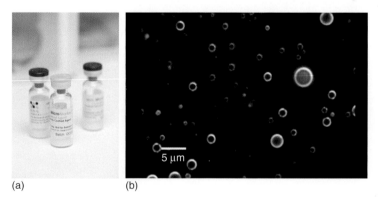

(a)   (b)

Figure 13.4 Effective blood pool tracers consisting of lipid encapsulated gas microbubbles (MBs) have been developed for clinical and preclinical ultrasound imaging over the past several decades. (a) MicroMarker contrast (VisualSonics) was developed specifically for use in mice. It has average particle size of about 2 μm and is injected intravenously in very small quantities of 50 μl containing ~10^7 MBs. (b) Dark field microscopy of microbubbles in solution.

13.4
Applications of Micro-Ultrasound in Studies of the Microcirculation

Doppler approaches enable visualization of vessels down to about 50 μm depending on frequency as described in Section 13.2.3. This information can be displayed in a number of formats including pulsed Doppler, color Doppler, and power Doppler. Pulsed Doppler is a measurement at a particular spatial location in which blood velocity is measured as a function of time. Therefore, it reports mainly on the hemodynamics of flow. Color Doppler encodes the mean velocity of flow and is presented as a color overlay on top of the grayscale image of anatomy. Flow toward the transducer is usually encoded in shades of red and flow away in shades of blue. Finally, power Doppler reports the integral of Doppler power and is a reflection of the number of moving scatterers (red blood cells) and is therefore a representation of blood volume. An example of a color flow and pulsed Doppler study of a mouse kidney is given in Figure 13.5. Here, a color flow image (scout image) clearly differentiates the renal vein and artery by means of its ability to color code flow direction and average velocity. By placing a cursor in the renal artery and aligning a direction vector with the flow axis, accurate flow velocity estimates based on Eq. (13.13) can be made and automatically displayed in a dynamic plot of the pulsed

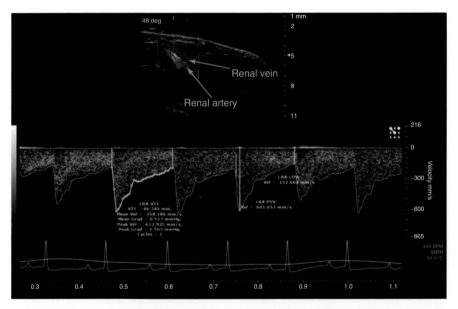

Figure 13.5 Color flow imaging (scout image above) clearly differentiates the renal vein of a mouse and artery by means of its ability to color code flow direction and average velocity. By placing a cursor in the renal artery and aligning a direction vector with the flow axis, accurate flow velocity estimates can be made and automatically displayed in a dynamic plot of the "Doppler" waveform. Here, the peak velocity is ~600 mm s^{-1}. Further analysis based on waveform measurements can then determine important indices that reflect the health of the organ.

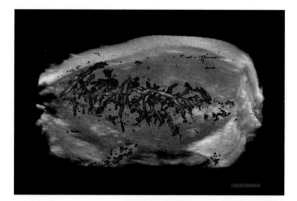

Figure 13.6 Three-dimensional image of an experimental tumor (KHT) growing in a mouse. Quantitative volumetric information is provided by the 3D image, while the morphology of the vascular supply is mapped by 3D power Doppler. Power Doppler reveals the vessels as small as 50–100 μm but does not show flow in the capillary microcirculation. Bar = 1 mm.

Doppler waveform. Here, the peak velocity is ~600 mm s^{-1}. Further analysis based on waveform measurements can then determine important indices that reflect the health of the organ. In Figure 13.6, a three-dimensional power Doppler image of an experimental tumor (KHT fibrosarcoma) growing in a mouse is given. The 3D image maps the morphology of the vascular supply to the tumor. Power Doppler reveals the vessels as small as 50–100 μm but does not show flow in the capillary microcirculation.

Doppler imaging tools for the microcirculation offer the potential to characterize disease progression and determine response to therapy, enabling timely modifications to the therapeutic strategy. A key component of studying cancer in

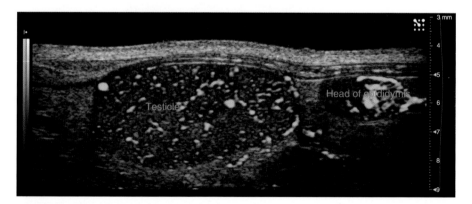

Figure 13.7 Power Doppler of a mouse testicle after injection of 50 μl of microbubble contrast agent shows a complex pattern of microvascular flow in the testis and head of the epididymis.

animal models is understanding how specific drugs affect angiogenesis. Studies by Goertz *et al.* [37] reported the first use of high-frequency micro-ultrasound 2D Power Doppler in studying the effects of an antivascular drug on blood flow. The authors reported a significant reduction in blood flow in superficial human melanoma MeWo tumors 4 h after injection of the tumor vascular targeting agent ZD6126 followed by a recovery of flow by 24 h after injection. Jugold and colleagues [38] investigated the effects of blocking VEGF-mediated pathways using a VEGF-R2 blocking antibody treatment. Using Power Doppler imaging, this study showed that after six days of treatment in subcutaneous tumors (spontaneously immortalized human skin keratinocytes) in nude mice, tumor vascularity significantly decreased. The studies of anti-VEGFR-2 treatment in MDA-MB-231 breast cancer tumors by

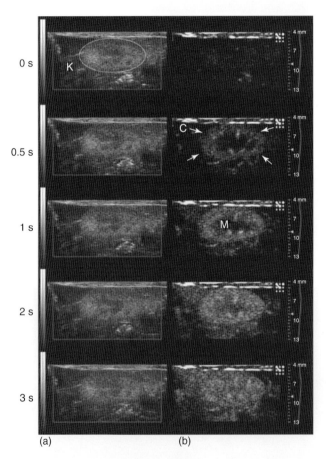

Figure 13.8 Nonlinear contrast imaging sequence at various instants during a contrast agent bolus in a female mouse kidney (K). B-mode images of the kidney (a) are displayed side by side with the nonlinear contrast images (b). At time zero, no contrast agent is present in the imaging plane. By 0.5 s, the cortex (C) of the kidney begins to fill with agent. After 1–2 s, the medulla (M) begins to fill, and by 3 s, the peak of the bolus enhancement has been reached. (Source: From Needles *et al.* [36] with permission).

Franco *et al.* concluded that sustained hypoxia and impaired vascular function were consistent findings in this model. The administration of antiangiogenic agents or signal blocking molecules does not always result in decreases of flow. Qayum *et al.* [39] showed this in a fibrosarcoma model following treatments that blocked oncogenic signaling molecules such as EGFR, PI3K, RAS, and AKT. Their work showed prolonged, durable enhancement of tumor vascular flow. This is relevant for treatment in that it may be desirable to increase flow to facilitate chemotherapeutic therapy. Olive *et al.* [18] examined this hypothesis in a study in which Gemcitabine was coadministered with a Hedgehog signaling inhibitor (IPI-926) in a mouse model of pancreatic cancer. Micro-ultrasound validated increases in perfusion and disease stabilization using this approach. Shaked *et al.* [19] used micro-ultrasound to examine a therapy consisting of sequential use of a vascular targeting agent (Oxy-4503, Oxygene Inc.) and anti-VEGFR-2 therapy (DC101, Imclone Inc.). Their results showed that the use of the antiangiogenic agent post antivascular treatment significantly impaired recruitment of circulating endothelial cells and subsequent revascularization of the tumor periphery. Micro-ultrasound is playing an increasing role in these evaluations of combination therapies.

13.4.1
Contrast Imaging

Following the imaging protocol of Section 13.3.1, the injection of contrast enables the visualization of the microcirculation right down to the capillaries. Processing of the contrast data to extract the contrast signal reveals details of the microcirculation as illustrated for a mouse testicle in Figure 13.7. Often, it is of interest to examine

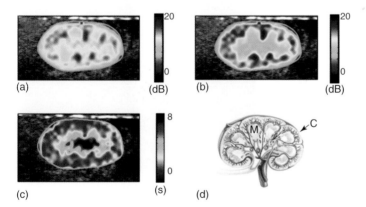

Figure 13.9 Parametric images of the whole mouse kidney depicting spatial variations in (a) peak enhancement, (b) wash-in rate, (c) and rise time. The images correlate visually with an anatomical illustration of the kidney (d), which differentiates the highly vascularized outer cortex region (C) from the inner pyramids, which collectively form the medulla region (M). (Source: From Needles *et al.* [36] with permission). Source: Copyright 2001 Benjamin Cummings, an imprint of Addison Wesley Longman, Inc.

the time course of contrast wash-in as this enables measurement of important aspects of the microcirculation such as relative perfusion and blood volume. An example of a wash-in in a mouse kidney following injection of MicroMarker contrast is given in Figure 13.8. Here, the filling of the kidney is observed with 20 MHz micro-ultrasound using an MS250 linear probe in nonlinear contrast mode as described by Needles *et al.* [36]. Over a 3 s period, contrast first fills the cortex and subsequently the medulla resulting in a more or less uniformly perfused organ. Further analysis on a pixel-by-pixel basis enables the creation of images that represent aspects of the wash-in curve. Generally, the slope of the wash-in is considered to be proportional to local perfusion, and the peak or plateau of this curve is proportional to blood volume. Figure 13.9 shows the analysis of the image data of Figure 13.8 analyzed in this manner. Overlaying the maximum slope and peak wash-in signal on the original grayscale image results in a "parametric"

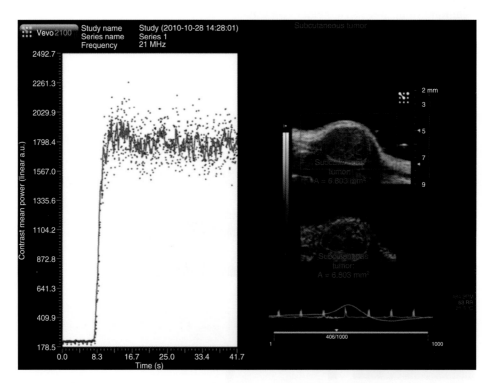

Figure 13.10 Tracing a region of interest allows the "wash-in" kinetics of contrast administration to be quantified. In this case, a small breast cancer tumor is under study. The vertical scale on left is detected microbubble power recorded inside the region of interest outlined in magenta on the images. The upper image is a B-scan through the center of the tumor, while, in the image below, the nonlinear signal from the contrast is displayed. The slope of the wash-in curve reflects the perfusion of the tissue, while the plateau is proportional to blood volume. The signals at bottom are the mouse's ECG (green) and breathing (olive) recordings.

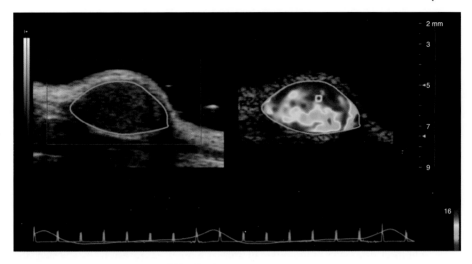

Figure 13.11 A parametric map of blood volume is superimposed over the grayscale image of this tumor. These maps readily reveal the heterogeneity of blood volume in this tumor.

image of perfusion and blood volume, respectively. Figure 13.9 shows significant differences in parametric behavior between the cortex and medulla of the kidney.

Contrast imaging can be effectively applied to cancer models in the mouse as well. This allows the noninvasive assessment of relative perfusion and blood volume without the need for tissue extraction, immunohistochemical staining, and vessel counting. An example of B-mode, and nonlinear contrast images of a mouse baring a Lewis Lung carcinoma, is given in Figure 13.10. The contrast image (lower panel) results from injection of 80 µl of Micromarker contrast into the tail vein of the mouse. Imaging is performed with a Vevo 2100 scanner using nonlinear contrast mode at 20 MHz. In this case, the kinetics show a rapid wash-in followed by a plateau in contrast intensity. A parametric image of another tumor is shown in Figure 13.11. In this case, the heterogeneity of blood volume is evident. The value of being able to report relative changes in perfusion and blood volume lies in the interpretation of biological responses to new therapies designed to manipulate the angiogenic microcirculations of growing tumors. The investigation of the effects of receptor tyrosine kinase inhibitors such as Sunitinib (Pfizer), antibodies such as Bevacizamab (Genentech), low-dose chemotherapy, and other antiangiogenic treatments are underway in many laboratories.

13.5
Conclusions

Micro-ultrasound has rapidly developed as a preclinical imaging technology over the past decade. This technology enables anatomical and functional aspects of the microcirculation to be visualized and quantified. The mechanical and array ultrasound technologies reported here extend the bandwidth of high-performance ultrasound imaging from 15 to over 50 MHz enabling significant improvement in resolution and image quality for preclinical applications. The established value of the mechanical high-frequency imaging systems is now augmented by new systems based on a 256 element linear array configuration with a 64 channel beamformer (Figure 13.2c,d). The architecture of the transducer and beamformer enable beam profiles that approach the diffraction limit and ensure high image quality. One of the major advances associated with the development of the high-frequency array-based micro-ultrasound is the ability to perform real-time color and power Doppler as demonstrated in Figures 13.5 and 13.6. The addition of MB contrast agents allows the true microcirculation to be probed. The wash-in kinetics of these agents offer information on perfusion and blood volume that can be superimposed as a parametric image on anatomical data as shown in Figures 13.9 and 13.11. In the preclinical arena, the new technology will find immediate application in a wide range of small animal biomedical research. In addition, the ability of micro-ultrasound to provide accurate measures of tumor volume and microcirculatory flow will allow rapid evaluation of new interventional therapies to be assessed. Other applications in cardiovascular disease, developmental biology, musculoskeletal disease, inflammation, atherosclerosis, and a wide variety of other mouse models of human disease are developing rapidly.

Finally, it should be noted that micro-ultrasound, having undergone dramatic expansion in the field of preclinical imaging, is now ripe to be exploited in clinical applications. Already efforts are underway to use the technology in prostate imaging, neonatal imaging, skin and ocular imaging, and a wide range of intraluminal imaging applications. The development of highly portable versions suitable for anesthesiology and other clinical activities is to be anticipated.

Acknowledgments

The author wishes to acknowledge funding from The Terry Fox Foundation, the Canadian Institutes of Health Research, the Ontario Research Fund, and VisualSonics. The author also extends thanks to the many staff and graduate students who helped expand the technology and applications of micro-ultrasound.

References

1. Rumack, C.M., Wilson, S.R., and Charboneau, J.W. (1998) *Diagnostic Ultrasound*, Vols. **1** and **2**, Mosbey, St. Louis, MO.

2. Cobbold, R. (2008) *Foundations of Biomedical Ultrasound*, Oxford University Press, New York.

3. Shung, K. (2005) *Diagnostic Ultrasound: Imaging and Blood Flow Measurements*, CRC Press, Boca Raton, FL, pp. 72–73.

4. Foster, F.S., Pavlin, C.J., Harasiewicz, K.A., Christopher, D.A., and Turnbull, D.H. (2000) Advances in ultrasound

biomicroscopy. *J. Ultrasound Med. Biol.*, **26**, 1–27.

5. Foster, F.S., Zhang, M.Y., Zhou, Y.Q., Liu, G., Mehi, J., Cherin, E., Harasiewicz, K.A., Starkoski, B.G., Zan, L., Knapik, D.A., and Adamson, S.L. (2002) A new ultrasound instrument for in vivo microimaging of mice. *Ultrasound Med. Biol.*, **28**, 1165–1172.

6. Phoon, C.K. (2006) Imaging tools for the developmental biologist: ultrasound biomicroscopy of mouse embryonic development. *Pediatr. Res.*, **60**, 14–21.

7. Zhou, Y.Q., Foster, F.S., Qu, D.W., Zhang, M., Harasiewicz, K.A., and Adamson, S.L. (2002) Applications for multifrequency ultrasound biomicroscopy in mice from implantation to adulthood. *Physiol. Genomics*, **10**, 113–126.

8. Nieman, B.J. and Turnbull, D.H. (2010) Ultrasound and magnetic resonance microimaging of mouse development. *Methods Enzymol.*, **476**, 379–400.

9. Kulandavelu, S., Qu, D., Sunn, N., Mu, J., Rennie, M.Y., Whiteley, K.J., Walls, J.R., Bock, N.A., Sun, J.C., Covelli, A., Sled, J.G., and Adamson, S.L. (2006) Embryonic and neonatal phenotyping of genetically engineered mice. *ILAR J.*, **47**, 103–117.

10. Pallares, P., Fernandez-Valle, M.E., and Gonzalez-Bulnes, A. (2009) In vivo virtual histology of mouse embryogenesis by ultrasound biomicroscopy and magnetic resonance imaging. *Reprod. Fertil. Dev.*, **21**, 283–292.

11. Li, Y., Garson, C.D., Xu, Y., French, B.A., and Hossack, J.A. (2008) High frequency ultrasound imaging detects cardiac dyssynchrony in noninfarcted regions of the murine left ventricle late after reperfused myocardial infarction. *Ultrasound Med. Biol.*, **34**, 1063–1075.

12. Liu, J., Du, J., Zhang, C., Walker, J.W., and Huang, X. (2007) Progressive troponin I loss impairs cardiac relaxation and causes heart failure in mice. *Am. J. Physiol. Heart Circ. Physiol.*, **293**, H1273–H1281.

13. Zhou, Y.Q., Foster, F.S., Nieman, B.J., Davidson, L., Chen, X.J., and Henkelman, R.M. (2004) Comprehensive transthoracic cardiac imaging in

mice using ultrasound biomicroscopy with anatomical confirmation by magnetic resonance imaging. *Physiol. Genomics*, **18**, 232–244.

14. Zhou, Y.Q., Zhu, S.N., Foster, F.S., Cybulsky, M.I., and Henkelman, R.M. (2010) Aortic regurgitation dramatically alters the distribution of atherosclerotic lesions and enhances atherogenesis in mice. *Arterioscler. Thromb. Vasc. Biol.*, **30**, 1181–1188.

15. Cheung, A.M., Brown, A.S., Cucevic, V., Roy, M., Needles, A., Yang, V., Hicklin, D.J., Kerbel, R.S., and Foster, F.S. (2007) Detecting vascular changes in tumour xenografts using micro-ultrasound and micro-ct following treatment with VEGFR-2 blocking antibodies. *Ultrasound Med. Biol.*, **33**, 1259–1268.

16. Goessling, W., North, T.E., and Zon, L.I. (2007) Ultrasound biomicroscopy permits in vivo characterization of zebrafish liver tumors. *Nat. Methods*, **4**, 551–553.

17. Graham, K.C., Wirtzfeld, L.A., MacKenzie, L.T., Postenka, C.O., Groom, A.C., MacDonald, I.C., Fenster, A., Lacefield, J.C., and Chambers, A.F. (2005) Three-dimensional high-frequency ultrasound imaging for longitudinal evaluation of liver metastases in preclinical models. *Cancer Res.*, **65**, 5231–5237.

18. Olive, K.P., Jacobetz, M.A., Davidson, C.J., Gopinathan, A., McIntyre, D., Honess, D., Madhu, B., Goldgraben, M.A., Caldwell, M.E., Allard, D., Frese, K.K., Denicola, G., Feig, C., Combs, C., Winter, S.P., Ireland-Zecchini, H., Reichelt, S., Howat, W.J., Chang, A., Dhara, M., Wang, L., Ruckert, F., Grutzmann, R., Pilarsky, C., Izeradjene, K., Hingorani, S.R., Huang, P., Davies, S.E., Plunkett, W., Egorin, M., Hruban, R.H., Whitebread, N., McGovern, K., Adams, J., Iacobuzio-Donahue, C., Griffiths, J., and Tuveson, D.A. (2009) Inhibition of Hedgehog signaling enhances delivery of chemotherapy in a mouse model of pancreatic cancer. *Science*, **324**, 1457–1461.

19. Shaked, Y., Ciarrocchi, A., Franco, M., Lee, C.R., Man, S., Cheung, A.M., Hicklin, D.J., Chaplin, D., Foster, F.S., Benezra, R., and Kerbel, R.S. (2006)

Therapy-induced acute recruitment of circulating endothelial progenitor cells to tumors. *Science*, **313**, 1785–1787.

20. Foster, F.S., Mehi, J., Lukacs, M., Hirson, D., White, C., Chaggares, C., and Needles, A. (2009) A new 15-50 MHz array-based micro-ultrasound scanner for preclinical imaging. *Ultrasound Med. Biol.*, **35**, 1700–1708.

21. Becher, H. and Burns, P.N. (2000) *Handbook of Contrast Echocardiography*, Springer, Berlin.

22. Burns, P.N., Powers, J.E., and Fritzsch, T. (1992) Harmonic imaging: a new imaging and Doppler method for contrast enhanced ultrasound. *Radiology*, **185(P)**, 142 (abstract).

23. Ferrara, K., Pollard, R., and Borden, M. (2007) Ultrasound microbubble contrast agents: fundamentals and application to gene and drug delivery. *Annu. Rev. Biomed. Eng.*, **9**, 415–447.

24. Borden, M.A., Qin, S., and Ferrara, K.W. (2010) in *Molecular Imaging* (ed. R. Weissleder), Peoples Medical Publishing House, Shelton, CT, pp. 425–444.

25. Hoff, L. (2001) *Acoustic Characterization of Contrast Agents for Medical Ultrasound Imaging*, Kluwer Academic Publishers, Dordrecht.

26. Hope-Simpson, D., Chin, C., and Burns, P.N. (1999) Pulse inversion Doppler: a new method for detecting nonlinear echoes from microbubble contrast agents. *IEEE Trans. Ultrason. Ferroelectr. Freq. Control*, **46**, 372–382.

27. Burns, P.N., Powers, J.E., Hope-Simpson, D., Uhlendorf, V., and Fritzsch, T. (1996) Harmonic Imaging: principles and preliminary results. *Angiology*, **47**, 63–73.

28. Burns, P.N. and Hope-Simpson D. (2000) Pulse inversion Doppler ultrasonic diagnostic imaging. US Patent 6,095,980.

29. Haider, B. and Chiao, R.Y. (1999) High order nonlinear ultrasonic imaging. *Proc. IEEE Ultrason. Symp.*, 1527–1531.

30. Eckersley, R.J., Chin, C.T., and Burns, P.N. (2005) Optimising phase and amplitude modulation schemes for imaging microbubble contrast agents at low acoustic power. *Ultrasound Med. Biol.*, **31**, 213–219.

31. Chomas, J., Dayton, P., May, D., and Ferrara, K. (2002) Nondestructive subharmonic imaging. *IEEE Trans. Ultrason. Ferroelectr. Freq. Control*, **49**, 883–892.

32. Forsberg, F., Liu, J.B., Shi, W.T., Furuse, J., Shimizu, M., and Goldberg, B.B. (2005) In vivo pressure estimation using subharmonic contrast microbubble signals: proof of concept. *IEEE Trans. Ultrason. Ferroelectr. Freq. Control*, **52**, 581–583.

33. Forsberg, F., Shi, W.T., and Goldberg, B.B. (2000) Subharmonic imaging of contrast agents. *Ultrasonics*, **38**, 93–98.

34. Shankar, P.M., Krishna, P.D., and Newhouse, V.L. (1999) Subharmonic backscattering from ultrasound contrast agents. *J. Acoust. Soc. Am.*, **106**, 2104–2110.

35. Shi, W.T., Forsberg, F., Hall, A.L., Chiao, R.Y., Liu, J.B., Miller, S., Thomenius, K.E., Wheatley, M.A., and Goldberg, B.B. (1999) Subharmonic imaging with microbubble contrast agents: initial results. *Ultrason. Imaging*, **21**, 79–94.

36. Needles, A., Arditi, M., Rognin, N.G., Mehi, J., Coulthard, T., Bilan-Tracey, C., Gaud, E., Frinking, P., Hirson, D., and Foster, F.S. (2010) Nonlinear contrast imaging with an array-based micro-ultrasound system. *Ultrasound Med. Biol.*, **36**, 2097–2106.

37. Goertz, D.E., Yu, J.L., Kerbel, R.S., Burns, P.N., and Foster, F.S. (2002) High-frequency Doppler ultrasound monitors the effects of antivascular therapy on tumor blood flow. *Cancer Res.*, **62**, 6371–6375.

38. Jugold, M., Palmowski, M., Huppert, J., Woenne, E.C., Mueller, M.M., Semmler, W., and Kiessling, F. (2008) Volumetric high-frequency Doppler ultrasound enables the assessment of early antiangiogenic therapy effects on tumor xenografts in nude mice. *Eur. Radiol.*, **18**, 753–758.

39. Qayum, N., Muschel, R.J., Im, J.H., Balathasan, L., Koch, C.J., Patel, S., McKenna, W.G., and Bernhard, E.J. (2009) Tumor vascular changes mediated by inhibition of oncogenic signaling. *Cancer Res.*, **69**, 6347–6354.

14
Studying Microcirculation with Micro-CT

Timothy L. Kline and Erik L. Ritman

14.1
Introduction

Micro-computed tomography (micro-CT) has emerged as a powerful modality for vascular exploration in intact small animals [1–5] and in corrosion casts and/or biopsies of larger animal specimens [6–8]. This is due to the fact that micro-CT provides high-resolution 3D volumetric data. The data are suitable for analysis, quantification, validation, and visualization of vasculature. As an example, interesting opportunities for highly quantitative 3D imaging studies of induced or implanted disease models can be studied [9, 10] and screening for anatomical abnormalities and detection and quantification of anatomical changes in live animals (or tissue samples) can be characterized [11]. The study of vascular development (such as mechanisms of neovascularization and evaluating pro- and antiangiogenic strategies) requires a complete and accurate characterization of the microvasculature. Thus, micro-CT, which is able to quantify anatomical information in three-dimensional nondestructively at a very high spatial resolution, is a great tool for studying questions related to microcirculation. Nonetheless, it is limited in its ability to convey metabolic and other cellular functions as compared to other methods such as radionucleotide imaging. However, such methods suffer from poor spatial resolutions and thus the information from multiple imaging methods should be used to provide a fully comprehensive analysis.

14.2
Micro-Computed Tomography

14.2.1
History

The development of CT imaging, as we know it today, developed in many different places, by researchers attempting to solve a wide range of problems. Interestingly enough, the mathematical foundation of CT was outlined by Johann Radon in

Microcirculation Imaging, First Edition. Edited by Martin J. Leahy.
© 2012 Wiley-VCH Verlag GmbH & Co. KGaA. Published 2012 by Wiley-VCH Verlag GmbH & Co. KGaA.

1917. Radon [12] proved that an object with *n*-components can be reconstructed from its (*n* − 1)-dimensional projections. Although Radon had little impact on the actual development of CT imaging, it was only after aspects of his transform had been independently developed some 60 years later that it was realized that Radon had already published such an approach. Some of the earliest works on digital tomographic imaging, however, were poorly disseminated due to mostly sociopolitical reasons. In the early 1950s, the Pole Josef Wloka [13] may well have been the first to use Radon's transform for generating tomographic images and was closely followed later that decade by the Russian Korenblyum and his colleagues [14]. In the early 1960s, the American William H. Oldendorf was interested in accurately estimating local concentrations of radiolabeled indicators within the brain. He developed an unfiltered back projection method to overcome the problem of superimposed radioactivity [15]. At the same time, Allen M. Cormack (a South African physicist) needed to make accurate estimates of the spatial distribution of therapeutic radiation absorption within the body. To do so, he developed an inversion formula [16] and is now credited for disseminating the possibilities Radon's mathematical formulation had for radiological applications [17]. Nearly a decade later, the Englishman Godfrey N. Hounsfield [18] solved the problem of discriminating white from gray matter in X-ray images of the brain by using an algebraic reconstruction algorithm. He patented the concept of a clinical CT scanner, and, in 1971, those CT scanners became available for clinical use. For their work, Cormack and Hounsfield shared the Nobel Prize for Medicine in 1979.

Since their clinical inception in 1971, CT scanners quickly became and have remained an important diagnostic tool for noninvasively imaging three-dimensional sections of the human body. Present day multislice CT scanners can image vascular trees by virtue of injected contrast agents. The smallest vessels imaged are about 1 mm in diameter. In general, the term microvasculature is used to describe

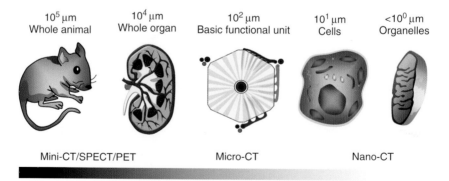

Figure 14.1 Illustration of the scales needed to image different sized specimens along with the corresponding tomographic scanners used for studying the orders of magnitude difference of specimen size. From left to right, the illustrations represent a small animal specimen (mouse), a whole organ specimen (kidney), the basic functional unit of the liver (lobule), a generic cell, and an organelle (mitochondrion).

vessel segments <1 mm in diameter, on down to the 5 μm diameter capillaries. Miniaturized versions of clinical scanners are termed *mini-CT scanners*. These scanners are capable of imaging entire small animal specimens. To image on down to the cellular level requires even higher spatial resolution capabilities, which are achievable by modern micro-CT scanners. The highest resolution scanners available today are known as *nano-CT scanners* and are able to image at and below the cellular level. Figure 14.1 illustrates the range of scales of specimens imaged by the various scanners.

Improving scanner resolution was initially driven by the bone research field. Bone is naturally well suited to CT imaging because of its large contrast from soft tissue. The first custom-made micro-CT scanners were built in the early 1980s, mainly for evaluating the three-dimensional microstructure of bone trabeculae [19]. In the early 1990s, the first commercially available micro-CT scanners became available and ever since, the capabilities of micro-CT imaging methods and the range of research investigations have been steadily growing. Figure 14.2 shows the result of a query of the PubMed database for publications related to micro-CT. The number of publications has seen an exponential growth in recent years. However, the study of microvasculature by micro-CT imaging comprises a small portion of the total research investigations ~16%), while bone-related research makes up over half (~58%).

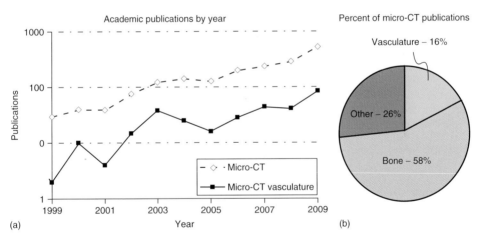

(a)   (b)

Figure 14.2 The increasing importance of micro-CT scanners is reflected in the rising number of micro-CT-based research papers published each year, as displayed in panel (a). The study of microvasculature, however, comprises a very small portion of micro-CT research investigations as shown in panel (b). The data were obtained through a query of the public database PubMed (MEDSUM tool). For the micro-CT publications, the mesh terms were X-ray microtomography *or* X-ray *and* microtomography *or* X-ray microtomography *or* micro *and* CT *or* micro-CT. The use of micro-CT for vasculature research had the same micro-CT mesh terms, along with the keywords: vessels *or* vasculature *or* microcirculation *or* circulation *or* blood. The micro-CT and bone data had the key terms: bone *or* bones (in addition to the micro-CT mesh terms).

14.2.2
Theory

The basis of all CT techniques is that X-ray projection data are collected in an ordered manner from multiple projection angles [20]. The projection data are related to how ionizing radiation interacts with matter. In the energy range (10–50 keV) typically used in micro-CT imaging, the so-called photoelectric effect is the main interaction mechanism [17]. At these energies, the attenuation of X-ray by the tissue decreases rapidly as photon energy increases. The attenuation in photon intensity is proportional to the third power of the element's order number and is inversely related to the third power of the photon energy. Thus, the actual attenuation depends on both the material as well as the energy spectrum of the X-ray source.

As an X-ray penetrates an object in transmission mode, the X-ray is exponentially attenuated by the material along its path. The attenuation law

$$I = I_0 e^{-\mu_t \cdot d} \tag{14.1}$$

relates the number of photons I reaching the system's detector to the number of photons I_0 incident on the specimen of thickness d. The energy-dependent material constant, μ_t, is called the *linear attenuation coefficient*. It represents the proportion that the radiation is attenuated by, for instance, 1 cm of the material. Thus, the final attenuation reflects the sum of all of these local linear attenuations along the X-ray beam's path. To produce a three-dimensional CT image, a whole collection of such two-dimensional projections is acquired. The two-dimensional projections can then be used to reconstruct a three-dimensional image. Finally, through the use of calibration phantoms, the CT grayscale values can be converted into physically meaningful values, such as the attenuation coefficients (cm^{-1}) or Hounsfield units, in which air is -1000, water is 0, and bone is of the order of 1000. At higher energies (50–150 keV), the interaction is predominantly Compton scattering so that the attenuation changes relatively little with photon energy variations.

14.2.3
Conventional Micro-Computed Tomography System

In the simplest sense, all micro-CT scanners are composed of three basic elements: (i) the X-ray source, (ii) the X-ray-to-electronic signal-converting imaging array, and (iii) a method for rotating either the specimen or the scanner around the specimen. To facilitate high spatial resolution, the scanners rely on various approaches. For example, there are systems that utilize a conventional cone-beam X-ray geometry such as that generated by Roentgen X-ray sources [21], or others that have a quasi-parallel beam geometry such as that generated by synchrotrons, or when the Roentgen source is a large distance from the object [1]. In addition, commercial scanners are available that are essentially scaled-down versions of their clinical CT scanner counterparts. For performing *in vivo* studies, additional design considerations are required and more complicated, rotating source–detector systems have been developed.

14.2.3.1 Specimen Stage Rotation Geometry

Micro-CT systems that physically rotate the specimen within the field of view of the scanner's X-ray path are the design of choice for isolated specimen imaging [4]. The benefits of rotating the specimen (as opposed to the source and detector) are that the design is robust, cost-efficient, and the system is an inherently simple design. Since there must be a high degree of precision in the system's mechanical components in order to facilitate high spatial resolution, a system with a reduced number of these components is far easier to build and maintain. One drawback to the rotating specimen geometry is that the specimens must be fixed to the sample stage in order to prevent motion blurring that makes this scanner geometry problematic for *in vivo* studies [22].

In Figure 14.3, the three main components, such as the X-ray tube, the object on a rotating stage, and the flat panel detector, are shown. Translational stages are used in order to change the magnification found in the subsequent image by varying the distance between source, object, and detector (a feature not commonly found in the source–detector rotation geometry). An example micro-CT image of the hepatic artery from a rat liver (Microfil contrast agent, 20 μm cubic voxels) is shown in Figure 14.4. This specimen was scanned with an in-house micro-CT imaging system [1]. The image is a maximum intensity projection (MIP) of the

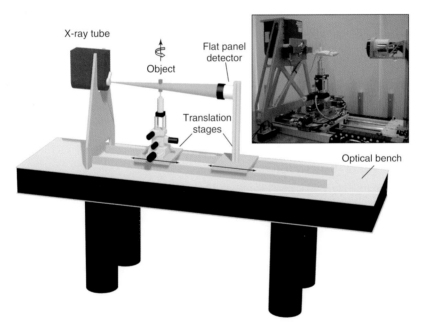

Figure 14.3 Illustration and photograph of a micro-CT imaging system with a rotating specimen geometry in which the object is physically rotated while the tube and the detector are stationary. The use of translation stages allows magnification settings to vary over a wide range. Scanners such as these can achieve very high spatial resolution and are most frequently used for *ex vivo* and *in situ* specimens. (Source: From Ref. [4]).

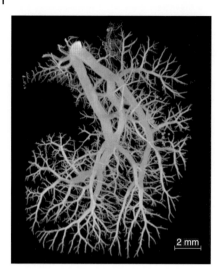

Figure 14.4 Maximum intensity projection of the micro-CT data (20 μm isotropic voxels) from the hepatic artery of a rat. The vasculature was filled with a contrast agent (Microfil) and was imaged *in situ*. Data such as this can then be used for measuring the geometry of microvasculature, such as the diameter and length of interbranch segments. With a resolution down to only a few micrometers, highly accurate quantitative anatomic information is obtained. This information can therefore be used to infer various physiological functions such as perfusion territories, local shear stresses on the vascular lumen wall, pressure distributions, and the magnitude of blood flow through the vascular tree's lumen.

volumetric data. To form an MIP image, "rays" are cast in the direction of the 3D volume (the angle of which depends on the desired angle of view), and each pixel of the image has a brightness corresponding to the maximum CT value found in the ray's path.

14.2.3.2 Source–Detector Rotation Geometry

Rotating source–detector systems are more complicated (than rotating specimen scanners) with regard to mechanical setup [4]. These are practically a requirement for performing *in vivo* studies. In *in vivo* studies, it is typically not feasible to rotate the object (although it should be noted that *in vivo*, rotating specimen scanners have been demonstrated [23]); thus, the specimen is kept stationary while the source and the detector are rotated [20]. An example of an *in vivo* micro-CT imaging system is shown in Figure 14.5. Magnification is frequently performed in such a system, by moving the X-ray source, specimen table, relative to the specimen stage, and detector. The spatial geometrical resolution depends mainly on the detector pixel pitch and the matrix size of the detector used as well as on the focusing mode of the X-ray tube [22]. Special care must be taken such that the varying gravitational forces do not change the rotation speed or the mechanical alignment of the source and detector relative to each other, as well as relative to the axis of rotation. An example *in vivo* micro-CT image of a rat's cerebral vasculature is shown in Figure 14.6 [3].

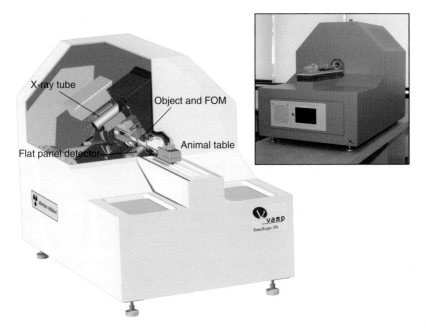

Figure 14.5 Illustration and photograph of a micro-CT imaging system with a rotating gantry geometry in which the X-ray source and detector are physically rotated while the specimen is kept stationary. Scanners such as these are typically used for *in vivo* scans. Since the X-ray source-to-specimen-to-detector distance is fixed, the degree of magnification in the image is not variable. (Source: From Ref. [4]).

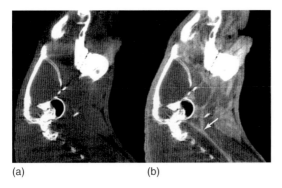

(a)   (b)

Figure 14.6 Sagittal sections computed from an *in vivo* micro-CT scan of a rat's head (voxel dimension: 170 μm). This figure highlights the importance of using contrast agents to enhance the visibility of vasculature. In panel (a), no contrast was used, but bone is clearly visualized because of its high X-ray attenuation. In addition, some general soft tissue features can be observed. In panel (b), the carotid arteries are indicated by the use of an injected contrast agent. The arrow indicates the carotid artery's bifurcation. (Source: From Ref. [3]).

14.2.4
Image Reconstruction

Cone-beam reconstruction [24] is the most common method used to convert the projection data collected by the micro-CT imaging system's detector into the stack of slices used to generate the three-dimensional volume data set [20]. This method of reconstruction is further extended into the method known as *filtered back projection*. This involves projecting the measured profiles back over the reconstructed image area along rays oriented according to the angles used for the projections. Before performing the reconstruction, filtering methods can be applied to remove artifacts and to enhance edges contained in the image (i.e., sharp CT grayscale changes). Other reconstruction methods exist such as iterative analytical and statistical methods. These methods produce superior reconstructed images (compared with filtered back projection); however, their computational demand has only recently become feasible with the advent of graphical processing unit (GPU) parallel programming techniques. For instance, utilizing GPU parallel programming techniques, several orders of magnitude speedups have been achieved [25], which means that the possibility of improved images, reconstructed in a practical amount of time, is realizable.

14.2.5
Image Quality

14.2.5.1 **X-Ray Dose**
Image quality is inherently related to X-ray dose, a concern that is particularly relevant for *in vivo* studies. High spatial resolution requires high doses. Reducing the dose causes higher image noise and reduced image contrast. Therefore, to achieve a certain image quality within a given voxel, a certain number of photons must impinge on that voxel (i.e., region within the specimen).

In the case of *in vivo* studies, the animal may suffer from the acute and/or chronic effects of radiation. In addition, issues pertaining to tumor growth (which could conceivably be modified by a micro-CT scan) and changes in cell population behavior (cells may behave differently after being irradiated) must be addressed when performing, in particular, longitudinal studies. Dose is also an issue in *in situ* studies since, at very high spatial resolutions, there is the potential for radiation damage to the specimen, thereby altering the physiology. A rule of thumb is that the radiation exposure must increase more than $(1 \text{ per voxel volume})^3$ if CT image signal to noise is to remain constant.

Besides specimen concerns, there also exist technological limitations related to X-ray dose. The X-ray tube has a maximum power which is related to the focal-spot size. High spatial resolution requires small focal-spot sizes.

14.2.5.2 **X-Ray Beam Hardening**
The X-ray energy from micro-CT scanners is inherently polychromatic, although synchrotron-radiation-based scanners (found at highly specialized national

laboratories) are able to generate nearly monochromatic X-ray beams (e.g., Brookhaven National Laboratories' beamline). Owing to the spectrum of energies, a phenomenon known as *beam hardening* is an important concern. Lower energy X-rays are attenuated more than higher energy X-rays when passing through an object, and the result is that the beam becomes more "hard" (i.e., less attenuating). This leads to an inaccuracy of the calculated attenuation coefficient of regions within the image and is particularly evident when the beam passes through a high attenuator (such as bone) and then induces a shift in the attenuation coefficient for the material that the X-ray beam passes through afterward. Streaking artifacts are a consequence, which are observable in the reconstructed image. Postprocessing methods can be applied to partially correct this problem, and X-ray filters (such as plates of aluminum or copper 0.5–1.0 mm thick) can also be incorporated into the scanner system to preferentially filter out low-energy X-rays before they reach the specimen.

14.2.5.3 CT Image Spatial Resolution

Another important parameter related to image quality is spatial resolution. This refers to the smallest resolvable distance between two structures that can be distinguished in an image. It represents the ability of the scanner to detect physical features and depends on many factors of the imaging system (i.e., source, detector, and scanner geometry). The modulation transfer function (MTF) of an imaging system is a common comparator for the micro-CT scanner's spatial resolution [20]. The MTF is a measure for how accurately the details of an object are represented by an imaging system. In any real imaging system, the MTF is nonideal in that the MTF values drop progressively at higher spatial frequencies. For the case of vascular research, this results in the apparent broadening of small vessel diameters and causes the CT value found in opacified small vessel lumens to decrease. This effect is illustrated in Figure 14.7 where the line profile (which represents the CT grayscale value across the diameter of the opacified vessel) is shown for different diameter vessel cross sections. Further improvements in scanner components have made bench-top nano-CT units feasible. These scanners have voxel resolutions on the order of 500 nm. However, the fact that the total volumes of the specimens that can be scanned are smaller and the requirement for even larger X-ray doses are considerations that must be addressed when using the higher resolution systems [26].

14.2.5.4 Physiological Gating

An additional concern for *in vivo* studies is motion artifacts resulting from cardiac and respiratory motion [23, 27, 28]. By monitoring either cardiac or respiratory cycles (i.e., with electrocardiogram or diaphragm monitoring, respectively), images can be reconstructed that acquire prospectively, or selected retrospectively, projections at approximately the same phase of the heart or lung motion. Another approach acquires scan data from multiple cycles so that different angles are acquired for completely different heart beats, but the scan data thus corresponds to the same phase of the cardiac cycle.

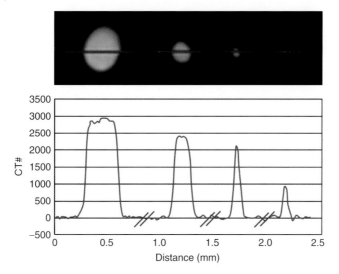

Figure 14.7 Line profile of the CT image gray scale values in opacified arterial branch segments of the indicated diameters. The y-axis is in the units of $1000\,cm^{-1}$. Larger diameter segments retain to a great extent the ideal square wave profile. As the branch segment decreases, significant reduction in peak gray scale occurs due to the blurring of the tomographic process. (Source: Modified from Ref. [25]).

14.2.6
Multimodality Imaging

No single imaging modality will provide all the necessary functional or anatomic information regarding microcirculation. The strength of micro-CT images lies in their quantitative anatomic information, which thereby allows for inferences regarding physiological function. Combining micro-CT image data with another imaging modality that provides complimentary information allows for an even more comprehensive evaluation of vascular structure-to-function relationships [29]. Important properties of different microscanner technologies are outlined in Table 14.1.

A necessary component of multimodality imaging methods is that spatial and temporal registration of the three-dimensional anatomy must be achieved. Where micro-CT may provide excellent high-resolution three-dimensional information pertaining to vascular branching geometry (for example), another imaging method may provide information related to the vascular tree's perfusion territories, information that may be used to gain additional insight into microcirculatory function. To perform image registration, a transformation or deformation field is applied to one volume, thereby allowing alignment with the other volume [5]. A three-dimensional grid phantom is one method for creating the spatial transformation matrix, which is used in conjunction with an imaging chamber that can be rigidly and reproducibly mounted on the different scanners (e.g., micro-PET (positron emission tomography) and micro-CT scanners) [30].

Table 14.1 Properties and comparison between different modality high-resolution scanners.

	Micro-CT		Micro-SPECT	Micro-PET	Micro-magnetic resonance imaging (MRI)
	Rotating state	Rotating scanner			
Resolution					
In plane	$\sim$1–100 μm	$\sim$50–100 μm	$\sim$1–2 mm	$\sim$1–2 mm	$\sim$100–200 μm
Slice thickness	$\sim$1–100 μm	$\sim$50–100 μm	$\sim$1–2 mm	$\sim$1–2 mm	$\sim$0.5–10 mm
Temporal	Minutes to hours	$\sim$150 ms – mins (gated)	Minutes (gated)	$\sim$0.5 s (gated)	$\sim$5–10 ms (gated)
In vivo	No	Yes	Yes	Yes	Yes
Provided information	Anatomical data, differentiation of contrast-enhanced vasculature, tissues, or structures	Anatomical and movement data, differentiation of contrast-enhanced vasculature, tissues, or structures	Functional information at molecular level, temporal, and spatial distribution of a radioisotope localize at a target	Functional information at molecular level, temporal, and spatial distribution of a radioisotope localize at a target	Structure, functional perfusion, cellular, and molecular events, differentiation of contrast-enhanced vasculature, tissues, or structures
Common applications to microvascular structure and function	Study of vascular branching geometry and connectivity, perfusion territories, perfusion defect regions, and organ tissue volumes	Organ perfusion, vascular leakiness, and heart wall motion	Regional heart wall motion and perfusion abnormalities, metabolism	Blood flow tracer distributions, metabolism	Measuring infarct size, perfusion, muscle/nerve fiber directions, and oxygenization status

14.2.6.1 **Micro-Positron Emission Tomography**

Scaled-down versions of clinical PET systems began surfacing in the early 1990s [31, 32]. Later that decade, reconstructed images with resolutions of 2.0 mm were produced and the term *micro-PET* was coined [33]. The larger scale clinical PET systems have long served as a powerful tool for noninvasively studying the physiology and biochemistry of the human body, thereby being an important diagnostic tool and, in addition, aid in guiding patient therapies [34]. Micro-PET is an imaging modality that can provide information pertaining to the function of living organisms [35]. It may also be used, for instance, to visualize and quantify angiogenesis *in vivo* [10]. Micro-PET provides 3D image volumes representing the temporal and spatial distribution of an indicator agent (radioisotope), which has localized to a specific anatomic or functional target [36]. The radioactive substance decays by positron emission. The emitted positron travels a very short distance (typically <2 mm) within tissue before it collides with an electron. On collision, the two annihilate each other and a pair of high-energy (511 keV) photons are emitted. The photons travel in almost opposite directions and are collected by detectors. The simultaneous detection of many such photon pairs localizes their point of origin somewhere along that line. A tomographic image can be created from such multiangular data.

Inherently, micro-PET has a very high sensitivity; requiring the use of very low amounts of radioisotopes for detecting physiological characteristics. In addition, since background radiation is very low, micro-PET has a very high signal-to-noise ratio. The targeting agents include metabolic substrates, small organic molecules, peptides, nanoparticles, and so on. Thus, micro-PET is capable of imaging essentially any type of target. Since micro-PET can reveal valuable insights into biochemical, physiological, and pharmacological processes, its major limitations are poor spatial resolution and the amount of ionizing radiation used. Micro-PET

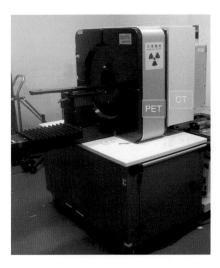

Figure 14.8 Illustration of a combined micro-PET/CT scanner [37].

is theoretically limited in spatial resolution to about 2 mm [35]. This is due to a combination of factors, most notably the finite range of the positron (distance before collision with an electron). When used in conjunction with micro-CT imaging, this problem is mitigated somewhat. Thus, high spatial resolution data, related to functional processes, is achievable through the use of a joint imaging modality such as micro-CT/PET. An example, combined micro-CT/PET system is displayed in Figure 14.8.

Figure 14.9 shows coregistered small-animal micro-CT/PET images [11]. Through the use of a novel radioligand tracer, tumor vasculature was noninvasively assessed in terms of how the vasculature responds to different treatments. Thus, the use of a multimodality imaging technique allows an enhancement for understanding various aspects of physiology and, in this case, an understanding of how different therapeutic strategies affect tumor vasculature.

14.2.6.2 Micro-Single Photon Emission Computed Tomography

Single photon emission computed tomography (SPECT) is the combination of both conventional radionuclide imaging and image reconstruction from projections. Conventional radionuclide imaging uses position-sensitive radiation detectors to measure X-ray photon emission from the three-dimensional distribution of

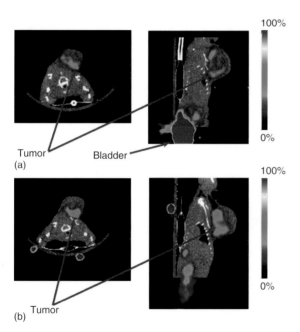

Figure 14.9 (a,b) Micro-CT image data (200 μm voxel size) is here shown coregistered with micro-PET data. High spatial resolution data, which is related to functional processes, is achievable through the use of the joint imaging modalities of micro-CT/PET. (Source: Figure modified from Ref. [11]).

radioactivity of radiolabeled biomarkers. This information forms a two-dimensional projection image. In SPECT, an image reconstruction method is applied to multiple 2D projection images to form a 3D image.

A commercially available combined nano-CT/SPECT imaging system is shown in Figure 14.10. Wietholt and colleagues [38] used micro-CT/SPECT fusion (registered) images to study circulation in rat lungs. Figure 14.11 shows the registered images for both the control group and a group of rats that had been subjected to a surgically induced occlusion of the left pulmonary artery. These transaxial slices (utilizing both micro-CT and micro-SPECT image data) allow the perfused regions within the specimen to be explored. In the case of the group of rats that had a surgical occlusion induced, the accumulation of the radiotracer occurred exclusively in the right (nonoccluded) lung of the animal, whereas the left (occluded) lung was not perfused via the pulmonary circulation.

A limitation of micro-SPECT is the low spatial resolution (in comparison to that of micro-CT imaging). Recent improvements in detector technologies and the incorporation of coated aperture (pinhole) geometry have allowed resolutions down to 1 mm to be achieved [39]. In addition to supplying high spatial resolution data, micro-CT data is also used as an attenuation correction for micro-SPECT data, which improves, for example, the uniformity of myocardial perfusion images [40] and thus allows micro-SPECT data to be useful quantitatively (not just qualitatively as merely a visualization tool). Thus, the full potential of SPECT functional imaging is realized by unambiguously assigning tracer uptake to organs or other anatomical features [41].

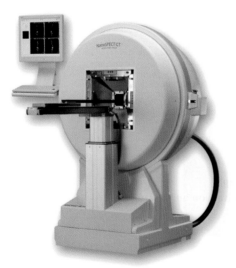

Figure 14.10 Combined nano-CT/SPECT imaging system offered by Bioscan (Washington, DC). This system uses a coded aperture to generate the scan data used for tomographic reconstruction.

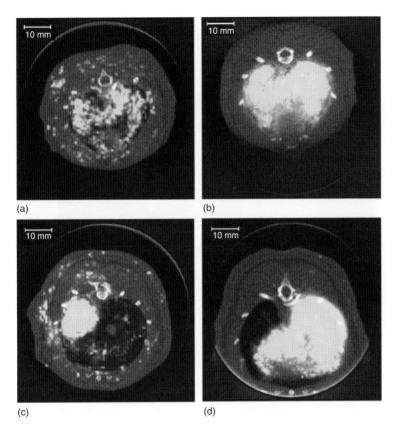

(a)   (b)

(c)   (d)

Figure 14.11 Transaxial slice through micro-CT/SPECT registered images for control rat group (a,b) and surgically occluded left pulmonary artery rat group (c,d), for both a left carotid artery injection (a,c) and a femoral vein injection (b,d). These transaxial slices (utilizing both micro-CT as well as micro-SPECT image data) allow the perfused regions within the specimen to be explored and related to anatomic structure. In the case of the group of rats that had a surgical occlusion induced, the accumulation of the radiotracer occurred exclusively in the right (nonoccluded) lung of the animal, whereas the left (occluded) lung is not perfused via the pulmonary circulation. (Source: This figure was modified from Ref. [38]).

14.2.6.3 Digital Subtraction Angiography
Combined micro-CT and digital subtraction angiography (DSA) have been incorporated into a single system recently [42]. Utilizing a blood-pool contrast agent (Fenestra VC), micro-CT imaging was used to assess the 3D vascular architecture of the tumor, while DSA imaging was used to assess tumor perfusion. The DSA data provides perfusion maps that can be combined (spatially coregistered) onto the micro-CT image data. An example from a combined micro-CT/DSA study is shown in Figure 14.12 [43]. The combination of micro-CT with DSA allows for morphological (in terms of accurately assessing 3D vascular architecture) and functional data (in terms of assessing tissue perfusion).

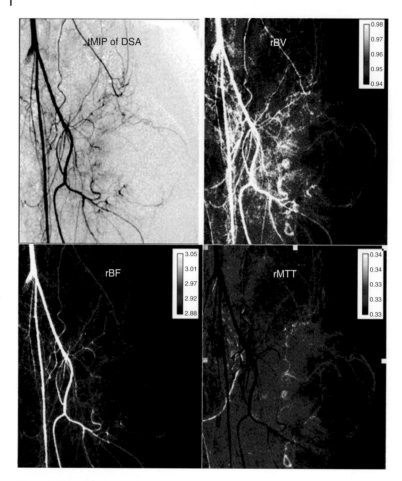

Figure 14.12 Maximum intensity projection (MIP) image and three perfusion maps (with a spatial resolution of 100 μm): relative blood volume (rBV), relative blood flow (rBF), and relative mean transit time (rMTT) are shown for a combined micro-CT/DSA study of the fibrosarcoma tumor in a rat. A conventional contrast agent, Isovue 370, was used in the DSA study and provided complementary functional information to the high spatial resolution micro-CT image data. (Source: This figure was modified from Ref. [43]).

14.2.6.4 Histology

One of the most common microscope-based imaging methods in use is histology, in which thin sections of tissue are imaged. Specific regions (such as particular cells) can be enhanced by specific stains that color particular regions. Histology is an inherently destructive imaging method, requiring bloodless biopsies of tissue to be extracted from a specimen. Micro-CT images have been shown to be able to acquire information somewhat similar to some aspects of histology (for example, micro-CT was shown to be feasible for the study of coronary arterial walls ([44], Figure 14.13), which is beneficial since micro-CT offers the possibility for nondestructive testing,

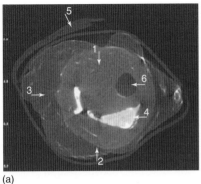

(a)

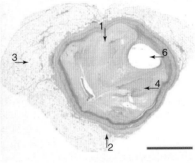

(b)

Figure 14.13 Advanced fibrocalcific atherosclerotic lesions were imaged by both micro-CT and histological sectioning (microscopic images of thin tissue samples). (a) Transverse micro-CT image. (b) Conventional histological image. The bar at the bottom right is 0.5 mm in length. Micro-CT is able to provide many anatomical structures with the same amount of detail as histology. This is beneficial since micro-CT provides fully 3D images, nondestructively. (1) Eccentric neointimal thickening, (2) boundary between media and adventitia, (3) adventitia, (4) calcification, (5) paraffin used to store coronary artery, and (6) vessel lumen. (Source: This figure was modified from Ref. [44]).

as well as analysis of much larger 3D tissue biopsies (where the histological sectioning process induces deformations in the samples). The information from histological sections can also be used to enhance micro-CT data by looking at cell differentiation in tissue.

14.3
Specimen/Animal Preparation

Unfortunately, the walls and contents of vasculature provide little inherent contrast from surrounding soft tissues for X-ray imaging. Specimen preparation is therefore an important step in micro-CT microcirculation studies so that the vasculature in the image can be visualized. To allow vascular visualization, contrast agents are injected into the vascular lumens, thereby causing the X-ray to be significantly attenuated by the vasculature. The considerations in specimen/animal preparation and contrast agent usage differ depending on the study.

14.3.1
Ex Vivo – Casting

Using a partially polymerized methyl methacrylate plastic (typically Batson's No. 17 corrosion casting compound), casts of vascular networks can be created. The details of this standard casting technique were outlined by Gannon [45]. The details of a recent study [46] where the cast of a rabbit's kidney vasculature was made and imaged by micro-CT are described next in order to outline the relevant steps involved.

A one-year-old female New Zealand white rabbit weighing 2.2 kg was euthanized by intravenous injection. Next, the animal's thoracic cavity was exposed by a ventral incision and the renal artery was cannulated. Heparinized saline solution was perfused through the vasculature using a three-way valve. This was performed to prevent blood clots from forming. Note that the perfusion pressure is an important consideration. Here, a pressure of 100 mmHg was used and 20–40 mmHg would have been used if performing venous perfusion (to prevent vessel wall rupture).

Once blood was cleared from the tissue, the valve was switched to perfuse a freshly prepared Batson's No. 17 solution. The Batson's solution was allowed to polymerize within the animal's tissue. With the specimen in an ice bath, the polymer took 2–3 h to cure. The use of an ice bath helps slow down the polymerization process that helps to minimize cast distortion during this exothermic reaction.

Once fully polymerized, the tissue was immersed in a 25% potassium hydroxide solution for 24–48 h. This solution corrodes away the tissue leaving only the polymerized plastic that represents the vascular tree lumens. The cast may then be imaged by micro-CT. The method of casting is clearly destructive but has the benefit of removing the surrounding tissue, which can cause potentially significant background noise in the subsequent micro-CT image. An image of both the created cast and the representative micro-CT image is depicted in Figure 14.14 [46].

14.3.2
In Situ – Contrast Agent Enhancement

In order to image the vascular lumens within intact specimens, a contrast agent such as Microfil is frequently used [1, 46–48] (latex- and gelatin-based contrast agents are also available [5]). The procedure is performed as discussed in the previous subsection; however, the Batson's No. 17 corrosion casting compound is replaced by the contrast agent. A contrast agent, such as Microfil, allows for the analysis of intact vasculature because of its high X-ray attenuation (2500–5000 HU) so that the perfused vasculature can easily be delineated from surrounding tissue. In contrast, the

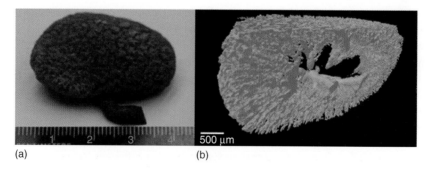

(a) (b)

Figure 14.14 (a) Vascular cast of a whole rabbit kidney (ruler is in centimeters). (b) 3D volume rendering of a portion of the vascular cast, imaged by micro-CT (35 μm voxel size). (Source: Modified from Ref. [46]).

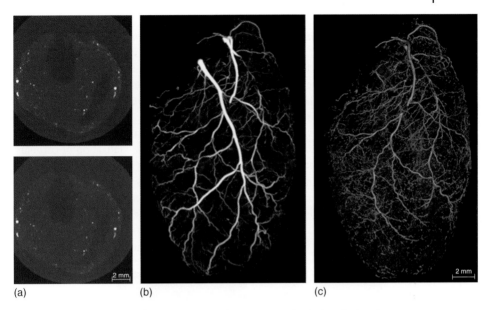

(a)   (b)   (c)

Figure 14.15 Micro-CT image data (20 μm isotropic voxels) of the vascular bed of a rat heart, which was filled with a contrast agent (Microfil) and was imaged *in situ*, is here displayed by different visualization methods. In panel (a), cross-sectional slices are shown for two different gray scale windowing levels. In panel (b), a maximum intensity projection (MIP) of the micro-CT data of the same vascular bed is displayed. Using a region-growing segmentation method, a fully connected vascular tree can be segmented, shown in red in panel (c). The vasculature in the image that are displayed as gray are either from the right myocardial arteries or are disconnected vessel segments due to the segmentation process or low contrast agent concentration.

corrosion casting method (discussed in the previous subsection) has relatively low attenuation (0–1500 HU) and thus requires that the surrounding tissue be removed.

Micro-CT image data (20 μm isotropic voxels) of the vascular bed of a rat heart, which had the coronary artery filled with a contrast agent (Microfil), then embedded in wax and imaged *in situ*, is displayed by different visualization methods in Figure 14.15. In panel (a), cross-sectional slices are shown for two different grayscale windowing levels. The windowing level assigns the color black to any pixel in the image with a CT value less than the lower threshold and the color white to any pixel with CT value greater than the upper threshold. In the top panel, the windowing level thresholds are [200 15 000], and, in the bottom panel, the windowing level thresholds are [−3000 15 000]. Pixels with CT values in the intermediate range are shown on a gray scale. Images such as these can be used, for instance, to manually define regions of interest within the images as well as measure various distances between different anatomical features. In panel (b), an MIP of the micro-CT data of the same vascular bed is displayed. It is shown here that the vasculature is easily delineated from the surrounding tissue because of the vasculatures' far higher CT values. Using a region-growing segmentation method, a fully connected vascular tree can be segmented, shown in red in panel (c). The vascular tree in this case is visualized by a technique known as *volume rendering*. In this case, the surface of the vessel tree is visualized and rendered with shading in order to give the structure a three-dimensional look. Properties of this segmented vessel tree such as the total vessel volume and surface area can then be measured, and local geometrical properties such as interbranch segment diameters and branching angles can be quantified.

Other contrast agents, such as osmium tetroxide (OsO_4), have also been used in micro-CT vascular research. Zhu *et al.* [49] showed how visualization of coronary arterial wall structure, early lesion formation, and changes in vascular permeability could be detected for the vasculature of porcine hearts by using OsO_4 as the contrast agent (Figure 14.16). First, the hearts were placed in formaldehyde immediately after harvesting. The unbound formaldehyde was then flushed from

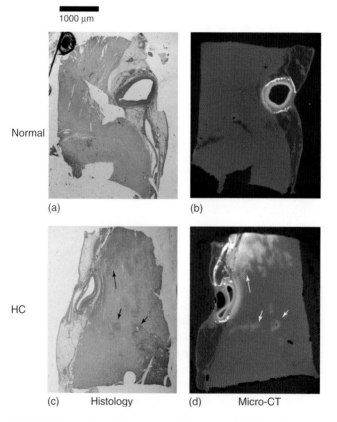

Figure 14.16 Representative myocardial immunohistochemistry of vascular endothelial growth factor (VEGF, a) and corresponding micro-CT image (b) of the same section. Note the similar distribution of VEGF (red, c) and perivascular OsO_4 (white, d). (Source: From Ref. [49]).

the vasculature by infusion of the coronary arteries with a 60 ml 0.9% saline, 10 ml 1% OsO$_4$ solution. This solution was hand injected in 1 ml increments into the artery every 6 min for 1 h. Finally, a portion of the distal epicardial coronary artery, which included a piece of the attached ventricular myocardium, was then sectioned, prepared, and scanned by micro-CT. The use of OsO$_4$ acts as a sort of cellular staining (e.g., its density distribution allows for some differentiation of the cells within vessel walls and myocardium).

14.3.3
In Vivo

The long scanning times of *in vivo* experiments (between 0.5 and 2 h) require intravascular contrast agents to either not leave the blood pool rapidly or be continuously infused into the vasculature [5]. Since contrast agents used for *in vivo* studies can be administered multiple times to the same animal, the possibility for longitudinal micro-CT studies exists.

Using a conventional iodinated vascular contrast agent (which is encapsulated within polyethylene glycol-stabilized liposomes), intravascular space was shown to be suitably enhanced for more than 3 h [50]. Iodinated triglycerides containing lipophilic cores of oil-in-water lipid emulsions (offered by Fenestra) provide long-lasting visualization of vascular systems with micro-CT. Kong *et al.* [51] used Pluronic F127 and a naturally iodinated compound (Lipiodol) to successfully form radiopaque nanoreservoir structures.

Shown in Figure 14.17 are the cerebral arteries of a mouse, which have been imaged by micro-CT *in vivo* [52]. Imeron 300, a conventional contrast agent, was used, which thereby allowed the cervical, extra-, and intracranial arteries and veins to be evaluated. With a reconstructed voxel resolution of 22 μm, vessels with a diameter >50 μm were successfully visualized.

14.3.4
Use of Probes

14.3.4.1 Nano-/Microspheres

As an example, microsphere embolization study [53], control, and "microsphere-simulated" embolization samples were obtained from a particular animal model. In this sense, the embolized specimens differed from the control in that an injection of nonradioactive microspheres into the left anterior descending artery was performed. Following the microsphere injection, the animal was euthanized and the hearts harvested. Next, the coronary arteries were infused with Microfil polymer at 100 mmHg infusion pressure and a nominal 2 cm^3 transmural biopsy of the myocardial region was collected after the Microfil injection. A micro-CT scanner was then used to generate the 3D specimen image data.

Comparison between control and embolized specimens was recently used [54] to study the volume loss of vessels below the size of the microspheres. This study essentially characterized the vascular consequences of microsphere embolization.

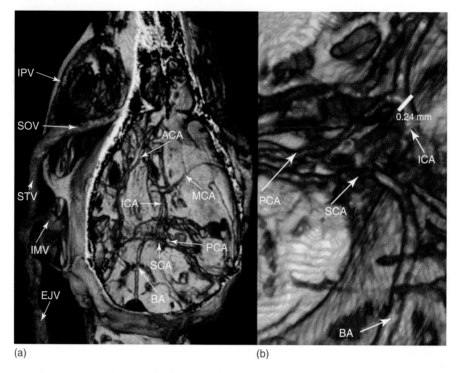

(a)   (b)

Figure 14.17 Volume-rendered images of the cerebral arteries of a mouse imaged by micro-CT *in vivo*. Imeron 300, a conventional contrast agent was used, which thereby allowed the cervical, extra-, and intracranial arteries and veins to be evaluated. With a reconstructed resolution of 22 μm, vessels with a diameter of 50 μm were successfully visualized. (a) Overview of the neurocranium with intracranial arteries and extracranial veins. (b) Magnification of the basal cerebral arteries with a white measurement bar placed over the ICA. Labels are ACA, anterior cerebral artery; MCA, middle cerebral artery; ICA, internal carotid artery; PCA, posterior cerebral artery; SCA, superior cerebellar artery; BA, basilar artery; IPV, infrapalpebral vein; SOV, supraorbital vein; STV, superficial temporal vein; IMV, internal maxillary vein; and EJV, external jugular vein. (Source: This figure is from Ref. [52]).

Microsphere embolization has shown how the perfusion defects due to blocked vasa vasorum could be studied for coronary vessel walls [6]. Also, local perfusion measurements were quantified in rat kidney vasculature [21] and pig myocardium [55] utilizing the method of microsphere embolization.

14.4
Image Analysis

A great challenge for the researcher studying microcirculation by micro-CT imaging is the postprocessing of the reconstructed image data. At the foundation of this challenge is the overall goal of accurately quantifying the microvascular structures' topology (i.e., connectivity or hierarchical nature) and its morphology (i.e., measurement of various properties, such as branch segment lengths, diameters, branching angles, vessel surface area, etc.). Being able to accurately characterize these properties of the microvasculature, flow patterns may be understood, optimal design principles may be exposed, and model systems may be fabricated.

The analysis of micro-CT images shares a great deal with other imaging modalities. Many algorithms, theories, and methods designed for different problems have been borrowed from other imaging methods and have seen success in their application to micro-CT images. Of course, the image analysis of micro-CT images continues to improve and contribute to the other imaging methods as well.

Many programs exist for performing image analysis, including the Analyze software program [56], Skyscan's (Kontich, Belgium) image analysis software, Matlab (Mathworks Inc.), and the software program Mimics by Materialise (Leuven, Belgium). Open source programs such as VTK can be used for visualization of micro-CT image data; also, ITK offers a whole host of image analysis algorithms for image registration as well as vascular segmentation and ImageJ is an excellent tool for performing various measurements of components within an image.

In the following subsections, methods pertaining to vascular segmentation, extraction of vascular centerlines, measurement of various geometrical properties, and modeling principles are discussed.

14.4.1
Segmentation

The task of delineating what is and what is not vasculature in an image has been studied by many research groups [8, 57, 58]. Typically, in microcirculation imaging studies, this is a two-phase problem, in the sense that we are interested in the vasculature and not interested in anything else (background). Owing to the use of contrast agents, the simple method of thresholding is the most common technique [47]. In this sense, the gray scale value of each voxel is considered and if it is within a certain range, it is set to being a vessel voxel (a one for instance), whereas if the voxel is outside of the specified range, it is not a vessel voxel (and set to zero). The process of image segmentation converts a gray scale volume data set into a binary data set, whereby the vasculature is easily represented as one distinct phase. A connected component analysis (region growing) can then be used to distinguish different vascular structures within the image. Shown in Figure 14.18 is a volume rendering of an intramyocardial cast from a human coronary artery. Here, the volume is rendered at four different CT gray scale thresholds. Clearly, significant differences in the vasculature are evident, which suggests that threshold choice is an important processing step and must be carefully chosen. Nonetheless, algorithmic approaches have been used to account for and alleviate the influence of threshold choice on subsequent vascular measurements.

The problem of segmentation is compounded by beam hardening, aliasing artifacts, partial volume effects, ring artifacts, and the nonideal MTF of the imaging

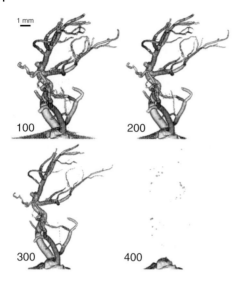

Figure 14.18 Micro-CT image data (20 μm isotropic voxels) of a corrosion cast of a human coronary artery. The material used to fix the specimen is seen at the bottom of each image. Here, volume renderings of the cast are displayed for different CT gray scale threshold choices. This threshold sets any voxel with a CT value greater than the threshold such that it is considered when creating the volume rendering (a rendering of the surface of the vasculature). All voxels with a value below the threshold are thus not visualized. The nonuniform nature of the CT gray scale is seen here, in particular, the lower values for branches with smaller diameters (since these are the first branches to be removed on raising the threshold). Also, it can be seen how all the branch segments become thinner as the threshold is increased. This results from the partial volume effect (whereby the vessel may only cross through part of a voxel and thus not attain as high of a gray scale value as those voxels that are fully within a vessel), as well as from blurring by the imaging system's modulation transfer function. This blurring has a larger effect on vessel segments with a small diameter than it does on larger diameter vessel segments.

system. This causes values of certain tissues (i.e., the lumen of vessel trees) to not be a specific value, but rather take on a range of values. Methods developed to overcome some of these problems include object tracking algorithms [57], local adaptive region-growing methods [8], active contours [59], as well as tubularity measure or Hessian-based filtering techniques [58]. The best approach depends on the quality of the micro-CT data in terms of how well the object stands out from the background and also just how complex the vascular structure is. For instance, Hessian-based filtering methods (which characterize the degree to which a voxel appears to pertain to a cylindrical type structure) have problems at bifurcation points since the vessel tree does not appear tubular in these regions. Also, active contour methods typically rely on user-specified parameters such as the number of iterations that the algorithm should run through, as well as various weighting parameters. Thus, a particular method should be chosen for each image analysis study, which is reliable and repeatable.

14.4.2
Centerline Extraction

Another preprocessing step for the subsequent characterization of vascular branching geometry is known as *centerline extraction*. The 3D segmented data set is used as the input for the extraction of the vascular tree's lumen centerline (also frequently termed, *skeleton*). The extraction of the vascular tree centerline allows for the simplification of the complex tree structure from which the branch segment location within the tree and its connection to the other branch segments is conveyed (essentially the first step in defining the vascular tree topology). Using locations along the centerline within the segmented image, the tree's hierarchical nature, branch lengths, branch diameters, and branching angles can subsequently be determined.

There exist many different methods for finding the centerline of vasculature. The three main categories are (i) iterative thinning [60] (i.e., peeling away surface voxels), (ii) mesh contraction [61] (i.e., shrinking), and (iii) methods based on "fast marching" [62, 63]. The different methods have been shown to each have strengths and weaknesses, and the different methods should be tested for their intended application. A successful centerline method will be robust, will follow closely the center of vessel lumens, and will not generate false branch segments ("whiskers").

14.4.3
Measurements

The measurement of length, diameter, and the connectivity relationship between interbranch segments lie at the foundation of most vascular geometry research [64, 65]. Other properties such as branching angle, vessel volume, and vessel wall surface area are also relevant parameters of vasculature, which can be produced with knowledge of the former. Accurately measuring vascular branching geometry is a task well suited to micro-CT image analysis. Manual-based methods can be performed, such as using a software program to measure cross-sectional widths of vessel tree lumens in two-dimensional slices. For high-throughput experiments, automated methods are desirable in order to generate large amounts of data in a relatively short amount of time. The data can therefore be reproducible and not constrained to the problems that occur from user subjectivity.

14.4.3.1 Segment Length
Once a vessel tree's centerline is extracted, measurements of the individual branch segments' length can easily be performed. The measurement of an individual branch segment's length can be determined by moving from one voxel to the next in the list of ordered centerline voxels, calculating the Euclidean distance between contiguous voxels, and summing the distances. This approximate method is known as the *sample-distance* method [66], where geometrically the interbranch segment's length is being approximated by the connected polygonal curve whose vertices are the branch segment's centerline voxels. Another method, that of simply

counting voxels [56, 67], can significantly underestimate interbranch segment length. Furthermore, smoothing of the centerline either through a moving average type of approach or curve fitting can further improve the accuracy of interbranch segment length measurements.

14.4.3.2 Segment Diameter

Several methods for measuring the branch diameter exist including distance map computation, cross-sectional area determination (brightness area product-based methods), and volume-based methods (where the diameter is calculated based on the segment's length and volume). Typically, these methods overestimate small vessel diameters. Hoffman *et al.* [68] compared the various techniques for determining vessel diameters. The main conclusion was that no technique perfectly characterized vessels over the full size range found in angiographic images; yet, it was suggested that a derivative-based technique was the most accurate for larger vessels. At a basic level, the convolution of a square wave function and a Gaussian blurring function results in an image that has a correct width at exactly half the original intensity (i.e., Full-width half-max (FWHM)). Therefore, the first-derivative edge detection as well as a thresholding technique of the local FWHM accurately characterize the input square wave's width (for vessels with diameters greater than two times the FWHM of the scanner's MTF). Additional considerations must be incorporated in order to accurately measure small interbranch segment diameters, which is typically done by using information pertaining to the imaging system's MTF.

14.4.4
Erode/Dilate Analysis

Micro-CT offers an excellent framework from which to analyze intact microvascular beds and a sequential "erode/dilate" technique [54, 69], which progressively eliminates branches of increasing diameter, is one approach that greatly reduces image analysis effort. By this method, the total luminal volume of different diameter branches is calculated. The method operates on a segmented image of the vasculature. The method uses the morphological operations of erosion and dilation [70, 71] whereby the segmented vascular bed is eroded and then dilated "n" times, where "n" is the iteration number (which can be related to the diameter of vessel segments lost at each iteration). Erosion involves removal of voxels from the surface of the lumen and dilation involves adding voxels to the surface of the lumens. After each iteration, the total vessel volume is measured. The results are then binned according to the vessel volume "V" that was lost (i.e., $V(n + 1) - V(n)$) by removing individual branches $2nh$ in diameter ("h" is the voxel size). This method has the benefit of being able to easily deal with highly complex structures, as well as images where multiple vascular trees exist.

As a few examples, the question of whether vasculature grows in proportion to the myocardium, as the rat heart develops, was studied by this erode/dilate method of analysis [69] and the results obtained were shown to compare accurately to the results of more complex methods, as well as indicate what diameter interbranch segments trap a microsphere of a given size [54]. In addition, Ohuchi *et al.* [72] used the morphological operation of dilation to deduce the volume of myocardial tissue perfused by selected arterioles.

14.4.5
Modeling

14.4.5.1 Analytical
The data regarding branching geometry can be investigated by analyzing the geometric properties of the vascular structures, in particular, with regard to the model derived by Murray [73] on the basis that the fluid transport system (vasculature) geometry is consistent with simultaneous minimization of both the power loss of laminar flow and a cost function proportional to the total volume of material needed to maintain the system (lumenal contents) – factors that have opposing geometric consequences. The vessel tree structures can be modeled as a binary tree in that, at each bifurcation, there exists one parent segment that divides into two branches. The "level" (or generation) of the branches is one higher than that of their parent branch segment.

The Hagen–Poiseuille equation [74] that describes laminar flow of an incompressible Newtonian fluid, through a pathway with a circular cross section, can also be used to calculate fluid flow resistance through different sections of vasculature, local shear stresses on vascular walls [65], and also the pressure distribution within vascular trees [48]. Shown in Figures 14.19 and 14.20 are the results of hemodynamic flow calculations of pressure distributions, fluid flow magnitudes, and shear stress distributions of vascular trees from placenta and lung vasculature of mice. These were computed by considering the vessel trees as networks of interconnected cylindrical pipes, taking into account the "pipes" series and parallel arrangements.

14.4.5.2 Computational Fluid Dynamics
More computationally demanding methods to characterize vasculature exist (Figure 14.21). These typically include fluid dynamic simulations. Owing to the computational complexity, simple structures, such as a single root segment, which bifurcates into two branches [75], or a mouse aorta composed of a main branch segment and a couple side branches [76], are typically characterized. Software programs such as ANSYS can be used to solve the Navier–Stokes equations. The modeling process involves defining inlets and outlets of the system, as well as other boundary conditions such as inlet flow magnitude and outlet pressure.

14.5
Summary and Future Developments

The important areas of scanner technologies (X-ray sources, geometries, and detectors), specimen preparation and scanning processes, image analysis techniques

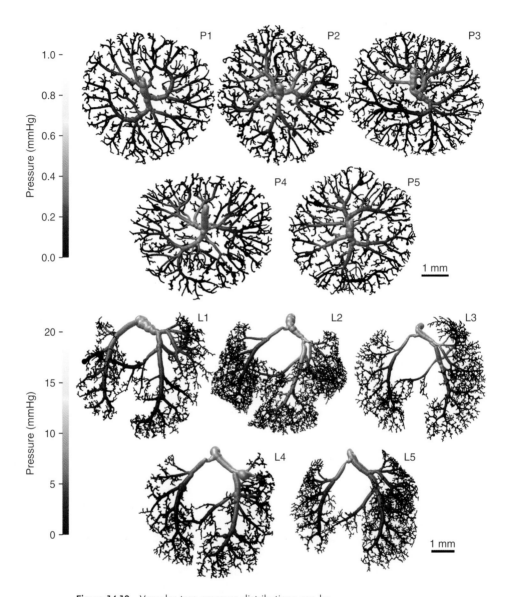

Figure 14.19 Vascular tree pressure distributions can be
determined analytically by modeling the vasculature as a
network of cylindrical pipes (connected in series and in parallel). Here, the computed pressure distributions for five
placenta (P1–P5) and five lungs (L1–L5) from mice specimens are shown. (Source: This figure is from Ref. [48]).

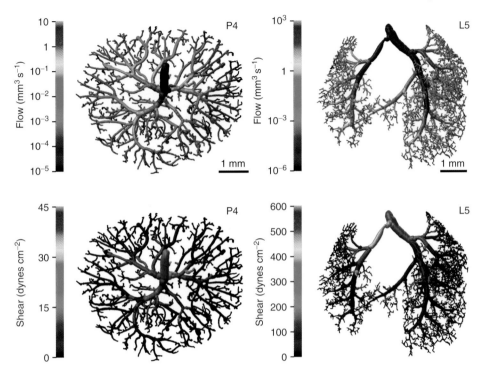

Figure 14.20 Vascular tree flow magnitudes and shear stress distributions can also be determined analytically by modeling the vasculature as a network of cylindrical pipes (connected in series and in parallel). Here, the computed fluid flow magnitude and shear stress distributions for a mouse placenta and lung specimen are shown. (Source: This figure is from Ref. [48]).

and simulations, as well as novel experimental designs are all fully open fields for micro-CT research.

The phase delay of X-rays can be used to provide higher tissue contrast than that achievable by attenuation-based X-ray imaging. Since X-rays travel at slightly different velocities through different tissues, interference patterns in the detected X-ray intensities develop, which can then be turned into actual phase delays that can be used for higher sensitivity tissue differentiation.

Novel detector arrays can make energy-selective X-ray detection a practical option for bench-top micro-CT imaging systems, and the capability of a detector to actually count individual photons, of the order of 10^4 photons per detector pixel per second, is also being realized.

The use of different contrast agents can be used to study vasculature in close proximity. For instance, the hepatic artery, portal vein, and biliary tree in the liver all follow essentially the same branching paths. By injecting different contrast agents and imaging at different photon energies, closely related vascular structures could be delineated and characterized.

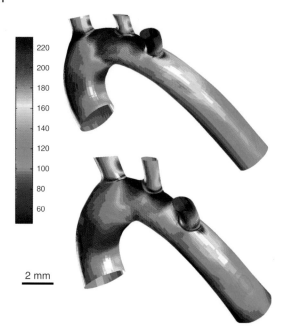

Figure 14.21 Wall shear stresses of vasculature can be computed through fluid dynamic simulations of the segmented vasculature. Here, the mean wall shear stress (in dynes cm^{-2}) for two different mouse aortas is shown. The wall shear stress vector magnitudes were averaged over the full cardiac cycle. Areas of relatively low wall shear stress are observed in the inner curvature of the aortic arch as well as the entrance orifice. The lateral surfaces of the ascending aorta and the region of the arch around the left common carotid artery are regions of high wall shear stress. (Source: This figure is from Ref. [76]).

The previously developed methods for performing a successful *in vivo* study have already had to work on overcoming problems related to motion artifacts, which will be useful for future *in vivo* longitudinal microcirculation studies. As an example, longitudinal study, the remodeling of microvasculature, as the dynamic process which it is, could be evaluated.

In addition, methods for cardiac gating could help answer the question of how well a micro-CT scan of a vascular tree (which is a snapshot in time) represents the "true" dynamic tree geometry.

For example, just how important is the diameter change caused by the contracting heart's pressure pulses? Many questions, like this one, can only be answered by doing *in vivo* scans at many time points within a single cardiac cycle.

Since physiological motion in a mouse (for instance) is 10× faster than in humans, special care is needed to reduce motion blur. For example, short exposure times with high fluency rates are needed; yet, lethal dose (or LD50) levels must be considered to allow for the feasibility of longitudinal studies. Clearly, *in vivo* micro-CT imaging is still in its infancy, which allows a great deal of room for future research investigations.

Fluid dynamic analysis of vasculature still has to overcome issues related to the definition of boundary conditions (a highly complex problem when dealing with hundreds or thousands of interbranch segments; a simulation which would involve just as many outlet pressures, for instance, to be defined) and applying physiologically realistic values to the simulation's initial conditions. In the past, these issues have required relatively simple structures to be characterized. Further, methodological improvements are needed to fully and accurately characterize the complex nature of fluid flow through vasculature.

The high spatial resolution data of micro-CT imaging is an important addition for many other imaging modalities, and further improvements in all the collaborative disciplines will help to further use micro-CT as a tool for studying microcirculation.

Acknowledgments

The authors would like to thank Ms Delories C. Darling for her help in the preparation of this chapter. This work was supported in part by NIH **Grant EB000305** and The Mayo Foundation.

References

1. Jorgensen, S.M., Demirkaya, O., and Ritman, E.L. (1998) Three-dimensional imaging of vasculature and parenchyma in intact rodent organs with x-ray micro-CT. *Am. J. Physiol. Heart. Circ. Physiol.*, **275** (3), H1103–H1114.

2. Paulus, M.J., Gleason, S.S., Kennel, S.J., Hunsicker, P.R., and Johnson, D.K. (2000) High resolution x-ray computed tomography: an emerging tool for small animal cancer research. *Neoplasia*, **2** (1–2), 62–70.

3. Seo, Y., Hashimoto, T., Nuki, Y., and Hasegawa, B.H. (2008) In vivo microCT imaging of rodent cerebral vasculature. *Phys. Med. Biol.*, **53** (7), N99–N107.

4. Kachelriess, M. (2008) *Micro-CT*, Springer-Verlag, Berlin, Heidelberg, pp. 23–52.

5. Zagorchev, L., Pierre, O., Zhen, Z., Karen, M., Mary, M.K., Michael, S., and Thierry, C. (2010) Micro computed tomography for vascular exploration. *J. Angiogenesis Res.*, **2** (1), 7.

6. Gössl, M., Malyar, N.M., Rosol, M., Beighley, P.E., and Ritman, E.L. (2003) Impact of coronary vasa vasorum functional structure on coronary vessel wall perfusion distribution. *Am. J. Physiol. Heart Circ. Physiol.*, **285**, H2019–H2026.

7. Zhu, X.Y., Bentley, M.D., Chade, A.R., Ritman, E.L., Lerman, A., and Lerman, L.O. (2007) Early changes in coronary artery wall structure detected by microcomputed tomography in experimental hypercholesterolemia. *Am. J. Physiol. Heart Circ. Physiol.*, **293**, H1997–H2003.

8. Le, H., Wong, J.T., and Molloi, S. (2008) Estimation of regional myocardial mass at risk based on distal arterial lumen volume and length using 3d micro-CT images. *Comput. Med. Imaging Graph.*, **32** (6), 488–501.

9. Savai, R., Langheinrich, A.C., Schermuly, R.T., Pullamsetti, S.S., Dumitrascu, R., Traupe, H., Rau, W.S., Seeger, W., Grimminger, F., and Banat, G.A. (2009) Evaluation of angiogenesis using micro-computed tomography in a xenograft mouse model of lung cancer. *Neoplasia*, **11** (1), 48–56.

10. Zagorchev, L. and Mulligan-Kehoe, M.J. (2009) Molecular imaging of vessels in

mouse models of disease. *Eur. J. Radiol.*, **70** (2), 305–311.

11. Morrison, M.S., Ricketts, S.A., Barnett, J., Cuthbertson, A., Tessier, J., and Wedge, S.R. (2009) Use of a novel arg-gly-asp radioligand, 18f-ah111585, to determine changes in tumor vascularity after antitumor therapy. *J. Nucl. Med.*, **50** (1), 116–122.

12. Radon, J. (1917) Über die bestimmung von funktionen durch ihre integralwerte längs. Gewisser Mannigfaltigkeiten, *Ber. Säch. Akad. Wiss.*, Leipzig, **69**, 262–277.

13. Wolka, J. (1953) Protokolle des seminars anwendungen der mathematic. (Lukaszewicz, Perkal, Steinhaus). der Universität Breslau. Tomografia.

14. Korenblyum, B.I., Tetel'baum, S.I., and Tyutin, A.A. (1958) About one scheme of tomography. *Izv VUZ Radiofiz*, **1**, 151–157.

15. Oldendorf, W.H. (1963) Radiant energy apparatus for investigating selected areas of the interior of objects obscured by dense material. US Patent 3106640.

16. Cormack, A.M. (1963) Representation of a function by its line integrals, with some radiological application. *J. Appl. Phys.*, **34** (9), 2722–2727.

17. Stauber, M. and Müller, R. (2008) Micro-computed tomography: a method for the non-destructive evaluation of the three-dimensional structure of biological specimens. *Methods Mol. Biol.*, **455**, 273–292.

18. Hounsfield, G.N. (1968–1972) A method of and apparatus for examination of a body by radiation such as x-ray or gamma radiation. UK Patent 1283915.

19. Feldkamp, L.A., Goldstein, S.A., Parfitt, M.A., Jesion, G., and Kleerekoper, M. (1989) The direct examination of three-dimensional bone architecture in vitro by computed tomography. *J. Bone Miner. Res.*, **4** (1), 3–11.

20. Sensen, C. and Hallgremsson, B. (eds) (2009) *Micro-Computed Tomography*, Springer-Verlag, Berlin, Heidelberg, pp. 301–318.

21. Marxen, M., Sled, J.G., Yu, L.X., Paget, C., and Henkelman, R.M. (2006) Comparing microsphere deposition and ow modeling in 3d vascular trees.

Am. J. Physiol. Heart Circ. Physiol., **291**, H2136–H2141.

22. Schambach, S.J., Bag, S., Scholling, L., Groden, C., and Brockmann, M.A. (2010a) Application of micro-CT in small animal imaging. *Methods*, **50** (1), 2–13.

23. Badea, C., Hedlund, L.W., and Johnson, G.A. (2004) Micro-CT with respiratory and cardiac gating. *Med. Phys.*, **31** (12), 3324–3329.

24. Feldkamp, L.A., Davis, L.C., and Kress, J.W. (1984) Practical cone-beam algorithm. *J. Opt. Soc. Am. A*, **1** (6), 612–619.

25. Kline, T.L., Zamir, M., and Ritman, E.L. (2010b) Accuracy of microvascular measurements obtained from micro-CT images. *Ann. Biomed. Eng.*, **38** (9), 2851–2864.

26. Langheinrich, A.C., Yeniguen, M., Ostendorf, A., Marhoffer, S., Dierkes, C., von Gerlach, S., Nedelman, M., Kampschulte, M., Bachmann, G., Stolz, E., and Gerriets, T. (2009) In vitro evaluation of the sinus sagittalis superior thrombosis model in the rat using 3D micro- and nanocomputed tomography. *Neuroradiology*, doi: 10.1007/s00234-009-0617-5.

27. Cavanaugh, D., Johnson, E., Price, R.E., Kurie, J., Travis, E., and Cody, D.D. (2004) In vivo respiratory-gated micro-CT imaging in small-animal oncology models. *Mol. Imag.*, **3** (1), 55–62.

28. Namati, E., Chon, D., Thiesse, J., Hoffman, E.A., de Ryk, J., Ross, A., and McLennan, G. (2006) In vivo micro-CT lung imaging via a computer-controlled intermittent iso-pressure breath hold (iibh) technique. *Phys. Med. Biol.*, **51** (23), 6061–6075.

29. Duvall, C.L., Robert Taylor, W., Weiss, D., and Guldberg, R.E. (2004) Quantitative microcomputed tomography analysis of collateral vessel development after ischemic injury. *Am. J. Physiol. Heart Circ. Physiol.*, **287**, H302–H310.

30. Chow, P.L., Stout, D.B., Komisopoulou, E., and Chatziioannou, A.F. (2006) A method of image registration for small animal, multi-modality imaging. *Phys. Med. Biol.*, **51**, 379–390.

31. Watanabe, M., Uchida, H., Okada, T., Yamashita, T., and Tanaka, E. (1992) A high resolution PET for animal studies. *IEEE Trans. Med. Imaging*, **11** (4), 577–580.

32. Bloomfield, P.M., Rajeswaran, S., Spinks, T.J., Hume, S.P., Myers, R., Ashworth, S., Clifford, K.M., Jones, W.F., Byars, L.G., Young, J., Andreaco, M., Williams, C.W., Lammertsma, A.A., and Jones, T. (1995) The design and physical characteristics of a small animal positron emission tomograph. *Phys. Med. Biol.*, **40** (6), 1105–1126.

33. Cherry, S.R., Shao, Y., Silverman, R.W., Meadors, K., Siegel, S., Chatziioannou, A., Young, J.W., Jones, W.F., Moyers, J.C., Newport, D., Boutefnouchet, A., Farquhar, T.H., Andreaco, M., Paulus, M.J., Binkley, D.M., Nutt, R., and Phelps, M.E. (1997) MicroPET: a high resolution PET scanner for imaging small animals. *IEEE Trans. Nucl. Sci.*, **44** (3), 1161–1166.

34. Schelbert, H.R. (2000) PET contributions to understanding normal and abnormal cardiac perfusion and metabolism. *Ann. Biomed. Eng.*, **28**, 922–929.

35. Holdsworth, D.W. and Thornton, M.M. (2002) Micro-CT in small animal and specimen imaging. *Trends Biotechnol.*, **20** (8), S34–S39.

36. Chatziioannou, A.F., Cherry, S.R., Shao, Y., Silverman, R.W., Meadors, K., Farquhar, T.H., Pedarsani, M., and Phelps, M.E. (1999) Performance evaluation of microPET: a high-resolution lutetium oxyorthosilicate pet scanner for animal imaging. *J. Nucl. Med.*, **40** (7), 1164–1175.

37. Jan, M.L., Ni, Y.C., Chen, K.W., Liang, H.C., Chuang, K.S., and Fu, Y.K. (2006) A combined micro-PET/CT scanner for small animal imaging. *Nucl. Instrum. Methods Phys. Res., A*, **569**, 314–318.

38. Wietholt, C., Molthen, R.C., Haworth, S.T., Roerig, D.L., Dawson, C.A., and Clough, A.V. (2004) Quantification of bronchial circulation perfusion in rats. *Proc. SPIE*, **5329** (1), 387–393.

39. de Kemp, R.A., Epstein, F.H., Catana, C., Tsui, B.M.W., and Ritman, E.L. (2010) Small-animal molecular imaging

methods. *J. Nucl. Med.*, **51** (Suppl. 1), 18S–32S.

40. Hwang, A.B., Taylor, C.C., VanBrocklin, H.F., Dae, M.W., and Hasegawa, B.H. (2006) Attenuation correction of small animal SPECT images acquired with ^{125}I-Iodorotenone. *IEEE Trans. Nucl. Sci.*, **53** (3), 1213–1220.

41. Kastis, G.A., Furenlid, L.R., Wilson, D.W., Peterson, T.E., Barber, H.B., and Barret, H.H. (2004) Compact CT/SPECT small-animal imaging system. *IEEE Trans. Nucl. Sci.*, **51** (1), 63–67.

42. Badea, C.T., Hedlund, L.W., De Lin, M., Boslego Mackel, J.F., and Allen Johnson, G. (2006) Tumor imaging in small animals with combined micro-CT/micro-DSA system using iodinated conventional and blood pool contrast agents. *Contrast Media Mol. Imaging*, **1** (4), 153–164.

43. Badea, C.T., Drangova, M., Holdsworth, D.W., and Johnson, G.A. (2008) In vivo small-animal imaging using micro-CT and digital subtraction angiography. *Phys. Med. Biol.*, **53** (19), R319–R350.

44. Langheinrich, A.C., Bohle, R.M., Greschus, S., Hackstein, N., Walker, G., von Gerlach, S., Rau, W.S., and Holschermann, H. (2004) Artherosclerotic lesions at micro CT: feasibility for analysis of coronary artery wall in autopsy specimens. *Radiology*, **231**, 675–681.

45. Gannon, B.J. (1978) *Vascular Casting*, vol. **6**, Van Nostrand Reinhold Company, New York, pp. 170–193.

46. Mondy, W.L., Cameron, D., Timmermans, J.P., Clerck, N.D., Sasov, A., Casteleyn, C., and Piegl, L.A. (2009) Micro-CT of corrosion casts for use in the computer-aided design of microvasculature. *Tissue Eng. Part C Methods*, **15** (4), 729–738.

47. Marxen, M., Thornton, M.M., Chiarot, C.B., Klement, G., Koprivnikar, J., Sled, J.G., and Henkelman, R.M. (2004) MicroCT scanner performance and considerations for vascular specimen imaging. *Med. Phys.*, **31** (2), 305–313.

48. Yang, J., Yu, L.X., Rennie, M.Y., Sled, J.G., and Henkelman, R.M. (2010) Comparative structural and hemodynamic analysis of vascular trees.

Am. J. Physiol. Heart Circ. Physiol., **298**, H1249–H1259.

49. Zhu, X.Y., Rodriquez-Porcel, M., Bentley, M.D., Chade, A.R., Sica, V., Napoli, C., Caplice, N., Ritman, E.L., Lerman, A., and Lerman, L.O. (2004) Antioxidant intervention attenuates myocardial neovascularization in hypercholesterolemia. *Circulation*, **109**, 2109–2115.

50. Mukundan, S., Ghaghada, K.B., Badea, C.T., Kao, C.Y., Hedlund, L.W., Provenzale, J.M., Johnson, G.A., Chen, E., Bellamkonda, R.V., and Annapragada, A. Jr. (2006) A liposomal nanoscale contrast agent for preclinical CT in mice. *Am. J. Roentgenol.*, **286**, 300–307.

51. Kong, W.H., Lee, W.J., Cui, Z.Y., Bae, K.H., Park, T.G., Kim, J.H., Park, K., and Seo, S.W. (2007) Nanoparticulate carrier containing water-insoluble iodinated oil as a multifunctional contrast agent for computed tomography imaging. *Biomaterials*, **28** (36), 5555–5561.

52. Schambach, S.J., Bag, S., Groden, C., Scholling, L., and Brockmann, M.A. (2010b) Vascular imaging in small rodents using micro-CT. *Methods*, **50** (1), 26–35.

53. Dong, Y., Malyar, N.M., Beighley, P.E., and Ritman, E.L. (2005) Characterization of sub-resolution microcirculatory status using whole-body CT imaging. *Proc. SPIE*, **5746**, 175–183.

54. Kline, T.L., Dong, Y., Zamir, M., and Ritman, E.L. (2010a) Erode/dilate analysis of micro-CT images of porcine myocardial microvasculature. *Proc. SPIE*, **7626**, 762620-1–762620-9.

55. Malyar, N.M., Gossl, M., Beighley, P.E., and Ritman, E.L. (2004) Relationship between arterial diameter and perfused tissue volume in myocardial microcirculation: a micro-CT-based analysis. *Am. J. Physiol. Heart Circ. Physiol.*, **286**, H2386–H2392.

56. Robb, R.A., Hanson, D.P., and Stacy, M.C. (1989) Analyze: a comprehensive, operator-interactive software package for multidimensional medical image display and analysis. *Comput. Med. Imaging Graph.*, **13** (6), 433–454.

57. Lee, J., Beighley, P., Ritman, E., and Smith, N. (2007) Automatic segmentation of 3d micro-CT coronary vascular images. *Med. Image Anal.*, **11** (6), 630–647.

58. Olabarriaga, S.D., Breeuwer, M., and Niessen, W.J. (2003) Evaluation of hessian-based filters to enhance the axis of coronary arteries in CT images. *Int. Cong. Series*, **1256**, 1191–1196.

59. Chan, T.F., and Vese, L.A. (2001) Active contours without edges. *IEEE Trans. Image Process.*, **10** (2), 266–277.

60. Lam, L. and Lee, S.W. (1992) Thinning methodologies – a comprehensive survey. *Pattern Anal. Mach. Intell.*, **14**, 869–885.

61. Schirmacher, H., Zockler, M., Stalling, D., and Hege, H.C. (1998) *Image and Multidimensional Digital Signal Processing*, IEEE, pp. 25–28.

62. Deschamps, T. and Cohen, L.D. (2000) Minimal path in 3d images and application to virtual endoscopy. *ECCV 2000*, **184**, 543–547.

63. van Uitert, R. and Bitter, I. (2007) Subvoxel precise skeletons of volumetric data based on fast marching methods. *Med. Phys.*, **34**, 627–637.

64. Zamir, M. (1998) Mechanics of blood supply to the heart: wave reflection effects in a right coronary artery. *Proc. Biol. Soc.*, **265** (1394), 439–444.

65. Op Den Buijs, J., Bajzer, Z., and Ritman, E.L. (2006) Branching morphology of the rat hepatic portal vein tree: a micro-CT study. *Ann. Biomed. Eng.*, **34** (9), 1420–1428.

66. Eberly, D. and Lancaster, J. (1991) On gray scale image measurements. *CVGIP: Graph. Mod. Image Proc.*, **53**, 538–549.

67. Soltanian-Zadeh, H., Shahrokni, A., and Zoroofi, R.A. (2001) Voxel-coding method for quantification of vascular structure from 3d images. *Proc. SPIE*, **4321**, 263–270.

68. Hoffman, K.R., Nazareth, D.P., Miskolczi, L., Gopal, A., Wang, Z., Rudin, S., and Bednarek, D.R. (2002) Vessel size measurements in angiograms: a comparison of techniques. *Med. Phys.*, **29**, 1622–1633.

69. Schaefer, H.M., Beighley, P.E., Eaker, D.R., Vercnocke, A.J., and

Ritman, E.L. (2009) Micro-CT analysis of myocardial blood supply in young and adult rats. *Proc. SPIE*, **7262**, 726225(1)–726225(6).

70. Haralick, R.M., Sternberg, S.R., and Zhuang, X. (1987) Image analysis using mathematical morphology. *IEEE Trans. Pattern Anal. Mach. Intell.*, **PAMI-9**, 532–550.

71. Gonzalez, R.C. and Woods, R.E. (2002) *Digital Image Processing*, 2nd edn, Prentice Hall.

72. Ohuchi, H., Beighley, P.E., Dong, Y., Zamir, M., and Ritman, E.L. (2007) Microvascular development in porcine right and left ventricular walls. *Pediatr. Res.*, **61** (6), 676–680.

73. Murray, C.D. (1926) The physiological principle of minimum work i. the vascular system and the cost of blood volume. *Proc. Natl. Acad. Sci.*, **12** (3), 207–214.

74. Sutera, S.P. and Skalak, R. (1993) The history of Poiseuille's law. *Annu. Rev. Fluid. Mech.*, **25**, 1–19.

75. Steinman, D.A. (2002) Image-based computational fluid dynamics modeling in realistic arterial geometries. *Ann. Biomed. Eng.*, **30**, 483–497.

76. Suo, J., Ferrara, D.E., Sorescu, D., Guldberg, R.E., Taylor, W.R., and Giddens, D.P. (2007) Hemodynamic shear stresses in mouse aortas: implications for atherogenesis. *Arterioscler. Thromb. Vasc. Biol.*, **27**, 346–351.

15
Imaging Blood Circulation Using Nuclear Magnetic Resonance

Christian M. Kerskens, Richard M. Piech, and James F.M. Meaney

Magnetic resonance imaging (MRI) is able to detect flow of all velocity regimes going from fast flow in arteries down to microscopic transport in cells. For imaging blood flow, methods can be divided into noninvasive and invasive methods. Noninvasive methods rely on changes in the longitudinal or transversal relaxation of the magnetization, which are always altered by flow. Those effects can be minimized to reduce flow artifacts, or they can be maximized to measure flow. In many cases, the signal change due to flow can be quantified. In contrast, invasive methods use indicators, which are injected into the blood stream. When they are passing the imaging plane, they can alter the MRI signal in several ways.

In this chapter, we start with the basic physical principles behind flow-sensitive MRI. After that, we focus on the main applications, which are MR angiography, MR perfusion imaging, and functional MRI (fMRI). We discuss various applications and limitations in clinical routine, medical, and cognitive research.

15.1
Introduction

Nuclear magnetic resonance imaging (NMRI) has revolutionized our world. Since the discovery of the nuclear magnetic moment, it has grown rapidly into a sophisticated technique with very wide applications in physical and organic chemistry, solid-state physics, biochemistry, biophysics, and medicine. In 1973, magnetic resonance imaging (MRI) was first suggested by Lauterbur [1] and, independently, by Mansfield and Grannell [2]. During the 1980s, it developed into an important tool for medical diagnosis, monitoring, and research. Most important applications are in oncology, cardiac, and neuroimaging. Since the 1990s, functional magnetic resonance imaging (fMRI) [3] measuring brain activations during specific tasks has become the most important tool for cognitive research.

Microcirculation Imaging, First Edition. Edited by Martin J. Leahy.
© 2012 Wiley-VCH Verlag GmbH & Co. KGaA. Published 2012 by Wiley-VCH Verlag GmbH & Co. KGaA.

15.1.1
The NMR Signal

Placed in a static magnetic field,[1] some atomic nuclei have an intrinsic property called *spin*, which aligns with the magnetic field. The nuclear spin has an intrinsic angular momentum that precesses with the so-called Larmor frequency Ω around its axis with $\Omega = \gamma^* B_0$, where γ is the gyromagnetic ratio and B_0 the static magnetic field. In protons, two states of alignment are possible, which have different energy levels in the magnetic field. Owing to the energy difference, a small excess of nuclei populate the lower state (Boltzmann statistic). This excess of spins accounts for the entire net magnetization, which is used in the NMR experiment (For further reading, see [6]).

Here for MRI, we consider the "bulk" magnetization **M** that arises from all of the magnetic moments in a sample, which can be treated classically. The classical description is based on the Bloch equations,[2] which are sufficient to understand the MR signal dependency for most imaging purposes. For a static magnetic field in *z*-direction, the Bloch equations become

$$\frac{dM_z(t)}{dt} = \gamma \left[M_x(t) B_y(t) - M_y(t) B_x(t) \right] - \frac{M_z(t) - M_0}{T_1} \tag{15.1a}$$

$$\frac{dM_x(t)}{dt} = -\gamma M_z(t) B_y(t) - \Omega M_y(t) - \frac{M_x(t)}{T_2} \tag{15.1b}$$

$$\frac{dM_y(t)}{dt} = \gamma M_z(t) B_x(t) + \Omega M_x - \frac{M_y(t)}{T_2} \tag{15.1c}$$

where T_1 and T_2 are the longitudinal (spin–lattice) and transversal (spin–spin) relaxation rates, respectively, and **B** is the magnet field. The indices *x,y,z* indicate vector components of the vectors **M** and **B**. For deeper understanding, we discuss two special cases:

1) For a very short applied radiofrequency (RF) field $\omega_x = \gamma B_x (B_y = 0$, pulse duration $\ll T_1, T_2$), we can neglect all relaxation terms in Eqs. (15.1a–c). The magnetization M' in the rotating frame, in which the transverse plane *x*–*y* rotates around the *z*-axis at the Larmor frequency, is

$$M_z'(t) = M_0 \cos(\omega_x t), \; M_y'(t) = M_0 \sin(\omega_x t), \; M_x'(t) = 0. \tag{15.1d}$$

---

1) The static magnetic field in MRI experiments serves a dual purpose, as both the polarizing field and the detection field. The sensitivity of NMR detection depends on both the magnitude of the magnetization and the frequency at which it precesses. Since both of these depend linearly on the magnetic field, higher fields mean substantially higher sensitivity [4]. Furthermore, as a susceptibility phenomenon, T_2^* blood oxygenation level – dependent (BOLD) effects are expected to increase with field strength [5]. This is important for cognitive studies as we see later.
2) For in-depth reading, see Ref. [7].

This solution shows the behavior of an RF pulse. It flips the magnetization by an angle $\alpha = \gamma B_x t_{RF}$, where t_{RF} is the pulse duration. An RF pulse can flip the magnetization into $x-y$ plane, but it can also refocus dephased magnetization in the transverse plane. This scheme is called a spin echo (SE). It consists of a $180°$ pulse that mirrors, in case of a pulse in the x-direction, the $x-y$ component around the y-axis. It enables to rephase static magnetization that was dephased by field variations.

2) In the absence of any applied RF pulse ($B_x = 0$ and $B_y = 0$), a simple solution can be found for the Bloch equations (Eqs. (15.1a–c))

$$M_z(t) = M_z(0) \exp\left(-\frac{t}{T_1}\right) + M_0 \left(1 - \exp\left(-\frac{t}{T_1}\right)\right) \tag{15.2a}$$

$$M_x(t) = M_0 \cos(\Omega t) \exp\left(-\frac{t}{T_2}\right) \tag{15.2b}$$

$$M_y(t) = M_0 \sin(\Omega t) \exp\left(-\frac{t}{T_2}\right). \tag{15.2c}$$

From Eqs. (15.2a–c), one can see that the longitudinal magnetization T_1 always returns back to M_0 while the transversal relaxation always decays to zero. Both processes influence the MRI signal and can be used to weight the image. Figure 15.1

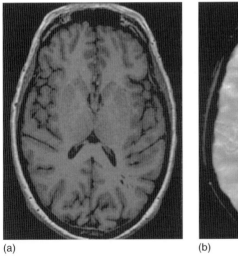
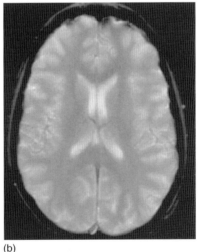

(a)   (b)

Figure 15.1 Comparison of T_1-weighted and T_2-weighted gradient echo sequences. (a) Axial T_2^*-weighted image of a human brain. (b) T_1-weighted image of a human brain with position of the slice geometry similar to (a). Different contrasts in cerebrospinal fluid (CSF) and gray and white matter are clearly visible. (From Ref. [8]).

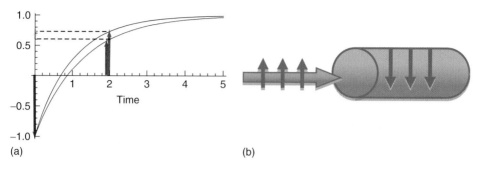

(a) (b)

Figure 15.2 (a) A time course of the MR signal after inversion of the magnetization via RF pulse (purple arrow) is shown (time = 0). The red line indicates the normal T_1 relaxation, while the blue line shows a faster decline due to a flow-induced shortening of the T_1 relaxation. The red and blue arrows are showing the signal differences 2 s after inversion. (b) A schematic drawing of noninverted magnetization flowing into a region of inverted magnetization is shown. The summation of all magnetization in the measuring plane then gives the total signal.

shows a T_1-weighted anatomical scan of a human brain. Gray and white matter can be easily differentiated because of the difference in their longitudinal relaxation (For introduction, see Bitar *et al.* [8]).

15.1.2
Mechanisms by Which Microcirculation Can Alter MRI Signal

Motion can influence the NMR signal in a similar way as the longitudinal and transversal relaxation, which we want to demonstrate using a simple example.

Let us consider a pipe containing water that flows with constant velocity into an imaging voxel.[3]

15.1.2.1 Time-of-Flight
The Bloch equation (Eq. 15.1a) can be expanded by a term $F/V_\lambda^* M_z$ that describes the amount of inflowing magnetization, where F is the volume flow per voxel volume V_λ. For a slice-selective inversion recovery experiment (where the inflowing magnetization is not inverted), we can solve this expanded Bloch equation and we find the following

$$M_z(t) = M_0 \left(1 - 2 \exp\left(-\frac{t}{T_{1f}} \right) \right) \tag{15.3}$$

where $1/T_{1f} = 1/(T_1 + V_\lambda F)$.

We can see from this Eq. (15.3) that an inflow of differently excited magnetization simulates a change in the longitudinal relaxation. As many MRI sequences are

3) For simplification, we will not consider that the water might also flow out of the voxel again.

T_1-weighted, flow effects play an important role in interpreting those images (Figure 15.2).

15.1.2.2 Phase Shift

Similar to the longitudinal relaxation, the transversal relaxation T_2^* can also be affected by flow. In order to make this happen, the protons of the fluid have to flow through a magnetic field that is not homogenous along the flow path. This is usually realized by so-called magnetic field gradients, which are part of every MRI scanner. These gradients are necessary for the spatial encoding of the NMR signal. Spatial displacements are turned into frequency displacement, which can be easily seen by expanding Eqs. (15.2b,c) with $\mathbf{B}_\zeta = \mathbf{B}_0 + \partial\mathbf{B}_i/\partial x_i^* x_i = \mathbf{B}_0\, G_i^* x_i$, where x_x with $i = 1, 2, 3$ represents the space coordinates. G_i is as defined a so-called magnetic field gradient, which is an essential part of every MRI sequence.

For a short gradient pulse, where we may neglect relaxations and transverse $\mathbf{B}$-fields, the solution for the Bloch equations in the rotation frame is

$$\mathbf{M}_{xy} = \mathbf{M}_{xy}(0) \exp\left(-i\gamma \int \vec{G}(t)\vec{x}(t)\mathrm{d}t\right) \tag{15.4}$$

where we have introduced complex numbers $\mathbf{M}_{xy} = \mathbf{M}_x - i\mathbf{M}_y$.

In our simple case, the space coordinate $x_1(t)$ is changing in time with $x_1(t) = v_1^* t$. This means that we find a velocity-induced phase change if a (so-called) dephasing gradient was applied for a duration T_G in flow direction. The phase change is

$$\mathbf{M}_{xy} = \mathbf{M}_{xy}(0) \exp\left(-i\gamma\, G_1 v_1\, T_D^2/2\right) \tag{15.4a}$$

which can be differentiated from the phase shift of static magnetization by applying a second, rephasing (flipped polarization) gradient. The static magnetization will be rephased if the time integral over the gradient is the same. This is called a gradient echo (GE). In contrast, we find a phase change for the flow as

$$\mathbf{M}_{xy} = \mathbf{M}_{xy}(0) \exp\left(-i\gamma\, G_1 v_1\, T_D^2\right) \tag{15.4b}$$

In common imaging techniques, this would lead to a spatial displacement of the pipe (flow artifacts). In specialized sequences, this information can be used for measuring flow and other motions (see below). In imaging sequences, the phase shift is also designed to relate it to spatial information (determined by phase encoding).

A bipolar gradient, whose positive and negative lobes are of equal importance, will have no effect on the phase of stationary spins (Figure 15.3a). On the other hand, we have seen that moving magnetization will cause a phase shift, depending on the velocity, and therefore will be poorly located and a motion artifact will be seen in vascular structures and moving fluids.

To avoid this artifact, so-called flow-compensative gradients can be introduced. This would avoid dephasing in flows at constant velocity. A flow-compensative gradient consists of polarizing gradient applied for T_G, flipped polarization for $2T_G$, and back flipped polarization for T_G (Figure 15.3b). A simple calculation using Eq. (15.4) reveals that the velocity component cancels itself out, as does the static for

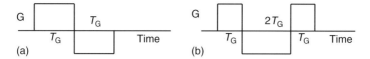

Figure 15.3 (a) Bipolar gradient pulse and (b) flow-compensative gradient.

the bipolar gradient. As the flow compensation consists of two bipolar gradients, the static phase is also not affected.

For flow compensation at variable velocity, gradient lobes have to be added on, resulting in a longer measurement time and a reduced signal. Flow-compensation gradients can be used in any sequence requiring the suppression of these artifacts, with the exception of phase contrast angiography (PCA).

15.1.2.3 MRI Indicator Methods

A third way to detect microcirculation is to change the signal inside the voxel through inflowing indicators, which can alter the signal.

15.1.2.3.1 Contrast Agents

Most common indicators are so-called MRI contrast agents that change the susceptibility. Tissue is more or less diamagnetic. A paramagnetic vascular contrast agent would change the environment around blood vessels and capillaries, which would then cause a change in T_1 and T_2* relaxation.

Most clinical examinations utilize one of several available contrast agents[4] that consist of paramagnetic ions such as Gadolinium (Gd) encased in a chelate molecule to minimize ion toxicity.

Following intravenous (IV) administration, extracellular fluid Gd contrast agents rapidly extravasate from the bloodstream into the interstitial space. An exception to this rule is the brain, where the blood–brain barrier (BBB) functions prevent the extravasations of contrast media from the blood vessels into the surrounding brain parenchyma.

Pathological conditions of the brain are often associated with BBB breakdown, leading on to leakage that permits subsequent diffusion of exogenously adminis- tered contrast material into the area of the lesion. For enhancing lesions, the use of Gd contrast agents provides important anatomical and functional information, including detailed depiction of lesion morphology, the overall extent of disease, and the hemodynamic properties of the perfused tissue.

In perfusion-weighted imaging, a rapid IV bolus administration of a Gd contrast agent achieves a high intravascular Gd concentration. With this delivery strategy, the effect of T_2^* relaxation outweighs the T_1/T_2 effects. T_2^* changes can be measured with fast imaging techniques that allow a read out of a contrast agent bolus with high temporal resolution.

4) A summary of the available contrast agents can be found in Ref. [9].

For quantification purposes, the relationship between concentration $C(t)$ and signal change $S(t)$ is important [87]. For most application, a simple relation is used

$$C(t) \propto \frac{1}{\text{TE}} \ln \left(\frac{S(t)}{S(0)} \right).$$

(15.5)

Unfortunately, susceptibility contrast agents such as gadolinium-DTPA (diethylene triamine pentaacetic acid) suffer from the fact that the relationship between measured signal and contrast is nonlinear and depends on parameters such as the field strength, shim of the magnet, and the constitution of the vessels [10]. Because of that and due to partial volume effects, correct scaling of the signal-to-concentration relation is mostly not possible. Altogether, this makes quantification troublesome, and in the general clinical practice, only a relative perfusion measure is possible [11].

15.1.2.3.2 Nanoparticles

During this past decade, science and engineering have seen a rapid increase in interest for materials with dimensions <100 nm, which lie in the intermediate state between atoms and bulk (solid) materials. Their attributes are significantly altered relative to the corresponding bulk materials as they exhibit size-dependent behavior such as quantum size effects (depending on bulk Bohr radius), optical absorption and emission, coulomb staircase behavior (electrical transport), superparamagnetism, and various other unique properties [12].

The magnetic nanoparticles have optimizable, controllable sizes enabling their comparison to cells (10–100 μm), viruses (20–250 nm), proteins (3–50 nm), and genes (10–100 nm). Scanning electron microscopy (SEM), transmission electron microscopy (TEM), atomic force microscopy (AFM), and X-ray photoelectron spectroscopy (XPS) provide necessary characterization methods that enable accurate structural and functional analysis of interaction of the biofunctional particles with the target bioentities [13].

For perfusion-weighted imaging, a rapid IV bolus administration similar to that in Gd contrast agent can be used, in combination with fast imaging techniques, to measure dynamic change due to perfusion. Similar problems regarding correlation between concentration and signal as with MR contrast agents occur.

15.1.2.3.3 Hyperpolarized Nuclei

NMR can be used to study many atomic nuclei, which have a nonzero spin quantum number, for example, ^{1}H, ^{3}He, ^{13}C, ^{15}N, and ^{129}Xe. However, at present, for reasons of sensitivity, clinical use of MRI is restricted to ^{1}H. ^{1}H, which is abundant in very high concentrations (circa 80 M) in biological tissue, has a higher sensitivity than any other nuclei in endogenous substances. The signal from a defined number of nuclear spins can be increased more than 100 000 times using hyperpolarization techniques. This enhancement of the signal allows *in vivo* imaging of nonproton nuclei (such as ^{13}C and ^{15}N) and their molecular distribution in a clinically relevant time frame.

Differing methods are available for hyperpolarization, producing polarization of up to 40% in some C-labeled substances [14]. Dilution in the vascular system causes the concentration of a hyperpolarized imaging agent to decrease. This effect can be cancelled out through hyperpolarization because the signal can be enhanced up to 10^6 times. This allows the imaging of changes in molecular structure, which would not have been previously possible (e.g., metabolic processes).

At present, the T_1 of the available ^{13}C and ^{15}N substances are short when compared with nuclei, such as ^{18}fluorodeoxyglucose (FDG), used in clinical PET procedures. This means that after polarization, advanced chemical synthesis cannot be performed. Clinically acceptable relaxation times may be attainable with an injectable water solution obtained through the application of a general polarization process to a wide range of small organic molecules. Developments in low-field MRI might enable longer relaxation rates *in vivo* [15].

Reported T_1 and T_2 values of the ^{13}C-containing molecules, used in *in vivo* imaging experiments, are typically 10–100 times longer than those of ^1H resulting in *in vivo* values of T_1 20–45 s and T_2 2–5 s [16, 17]. Because the signal from thermal equilibrium polarized ^{13}C nuclei is far below the limit of detection, following an administration of hyperpolarized ^{13}C, the MR signal that is detected can only come from the injected substance. This differs from standard proton imaging where the contrast substance injected affects the relaxation times of protons in proximity to the paramagnetic molecules. Hyperpolarized ^{13}C imaging has no background signal apart from patient and coil/receiver system noise, making subtraction of images unnecessary. The T_1 value of a given substance dictates the expected signal amplitude in the area of imaging at a defined time after injection. Imaging pulse methods take advantage of the long T_2 values for multiecho imaging strategies; however, the imaging agent and the clinical application are the determining factors in selecting the applied pulse sequence.

As hyperpolarized ^{13}C MRI gives direct information regarding the molecule, to which hyperpolarized atoms are attached, it makes tissue and cell viability research possible. NMR's capacity for distinguishing signals from the tracer in different molecules [16, 17] has more potential for direct molecular imaging than SPECT or PET, which are limited to imaging only the distribution of the active nuclei. The visualization of differing molecules containing ^{13}C with chemical shift imaging makes it feasible to generate frequency and spatial information simultaneously.

15.2
MR-Angiography

In the early days of MRI, the signal from flowing blood was considered a nuisance as it generated frequent artifacts, which detracted from image quality. It was some time before it was realized that the signal could be exploited to generate diagnostic quality images of blood vessels. Although magnetic resonance-angiography (MRA) is frequently regarded as a specific subdiscipline, it is important to remember that blood vessels can be identified on virtually all MR images.

15.2.1
MR-Angiography Techniques

In the following sections, we describe the important techniques used in MRA.

15.2.1.1 Time-of-Flight MR Angiography (TOF MRA)

In time-of-flight magnetic resonance-angiography (TOF MRA), flow-compensated GE imaging sequences are optimized to favor the vascular signal over that of the surrounding tissue. This can be achieved by using RF pulses with a high flip angle while using a short repetition time (TR). The stationary tissue signal will get saturated due to short TR because the longitudinal magnetization does not have time to relax back to equilibrium magnetization. The signal in a train of RF pulses reduces to a low steady state of magnetization.[5]

At the same time, this method favors the inflow effect because the blood flowing into the imaging plane has not been affected and its longitudinal magnetization is maximal. The signal from the nonsaturated blood flow is higher than that of the saturated tissues.

The signal in TOF MRA depends on hemodynamic, geometrical, and tissue conditions as well as sequence parameters. The hemodynamics of the inflow alter the amount of nonsaturated magnetization entering the imaging region. Complex or turbulent (stenosis) flow, which is linked to spin dephasing and slow flow, limits the TOF MRA sensitivity.

The length and orientation of the vessel is an important factor in the display of blood vessels. The vascular signal will be optimized by placing the slice perpendicular to the axis of the vessel, while vessels oriented parallel to the slice plane may not be discernable due to saturation effects. Either arteries or veins can be selectively visualized by placing a presaturation band on one side of the imaging slice, thus suppressing unwanted arterial or venous flow. The suppression of static tissue signal can be improved on with preparation pulses. These employ magnetization transfer (MT) saturation, which affects mainly tissue as it contains more large molecules or selective excitation of the water or fat saturation. Poor suppression of the signal from stationary tissues can happen in tissue with short T_1 relaxation, for example, those containing fat, atheroma, hematoma, and thrombi. The sequence parameters available to optimize contrast between static and flowing magnetization are TR, flip angle, echo time (TE), and slice thickness. Two imaging modalities are used for TOF MRA: 2D and 3D imaging. In 2D acquisition, time-of-flight imaging allows the use of a set of thin slices. Thin slices have better sensitivity to slow flows (which do not remain in the slice for long and will therefore

5) In many applications, fast MRI methods are used to achieve high temporal and spatial resolution. In order to achieve this, the repetition time has to be decreased. The repetition time has an impact on the signal intensity. To optimize the signal for this purpose, one can use the so-called Ernst angle [18]. This repetitive excitation with RF pulses leads to a steady state of longitudinal magnetization. The Ernst angle is derived by optimizing TR, T_1, and the flip angle relative to each other. One finds for the Ernst angle $\alpha = \arccos(\exp(-TR/T_1))$. The Ernst angle is generally important in achieving good S/N ratio.

not be saturated). It also gives the possibility of using high flip angles (giving better stationary tissue saturation and an increased vascular signal). However, this has the disadvantage of poor spatial resolution along the axis of the slice stack as they are stacked up to reconstruct a pseudo-volume.

On the contrary, 3D TOF MRA gives good spatial resolution in all three spatial directions, with a better signal-to-noise (S/N) ratio for fast flow. However, each repetition excites the total volume, producing a progressive saturation of the flows, even more so when they are slow. The slowest flows may even disappear entirely due to saturation. Flow saturation can be reduced as it passes through the explored volume by dividing 3D acquisition into slabs and by using ramped RF excitation, a technique that progressively the flip angle changes from one side of the imaging volume to the other [19].

15.2.1.2 Phase Contrast Angiography

PCA describes a method whereby phase shifts are experienced by protons moving through a bipolar gradient. For a bipolar gradient of an imparted length and strength, the moving spins dephase in proportion to their velocity v_{enc} as shown in Eqs. (15.4a,b). The potential values of the phases range from $-\pi$ to $+\pi$. However, beyond this range of possible values, aliasing occurs, which causes the velocity to be poorly encoded. Hence, the characteristics of the encoding gradient only encode flows within specific velocity parameters from $-v_{enc}$ to $+v_{enc}$ as defined by the user. PCA consists of two imaging sequences, both containing bipolar velocity-encoding gradients. They differ by the polarity of the gradients. This results in two images with opposite phase encoding, which allows differentiation between flowing and static magnetization. The acquisition in 2D PCA imaging is fast, making it useful for testing differing encoding speeds. The slice plane is perpendicular to the flow direction for the quantitative study of flows. In 3D PCA imaging, each partition is encoded in three directions, which results in better quality images than in 2D PCA due to reconstruction of the images in maximum intensity projection (MIP). Three-dimensional PCA is a more sensitive imaging technique for slow flows than

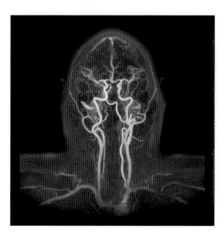

Figure 15.4 Carotids – MIP of the whole data set showing normal appearance of the head and neck arteries on contrast-enhanced MRA.

TOF where there is a tendency toward saturation. Parallel imaging can reduce the scan time of these sequences enormously [20].

15.2.1.3   Contrast-Enhanced MR-Angiography (CEMRA)

Contrast-enhanced methods have better signal-to-noise ratios and are faster than noncontrast agent injection techniques. There are many benefits in Gadolinium chelate-induced T_1 shortening, such as marked increase in the vascular signal that is independent of inflow effects and virtual complete of saturation of the blood signal that allows larger volumes to be examined in any plane. Furthermore, turbulent flow imaging is improved. A 4D dynamic MRA is also possible, enabling an injected bolus to be observed while flowing through the system. However, accurate timing is necessary when injecting the bolus if the acquisition is to occur simultaneously with the intravascular passage of the contrast agent. Inaccuracy in the timing can lead to either ringing artifact if central k-space data are acquired too early while the T_1 value is rapidly changing or contamination by venous signal if acquired too late (Figure 15.4).

15.2.1.4   Choice of the Underlying Technique

Blood vessels are usually recognized as a function of the presence and velocity of flowing blood contained therein, which present a characteristic signal on MR images. In the case of SE images, blood usually appears dark, while on GE images, vessels usually appear bright. Alteration of the contour of the vessel, the presence of abnormal intraluminal content, and alterations in blood flow velocities compared to adjacent or paired vessels disrupts the normal signal from flowing blood and usually gives information about the state of the blood vessel. GE sequences that demonstrate bright blood vessels (bright blood MRA) form the basis of most MRA approaches looking at the vessel lumen. However, there are exceptions to this generalization, for example, for delineation of pathology in the blood vessel wall where SE images play a larger role. Similarly, dark blood images are routinely used to accurately delineate the cardiac wall in patients in whom abnormality of the cardiac muscle is suspected.

15.2.1.5   Fast Imaging

Since most MRA techniques employ fast acquisitions, systems equipped with fast gradients are necessary. Progressive improvements in gradient performance, parallel imaging, partial k-space (e.g., keyhole imaging), time-resolved imaging, (e.g., TRICKS), and so on have resulted in scanning techniques with sufficient spatial and temporal resolution to address most clinical issues.

15.2.2
Clinical Applications

15.2.2.1   Different Diseases Usually Affect Arteries and Veins

Although many different disorders can affect blood vessels, diseases usually affect arteries by causing stenosis (narrowing) within them or by causing abnormal dilatation of the vessel (aneurysm formation). Although the pathology causing these end effects usually starts within the blood vessel wall, the wall is usually too thin to image reliably and a "road map" of the lumen of the vessel is acquired. This is usually performed by acquiring relatively thin cross-sectional images of the blood vessel by using a technique that portrays the blood vessel as the brightest structure on the image, and then usually a computer-based algorithm such as MIP to reproject the relatively large number of slices into a (pseudo) three-dimensional image that portrays the arterial tree as if it were extracted from the other anatomy. As a high degree of vessel to background contrast improves the efficiency of this extraction algorithm, efforts are aimed at boosting intravascular signal while minimizing background signal. Although imaging of the blood vessel wall, and particularly the factors that lead to narrowing of the lumen are highly sought after prizes, delineation of the components of atherosclerosis (the most common cause of narrowing) remains elusive. Improvements in wall delineation will depend on development of improved surface coils, higher resolution, and better methods for flow-related artifact and motion correction.

15.2.2.2 Requirement for MR Imaging of Blood Vessels

As MRI employs neither ionizing radiation nor invasive arterial catheterization, it potentially offers an ideal or near ideal modality for blood vessel imaging. However, in the early days of MRA when techniques were limited to TOF and PCA methods, it rapidly became apparent that long examination times and frequent artifacts would limit widespread use of MRA in clinical practice despite the fact that the study was virtually devoid of side effects (occasional contraindications of claustrophobia and the presence of implanted devices excepted). The introduction of contrast-enhanced techniques into clinical practice overcame many of the limitations of TOF and PCA. The benefit of contrast-enhanced magnetic resonance-angiography (CEMRA) lay in the fact that intravascular signal was no longer dependent on flow characteristics (which varied between patients and between different vessels in the same patient), and blood flow velocities that frequently declined with a parallel decline in intravascular signal now became largely irrelevant. Intravascular signal relied primarily on the degree of T_1 shortening which was determined by the injection rate of gadolinium. CEMRA became the standard bearer for MRA because of its inherent high vessel contrast, unrivalled CNR, freedom from artifacts, and speed of performance.

For CEMRA, images are acquired during first arterial passage of an intravenously injected bolus by synchronizing peak arterial enhancement with central k-space data. As the arterial phase (before circulation of the contrast agent into the veins) is relatively short, this mandates that image data is rapidly collected at the correct time. This is facilitated by either measuring the circulation time before the MRA with a test bolus or using "bolus detection," a term to denote the process whereby the circulation of contrast into the region of interest (ROI) can be visualized in real time by acquiring a low-resolution thick-slice image that is reconstructed and displayed in real time on the monitor, which allows the operator to commence the 3D scan immediately on arrival of the contrast agent within the artery of interest.

Even by exploiting fast 3D GRE acquisitions with acceleration techniques (parallel imaging), the acquisition time may extend well beyond the imaging window (often as short as 10 s) of arterial enhancement. However, the unique nature of k-space data facilitates the development of "pure" arteriograms despite this fact by synchronizing the contrast-defining central k-space data with the arterial phase of contrast enhancement.

Since it was so widely believed that gadolinium-based contrast agents were almost devoid of serious side effects, the penalty of intravenous cannulation and the minimal risk of adverse reaction to the injected contrast agent were dismissed as largely irrelevant. The fact that gadolinium-based contrast agents were substantially safer than iodinated contrast agents (injected for X-ray catheter angiography and computed tomographic angiography – CTA – the main competitor to MRA) was noted. For these reasons, CEMRA proliferated widely in clinical practice at the expense of noncontrast techniques that were used less often. However, increasing awareness of the rare but potentially fatal condition of nephrogenic systemic fibrosis (NSF), which is strongly associated with high-dose gadolinium usage especially in patients with kidney failure, has prompted renewed interest in noncontrast MRA techniques.

15.2.2.3 Difference in Gadolinium Contrast Agents

When intravenous contrast agents are injected for MRA, it is important to remember that there are some differences between the agents, the majority of which are gadolinium-based. Different contrast agents for MRA differ in their relaxivity, formulation strength, and degree of protein binding. The "standard" contrast agents are formulated at $0.5 \, mmol \, l^{-1}$ and are well proven as effective agents in clinical practice. A single agent (Gadovist, Berlex) is formulated at $1.0 \, mmol \, l^{-1}$. Also, different contrast agents differ in their degree of protein binding, which affects the relaxivity. For example, one of the "standard" $0.5 \, mmol \, l^{-1}$ agents exhibits weak protein binding (most of the other agents have essentially no protein binding), which improves its' relaxivity and therefore gives greater T_1 shortening on a volume comparison with other agents (Multihance, Bracco). More recently, a contrast agent with strong protein binding has been introduced into clinical practice. Because of the strong protein binding in plasma, it does not rapidly diffuse into the tissue and thus persists for a long period within the circulation. The long intravascular persistence of agents such as MS325 (the only one launched as a clinical product) leads to its classification as a blood-pool contrast agent (Ablavar, Lantheus).

15.2.2.4 Noncontrast MRA in Clinical Practice

TOF and PCA methods have been rapidly displaced by CEMRA for many applications. In some instances, for example, for evaluation of the intracranial arteries, TOF techniques remain the approach of choice (Figure 15.6). Also, although results have been variable in clinical practice, coronary MRA remains the preserve of noncontrast approaches to date. For the majority of vascular territories where CEMRA had become the technique of choice, renewed interest in noncontrast techniques was driven by concerns about safety of the contrast agent (gadolinium) injection.

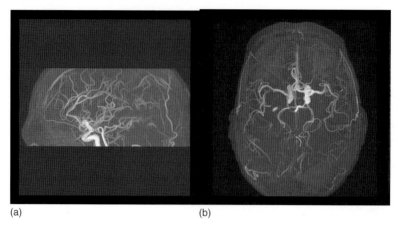

(a)   (b)

Figure 15.5 (a,b) TOF MRA in two orthogonal planes demonstrating normal appearance of the intracranial arteries at 3.0 T in (a) lateral and (b) craniocaudal projection.

Although a noncontrast technique to replace CEMRA as the prime technique for noninvasive vascular assessment has not been found, steady progress in newer noncontrast techniques has resulted in some competing techniques that may adequately allow decision making in clinical practice. For example, ECG-gated 3D partial-Fourier fast spin echo (FSE) methods and 3D balanced steady-state free precession (SSFP) methods have been reported for imaging of the larger vessels (thoracic aorta and pulmonary arteries). Data from the peripheral circulation suggest that delays in vascular enhancement on noncontrast time-resolved images may reflect stenosis severity. In addition, although time-resolved imaging is traditionally thought as the preserve of fast contrast-enhanced techniques, ECG-gated partial-Fourier FSE method, and adiabatic fast passage (AFP) inversion at 3 T (longer T_1 relaxation times at 3 T benefit AFP by prolonging the duration of tagging effect) with SSFP offer a promising noninvasive MR angiographic method for time-resolved MRA.

15.2.2.5 From Anatomy to Function: MRA as Part of a Multisequence Approach

Usually, MRA depicts the blood vessel lumen adequately and in many instances this is sufficient for clinical management. However, in many instances, it is important not only to detect the degree of vessel wall narrowing (usually by CEMRA) but also to detect the effect that the stenosis is having on the organ being supplied by the abnormal vessel. Although there is some correlation between the degree of narrowing of the vessel and the impairment in flow to the organ beyond, because of many physiological compensatory mechanisms, the effect is often not well correlated with the degree of narrowing. As a result, many methods have been proposed to measure flow into organs. For example, in the case of narrowing of the arteries supplying the kidneys, flow can be measured by 2D and 3D PCA methods

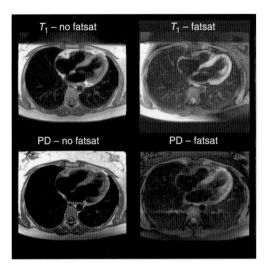

Figure 15.6 Dark blood imaging of the heart using spin-echo T_1 and proton-density-weighted imaging without and with fat saturation.

and also by measuring excretion of a small amount of the contrast agent injected before the MRA (Figure 15.6).

In other instances, for example, in patients with suspected stroke, MRA is part of a wider imaging workup. For example, the detection of the findings of infarction on SE imaging (T_2 and FLAIR) and diffusion-weighted imaging triggers a search for an abnormality within the arterial tree, the occlusion of which could be responsible for the infarct. Under such circumstances, anatomical imaging (usually SE and diffusion-weighted imaging) is typically combined with vascular imaging (e.g., TOF MRA of the intracranial arteries) and possibly with perfusion imaging to detect the degree of insult to the brain parenchyma. Although this has traditionally been performed by susceptibility imaging following injection of the contrast agent, the requirement to scan dynamically in the arterial phase precludes first-pass MRA of the carotid and vertebral arteries. However, by adding techniques such as arterial spin labeling (ASL) to detect cerebral blood flow (CBF), comprehensive assessment of the arterial tree and the effect of arterial narrowing become possible during a single examination.

15.2.2.6 Effect of Field Strength: 1.5 T vs. 3 T

As the difference between parallel and antiparallel protons is 10 per million at 3 T compared to 5 per million at 1.5 T imaging at 3 T anticipates a doubling of SNR over 1.5 T. However, as a host of additional interrelating factors, such as T_1, T_2, and T_2^*, affect SNR in addition to field strength SNR increases of less than double ($\sim$1.70–1.8) can be anticipated at 3 T. CEMRA at 3 T imaging benefits not only from the inherent improved SNR but also from the ability to use higher acceleration factors and from the fact that T_1 values are longer at 3 T, so that for any dose

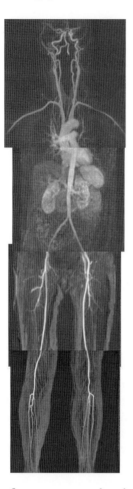

Figure 15.7 Whole-body MRA using a multistation stepping-table approach following a single injection of contrast agent.

of contrast agent the observed tissue contrast (difference between unenhanced and contrast agent-enhanced images) is better at 3 T compared to 1.5 T. From a practical viewpoint, the anticipated SNR boost at 3 T can be expected to improve image quality, improve temporal, or spatial resolution using the same volume (and injection rate) of contrast agent, or alternatively, a smaller volume of contrast agent can be injected for a similar effect as achieved at 1.5 T.

15.2.3
Conclusion

Many methods have been validated in clinical practice to evaluate the vascular tree noninvasively. Contrast-enhanced (Figure 15.7) techniques offer unrivalled spatial and temporal resolution and speed of performance. In some clinical instances and where it is inadvisable to use gadolinium-based contrast agents, there are many noncontrast techniques that can be exploited to good effect.

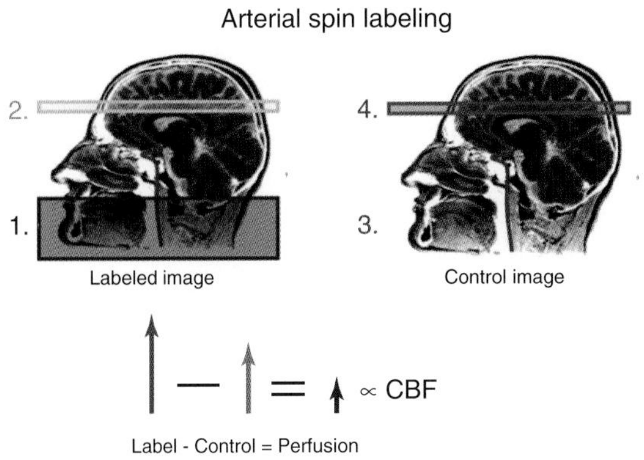

Arterial spin labeling

Label - Control = Perfusion

Figure 15.8 Generalized schematical drawing of an ASL areas. (1) Labeling plane (labeling of inflowing blood by inversion), (2) imaging plane (labeling), (3) repeat experiment without labeling, (4) imaging plane same position as in (2) but without labeling, and (5) subtracting results in an image with signal intensity depending on CBF. (Picture is taken from *http://www.umich.edu/fmri/asl.html*). (Source: Images Courtesy of University of Michigon (Educational Resources).)

15.3
Perfusion Imaging

Blood vessels and capillaries, which are beyond the resolution of normal MRI sequences, can be visualized as the so-called perfusion images, where the signal intensity in a voxel is related to the amount of flow and volume of those small vessels. In this section, we discuss the most common approaches.

15.3.1
Time-of-Flight Perfusion Imaging

The TOF methods primarily optimized to measure perfusion are called *arterial spin labeling* or arterial spin tagging (AST) techniques. These techniques can be divided into two groups, which are referred to as *continuous and pulsed ASL.*

15.3.1.1 Continuous Arterial Spin Labeling (CASL)
In 1992, this technique based on an idea for MRA [21] was used for the first time for imaging brain perfusion [22, 23]. In continuous arterial spin labeling (CASL), an inversion slice or labeling plane is located proximal to the imaging plane. The location is chosen in such a way that the slice cuts through big arteries. For a few seconds, magnetization flowing through this plane is continuously inverted by the principle of a flow-driven version of the AFP[6] [21]. The inverted magnetization leaves the labeling plane flowing into the imaging plane, where it can be detected with MRI. A number of pulse sequences can be used as the imaging sequence,

6) The principle of AFP is explained in Ref. [6].

including SE [23], echo-planar imaging (EPI) [24], and fast low-angle shot (FLASH) [25]. Since the imaging plane contains magnetization from static tissue, a second control image is acquired to subtract the tissue component (Figure 15.8).

The flow-driven AFP will not only invert flowing magnetization but also static tissue due to MT [26]. To take this effect into account, a flow-driven AFP pulse is also applied before the control image. The labeling plane is then positioned mirrored to the imaging where no arteries can be expected. The flow-driven AFP consists of an RF pulse and an accompanying magnetic field gradient, G, along the direction of arterial flow [21]. RF pulse durations of several seconds are needed to achieve CASL.[7] The off-frequency f_{lab} to provide a labeling location, Δr, a small distance away from the imaging plane is for a given gradient strength, G, as follows [27]:

$$f_{lab} = \gamma G \Delta r / 2\pi \tag{15.6}$$

The gradient strength also plays an important role for the flow-driven AFP. For spins moving with a velocity, v, parallel to the gradient, G, the effective magnetic field is changing in time according to $B_{eff} = \gamma G v t$.

When this dependency is combined with the AFP condition, we arrive at the adiabatic condition for flow-driven adiabatic inversion [23, 28]

$$\frac{1}{T_1}, \frac{1}{T_2} << \left| \frac{\vec{G} \cdot \vec{v}}{B_1} \right| << \gamma |B_1| \tag{15.7}$$

A more elegant way to find the degree of inversion is possible with a quantum mechanical approach given by Zhernovoy [29]. He leads to the following expression for $\boldsymbol{M}_z$ in terms of the $\boldsymbol{B}_1$ field

$$\boldsymbol{M}_z = \boldsymbol{M}_0 \left(2 \exp(-\frac{\pi \gamma B_1^2}{2\vec{G} \cdot \vec{v}}) - 1 \right) \tag{15.8}$$

In practice, the degree of the inversion achieved by the flow-driven adiabatic inversion scheme depends on the velocity of the blood, the orientation of the vessels relative to the labeling plane, the RF power and gradient strength. It is typically in the range of 80–95% [30–33]. Following the long labeling pulse, a spoiler gradient is often introduced to remove any transverse magnetization formed by imperfections in the inversion pulse.

As we mentioned, AFP also produces another contrast in MRI, which is MT. MT effects are problematic as they cause saturation at the imaging plane. These effects cause signal loss in the perfusion-weighted images that leads to errors in the subsequent quantification step.

The MT effects arise due to off-resonance excitation. Protons that are bound to macromolecules in the tissue have extremely short T_2 relaxation times and are therefore invisible to most imaging sequences. These protons are saturated over the entire duration of the ASL pulse. Owing to their broad RF absorption spectrum,

---

7) Long RF pulses can easily exceed regulatory limits on specific absorption rate (SAR) and the capability of the RF amplifiers.

protons bound to macromolecules at the imaging plane are saturated, while free water protons are largely unaffected at the imaging plane because of their narrow RF absorption spectrum. Subsequent chemical exchange between protons from macromolecules and free water results in MT. This culminates in a reduced signal from the free water pool at the imaging plane.

MT is not a symmetric function of frequency. However, there have been several schemes proposed in order to compensate for this source of error [34, 35]. The best way to reduce MT is the use of dedicated labeling coil, which is actively decoupled from the imaging receive coil. The labeling coil is typically small and placed far away from the imaging plane. Owing to the small sensitive region of the labeling coil, no saturation of macromolecules at the imaging plane occurs and this proves particularly useful when multislice perfusion imaging is required.

15.3.1.2 Pulsed Arterial Spin Labeling (PASL)
In pulsed arterial spin labeling (PASL), short RF pulses inverting a defined volume of blood perform the labeling of blood. From a mathematical view, one can say this labeling method establishes an initial condition, which will then evolve in time. This stands in contrast to CASL where we define a boundary condition at the labeling plane. For effective saturation or inversion of flowing magnetization, the usage of adiabatic RF pulses is of advantage. These can, in combination with gradients, select any chosen defined volume. The labeled volume then flows into the imaging plane for detection. Again, for separation of static and flowing magnetization, a control imaging is required.

In the following, a short summary of different PASL techniques is given

1) Echo-planar imaging and signal targeting with alternating radio frequency (EPISTAR) [36]. The labeling phase uses a slice-selective saturation pulse to saturate magnetization at a defined ROI. Imaging occurs after a short period of around 1 s to allow inflow of saturated magnetization. Afterward the control image is acquired without any additional preparation.

2) Transfer insensitive labeling technique (TILT) [37]. The drawback with EPIS-TAR is that it suffers from MT effects during the labeling phase. The TILT labeling technique uses an inversion scheme. The inversion pulse consists of two consecutive 90° RF pulses of the same phase. The control phase also uses two 90° RF pulses but now with an opposite phase. The second 90° pulse turns the magnetization back to the nonexcited state. MT similarly influences both images.

3) Flow-sensitive alternating inversion recovery (FAIR) [38]. This labeling scheme consists of a slice-selective inversion pulse for the labeling phase and a nonselective inversion for the control phase. Again, imaging occurs after a short inflow period. FAIR is less sensitive to MT effects than EPISTAR because it does not use off-resonance RF pulses with respect to the imaging slice. This allows multislice perfusion-weighted imaging.

15.3.2
Quantification

Attempts to quantify microcirculation are as many as there are sequences. Here, we offer a critical overview of the basic principles. They can be divided into three principles, where two of those principles are adaptations of other medical tracer methods.

15.3.2.1 Modified Fick' Law

Detre and Williams [22, 23] modified the Bloch equation by adding in- and outflow terms as introduced by Kety and Schmidt [39] in 1948. With this approach, a monoexponential decay can be found to describe the tissue response function. In the longitudinal direction, where the signal is altered by inflowing magnetization, the modified Bloch equation then takes the following form [22, 23]:

$$\frac{dM(t)}{dt} = fM_a(t) - \frac{f}{\lambda}M(t) + \frac{M_0 - M(t)}{T_1} \tag{15.9}$$

where f is defined as the blood flow (ml g^{-1} s^{-1}), λ is the blood/brain partition coefficient for water (the ratio of the quantity of water per gram of blood to the quantity of water per gram of brain), T_1 is the spin–lattice relaxation time of blood water, M is the longitudinal magnetization per gram of brain tissue, M_0 is M under fully relaxed conditions, and M_a is the longitudinal magnetization per milliliter of arterial blood. Using this equation, Detre *et al.* [22] found for a CASL experiment, with a full saturation of the imaging plane, the following results

$$f = \frac{\lambda}{T_{1app}} \frac{M^{ctrl} - M^{lab}}{2M^{ctrl}} \tag{15.9a}$$

where T_{1app} is the relaxation time that describes the exponential decrease in M_b due to the T_1 relaxation time of brain water and a flow and exchange term ($1/T_{1app} = 1/T_1 + f/\lambda$), M^{ctrl} is the image intensity in the control image, and M^{lab} is the image intensity in the labeled image. However, a discussion of Eq. (15.9) reveals the weakness of the model. The arterial magnetization does not have a T_1 relaxation dependency, although Calamante *et al.* [40] addressed this problem by incorporating T_1 blood relaxation. Another problem related to T_1 relaxation is the transit time from the labeling position to the imaging slice. Magnetization change due to transit time was introduced by Kwong *et al.* [38].

15.3.2.2 Indicator-Dilution Model

Buxton [41] proposed a general kinetic model, where the magnetization difference between the labeled and control images is described using a convolution integral. This method was first proposed for tracer methods by Meier and Zierler [42]. The convolution allows separation of the various physical processes involved. Buxton described the following time-dependent functions: (i) the delivery function (or fractional (arterial input function, AIF)) $c(t)$, which is the normalized concentration of labeled water arriving at the ROI at time t; (ii) the residue function $r(t,t')$, that fraction of labeled water molecules, which arriving at the ROI at a time t' is still

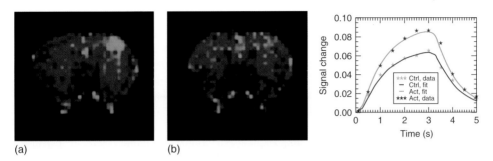

(a)   (b)

Figure 15.9 (a) ASL perfusion map acquired during electrical stimulation of a rat's forepaw. The corresponding increase in cerebral perfusion in the right somatosensory cortex can be clearly identified. (b) ASL perfusion map acquired in resting state. The graph shows a least-squares fit of the bolus-tracking ASL data (yellow and red asterisks for control and activation experiments, respectively) to theoretical model (blue and green solid lines for control and activation experiments, respectively) for the right somatosensory cortex.

present at time t; and (iii) the magnetization relaxation function $m(t')$, describing the fraction of the original longitudinal magnetization associated with labeled water molecules, which arrives at time t' and is still present at time t.

$$\Delta M \propto \int^{t} c(t') \cdot r(t - t') \cdot m(t - t') \mathrm{d}t' \tag{15.10}$$

Buxton based the model on a number of assumptions, which lead to a residue function of the form, $r(t) = \exp[-ft/\lambda]$. Parkes [43] showed that, with the choice of this residue function, Buxton's approach is the equivalent of the modified Bloch equation (15.9). The fundamental assumption of the modified Bloch equation is that water undergoes rapid exchange across the capillary walls. It is generally accepted that this assumption is false and that labeled blood water actually remains within the vessel for a time period relaxing with T_{1a} before it exchanges across the capillary wall into the extravascular (EV) water [43]. Therefore, some authors introduced models with two compartments [43–46]. However, by addressing the many physical processes involved while the labeled water is flowing from arteries into capillaries and tissue, the models became so complex with many variables that quantification with ASL is not possible at all.

In summary, we have seen that the Eq. (15.9) has been modified in many ways to compensate for the inability to describe blood flow with ASL. The underlying problem is simple. All ASL techniques are defined in space and time. The spatial encoding through the labeling plane for CASL or the inflow volume in PASL cannot be expressed with the Eq. (15.9) as there are no spatial variables present in this equation. This problem has been identified using a different approach based on the Fokker–Planck equation [28, 47].

15.3.2.3 Fokker–Planck Approach

The Kety and Schmidt approach [39] was derived from 1. Fick's law. They assumed that inflow and outflow must be equal. In steady-state conditions, we know that the same amount of blood that flows in must flow out again. But we also know a concentration of tracer flowing in will be diluted when it flows out again. Therefore, the description of Kety and Schmidt was well chosen for their experiment where they observe in- and outflow. For ASL, this is not sufficient. We cannot observe the outflow and the concentration of labeled blood gets lost due to T_1 relaxation. But why is the concentration changing? The answer is simple: dilution. The blood volume increases by a factor of around 100 when flowing from artery vessels into capillary and brain tissue. Hereby, a tracer will be diluted by distortion and diffusion processes, which can mathematically summarized and described with a diffusion term. Fick's law can then be expanded to a Fokker–Planck equation as follows

$$\frac{\partial c}{\partial t} = -F\frac{\partial c}{\partial V} + P\frac{\partial^2 c}{\partial V^2}\frac{\partial c}{\partial t} = -F\frac{\partial c}{\partial V} + P\frac{\partial^2 c}{\partial V^2} \tag{15.11}$$

where the first term describes the transport and the second the diffusion and distortion processes.

When we consider the Fokker–Planck equation with constant parameters F and P, this approach could be generalized. With F and P as function of space and time, every thinkable hemodynamic process could well be approximated. The Eq. (15.11) is a familiar equation in physics but not commonly used in medicine and biology.

The Fokker–Planck equation (Eq. 15.11) was used to expand the Bloch equation (Eq. 15.1a) [28, 47].

$$\frac{\partial c}{\partial t} = -F\frac{\partial c}{\partial V} + P\frac{\partial^2 c}{\partial V^2} - \frac{c}{T_1} \tag{15.12}$$

To show the advantages of this approach, we will consider a simple case. Let us bear in mind the original CASL experiment again. The blood in the imaging voxel gets saturated with labeled blood and reaches an equilibrium. The magnetization change in time is then $\partial c/\partial/\partial t = 0$. Equation (15.12) can now easily be solved. We find

$$c(V) = C_0 \exp\left(\frac{1}{2}\frac{F}{P}\left(1 - \sqrt{1 + \frac{4P}{T_1 F^2}}\right)V\right) \tag{15.13}$$

This results shows that the signal depends on blood volume and flow. It can also be shown that the exponent only depends on the transit time (MTT, CTT) defined below. One other important test is the case $T_1 \rightarrow \infty$. In this situation, the magnetization found reaches the starting magnetization of the inversion C_0 (full saturation). If we were to change the position of the labeling plane, the MTT would change and with that the signal.

For the PASL solution, we take into account an initial value problem. The concentration of excited magnetization at every point in the volume V is given by $c_0(V', 0)$ for $t = 0$, where V' is some known function of the volume. Under this condition, the Fokker–Planck equation (Eq. (15.12)) can be solved using a Fourier transformation as follows:

$$c(V, t) = \frac{\exp(-t/T_1)}{\sqrt{4\pi\, Pt}} \int_{-\infty}^{\infty} c_0(V', 0) \exp\left(-\frac{(V - V' - Ft)^2}{4Pt}\right) dV' \tag{15.14}$$

This formula determines the distribution of any contrast agent ($T_1 \to \infty$) in terms of the given initial distribution. Considering the EPISTAR experiment, where only arterial blood is tagged, we can assume that the initial distribution is approximated by a delta function, $\delta(V)$ (arterial blood volume and capillary blood volume). The integration of Eq. (15.14) leads to the solution for EPISTAR:

$$c(V, t) = C_0 \frac{\exp(-t/T_1)}{\sqrt{4\pi\, Pt}} \exp\left(-\frac{(V - Ft)^2}{4Pt}\right) \tag{15.15}$$

This condition would be related to the experimental condition of EPISTAR. Other experimental conditions can be found by adjusting the integration limits to a defined blood volume.

CASL, where the labeling is applied for a defined duration, is a boundary-value problem. The magnetization labeled at the labeling plane, $V = 0$ (where V is being used here as a coordinate to denote location in relation to the labeling plane), enters the imaging plane as time progresses. However, at $t = 0$, the concentration of excited spins in the brain is zero. This leads to the following result for all CASL experiments

$$c(V, t) = \int_0^t c_0(\tau) \frac{\exp(-t/T_1)}{\sqrt{4\pi\, P(t - \tau)}} \frac{V}{(t - \tau)} \exp\left(-\frac{(V - F(t - \tau))^2}{4P(t - \tau)}\right) d\tau$$

$$\tag{15.16}$$

where $c_0(t)$ is the input function.

What is interesting is that by defining the mean transit time, $MTT = V/F$, and a capillary transit time, $CTT = P/F^2$, the dependent variables of the solutions can be reduced by one. The signal curve of a bolus-tracking ASL experiment will then only depend on times, the only physical unit that is directly measurable in ASL experiments. To quantify flow or volume, the signal intensity has to be related to the actual blood volume in the imaging voxel.

For comparison with conventional bolus-tracking methods, we let $T_1 = \infty$. Then, we find that the MTT is equivalent to an MTT defined for indicator-dilution approaches [22, 29]. Simplified for a delta function input, $\delta(t)$, the first moment is given by

$$MTT_{\text{Zierler}} = \frac{\int_0^\infty t \cdot r(V, t)dt}{\int_0^\infty r(V, t)dt} = \frac{V}{F} \tag{15.17a}$$

where $c(V, t)$ is the solution of the Eq. (15.16) for the initial conditions $\delta(V)$, $T_1 \to \infty$, which can be interpreted as tissue response function. Similarly, the second moment is given by

$$CTT = \frac{1}{2} \frac{\int_0^\infty (t - \bar{t}_1)^2 \cdot r(t)dt}{\int_0^\infty t \cdot r(t)dt} = \frac{P}{F^2} \tag{15.17b}$$

which has been interpreted as the time taken for the bolus to be distributed at an ROI [48, 49]. These definitions are in agreement with the hypotheses that a bolus is transported to the ROI due to bulk flow, F, and is then dispersed at the ROI due to random effects within the microvasculature.

Further analysis of the solution (Eq. (15.16)), which describes the bolus-tracking ASL solution, reveals the conventional structure of a residue detection experiment with bolus dispersion [48]. Equation (15.16) can be rewritten as follows:

$$c(V, t) = \int_0^t \underbrace{c_0(t)}_{\text{AIF}} \underbrace{\exp\left(\frac{-t}{T_1}\right)}_{m(t)} \underbrace{\frac{V}{\sqrt{4\pi P(t - \tau)^3}} \exp\left(-\frac{(V - F(t - \tau))^2}{4P(t - \tau)}\right)}_{r(t-\tau)} d\tau$$

(15.18)

From this equation, it can be seen that the solution is equivalent to a convolution described by

$$c(V, t) = \text{AIF} \otimes r(t) \otimes m(t) \tag{15.19}$$

where AIF is the arterial input function, $m(t)$ is the relaxation function, and $r(V,t)$ is the residue function, as shown in the Eq. (15.18).

15.3.3
Perfusion Imaging Using Phase Shift

In the longitudinal direction, the signal is altered by inflowing magnetization. In transverse directions, the inflow does not change the relaxation directly. However, motion can be influenced in this domain indirectly by local magnetic field differences, which can be present in the imaging sample (for example in paramagnetism) or which can be introduced by MRI sequence with magnetic field gradients. The application of gradients allows the measurement of blood flow for different purposes.

The IntraVoxel Incoherent Motion (IVIM) method developed by Le Bihan et al. [50] is based on the use of diffusion-sensitizing gradients and used to detect the movement of water within biological tissue containing flowing blood. It also differentiates between diffusion and flow contributions. IVIM has its basis in the assumption that an image voxel of tissues contains a large number of capillary segments. Because of this large number, it is assumed that it is possible for the water molecules in the capillary network to move in differing directions at a distribution of speeds. At the voxel scale, microcirculation can be, therefore, viewed as a collection of random movements modeled as a (distributed and incoherent) pseudo-diffusion process. Such random motion can be amplified, with a motion-sensitive MRI sequence, as a phase incoherence of the spins that causes a loss of intensity of image. The blood flow-driven motion is several times higher than Brownian motion; therefore, the intensity attenuation contains a separate fast and slow component. The fast component correlates to the pseudorandom microcirculation. The slower component corresponds to Brownian motion.

The dependence of the MR signal S_{IVIM} on the diffusion-weighting b-value[8] can be approximated as a biexponential relation: $S_{IVIM}/S_0 = (1 - f)\exp(-bD) + f \times \exp[-b(D + D^*)]$, where S_0 is the signal intensity for $b = 0$, f is the vascular volume fraction, D is the molecular diffusion coefficient, and D^* is the flow index. This allows both forms of movement to be measured in all three spatial directions.

15.3.4
Perfusion Imaging with Tracers

This approach uses ultrafast imaging techniques with high temporal solution to measure a tracer bolus flowing through the tissue. An administered bolus of tracer defines the AIF, which is the time-dependent function of the trace at the supply artery. The AIF can be estimated by measuring signal changes in and around a major blood vessel [51]. Measurement of both the AIF and the time course of tracer concentration in the tissue allows the quantification of cerebral blood volume (CBV) and CBF using the Meier and Zierler indicator-dilution method [42, 52, 53].

15.3.5
Applications

In 1991, Belliveau *et al.* [3] used an MRI contrast method to demonstrate for the first time that MRI has the ability to image functional activation in the brain. Edelman *et al.* [36] (for PASL) and Kerskens *et al.* [25] (for CASL) showed that ASL can provide results as accurate as contrast techniques. Recently, Kelly *et al.* [47] used a new ASL technique that enabled them to quantify blood flow-related parameters during brain activation (Figure 15.9a) [54]. In clinical application, it has been found that ASL measurements are highly accurate in detecting lesion laterality in temporal lobe epilepsy, stenotic–occlusive disease, and brain tumors. At the moment, conclusions about the utility of ASL in clinical routine are limited by the small sample sizes of studies currently in the literature [55].

15.4
Blood Oxygenation Level-Dependent (BOLD) Contrast

Blood oxygenation level–dependent (BOLD) contrast [56–58] is derived from the fact that deoxyhemoglobin is paramagnetic while the brain tissue is diamagnetic. Changes in the local concentration of deoxyhemoglobin within the brain lead to alterations in the MR signal. The contrast mechanism is similar to those discussed for contrast agents.

---

8) The b-value includes the sequence-specific parameter of spin-echo diffusion experiment [51].

15.4.1
BOLD Contrast Mechanism

BOLD contrast has become very important as the contrast changes during brain stimulation. It allows the use of MRI in noninvasively mapping of areas with increased neuronal activity in the human brain without resorting to an exogenous contrast agent [59–61]. This revolutionary development of the past two decades is called *functional magnetic resonance imaging* (fMRI). The contrast mechanism is based on the fact that neuronal activation induces an increase in regional blood flow without a commensurate increase in the regional oxygen consumption rate ($CMRO_2$) [62]. Therefore, the amount of oxygenated hemoglobin that is delivered to the tissue is greater than the oxygen extracted by the activated neurons. The net effect is a local increase in oxyhemoglobin (diamagnetic) and a local decrease in deoxyhemoglobin (paramagnetic). Consequently, the decrease in paramagnetism leads to an increase in transversal relaxation rate T_2^* and T_2, which can be detected with optimized MRI sequences. The optimum TE_{opt} to detect changes in the transversal relaxation is given by

$$TE_{opt} = \ln\left(\frac{T_{2c}}{T_{2a}}\right)\left(\frac{1}{T_{2a}} - \frac{1}{T_{2c}}\right)^{-1} \tag{15.20}$$

where T_{2a} and T_{2c} denote the relaxation time during activation and control, respectively. For small changes in T_2/T_2^*, the optimum TE to maximize signal changes is found to be equal to T_2/T_2^* [5]. The assumption of small activation-induced changes in T_2/T_2^* might generally be true for the EV compartment, but, for example, the T_2 of venous blood can change significantly during activation. The consequence of this is that at lower field strengths, the T_2 of venous blood is longer than that of the tissue and its contribution to the BOLD signal change will be overweighted. At very high-field strengths, T_2 is very short, and at the optimum TE for tissue, the intravascular signal may be neglected [5].

For cognitive science, it is desirable to have a high sensitivity and specificity of the activation map. Since the BOLD contrast is an indirect measurement of the neuronal response, a discussion about the origin of signal changes is important.

First, one can divide the signal contributions into extravascular (ev) and intravascular (iv) components and, secondly, into dynamic and static dephasing of magnetization in the susceptibility gradient of the magnetic dipole of the hemoglobin iron complex [5, 63]. The static case is detectable with GE sequences sensitive to local frequency offsets, while SE sequences refocus this offset. In the dynamic case, the frequency offset becomes dependent on motion and diffusion. These dynamic effects are detectable with both GE and SE sequences. Static dephasing is the dominant extravascular mechanism for vessels of a diameter greater than about 20 μm [64], while dynamic dephasing is the most important mechanism for capillaries and smaller postcapillary vessels.

15.4.2
fMRI

The BOLD contrast has been extensively used to investigate questions within classic cognitive neuroscience, including issues pertaining perception, attention, and memory. The rationale of most of those studies is that the BOLD signal shows localized levels of neuronal activity, which, in turn, reflects cognitive processes. To circumvent the fact that the entire brain is always active to some degree, the subtraction paradigm has been applied. For the subtraction paradigm, a participant performs a task with two very similar conditions. One condition has exactly one feature (or putative process) more than the other, the process one wants to investigate. Subtracting brain activity in one condition from the other (called a *contrast*) produces a map of activity reflecting the process of interest. Using the subtraction paradigm, Downing and colleagues [65] established the existence of a cortical area specific to visual processing of the human body. Their participants viewed images of bodies and body parts in one condition and other objects and object parts in one of the control conditions. The difference between the conditions was particularly large in a part of the ventral visual stream of the cortex, in what they termed the extrastriate body area (EBA).

In such experiments, the conditions can principally be arranged in two ways. One condition can be repeated many times over, before a break, after which the next condition is repeated many times. Clustering events of the same kind in this manner is referred to as a *block design*. Then, the analysis involves comparing brain activity across blocks. Such designs are relatively simple and statistically powerful; that is, they are sensitive to detect activity. On the other hand, they are susceptible to confounding factors, such as drifts or movements, related to time. Crucially, they can only be used to investigate processes that can be repeated many times in sequence: any process related to novelty will be difficult to study with a block design. The alternative to it is to mix trials of different conditions in a nonpredictable, often random, way. The analysis then involves averaging single trials specific to one condition. Such studies are called *event-related design* and offer great experimental flexibility but sacrifice statistical power.

15.4.2.1 The fMRI Setup
A person participating in an experiment is located on a tray in the bore of an MRI magnet. The participant's head is gently fixed within an RF coil, a device that resembles a helmet. To perform the tasks necessary for a given experiment, participants can see a computer screen (through goggles or a mirror system), which displays instructions and stimuli; they can hear stimuli through headphones, and smell or taste stimuli through tubes. Robotic devices can be introduced to produce tactile sensations and record motor actions. Participants typically respond with small, handheld keyboards (Figure 15.10).

Stimulation setup

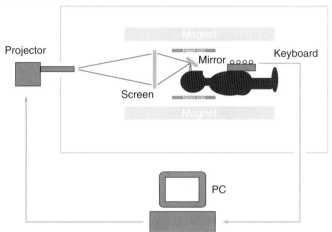

Figure 15.10 Schematic drawing of an fMRI experiment.

15.4.2.2 fMRI Analysis

Data acquired from an fMRI session generally takes the form of a time series of three-dimensional matrices. Within these matrices, each value – known as a *"voxel"* – corresponds to the BOLD signal acquired from a small cuboid region of space at a point in time. The number of data points resulting from a single participant's session can therefore be in the order of millions and requires a lengthy and computationally intensive analysis.

A typical analysis includes preprocessing steps aimed at transforming data into a standard format and detecting and removing imaging artifacts. This includes a slice-timing correction (data are acquired sequentially in slices, so the top slice will be recorded earlier than the bottom slice) and a realignment of scans within participants, as they move slightly during the experiment. As brain morphology differs considerably between people, the brain of any participant needs to be aligned to what is considered a "standard" brain template. (What constitutes a good template is an issue of contention, but most researchers agree that it should be derived by averaging the neural anatomy of many people.)

At the next stage of the analysis, regressors are generated describing the time course of the experiment, which are then compared to the time course of the BOLD signal from all voxels. The regressors are then combined to create a general linear model (GLM) with conditions relating to experimental manipulation and regressors of no interest (e.g., movement parameters). The GLM allows an estimate at each voxel of the relationship between each regressor and the BOLD signal. This results in differences of strength of relationship between conditions for each voxel of the brain. To obtain statistically confirmed statements about the location of activity, the parameter estimates at each voxel are then subject to statistical tests.

The results of fMRI studies are frequently displayed as heat maps, superimposed on an image of brain anatomy (Figure 15.11). The colors of the heat map correspond

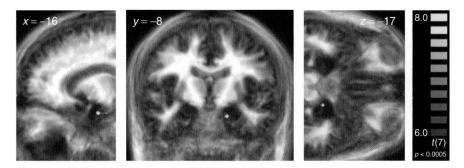

Figure 15.11 Activation within the amygdala during the reading of palatable food descriptions. The color bar indicates each voxel's result of the statistical test, in this case a *t*-value. (From Piech *et al.* [74], their Fig. 1).

to *t*-values of each displayed voxel (*t*-values are statistical values indicating how much the activity in a voxel is related to one experimental condition). Since separate statistical tests are conducted for each voxel, the result must be corrected for multiple comparisons.

To further characterize the activity of a region thought to be related to the experimental manipulation, the raw BOLD signal in that ROI can be extracted at specific time points. Figure 15.12 shows such an analysis. In that example, the authors extracted signal from an area associated with reward while participants were tasting wine. The separate plots correspond to conditions in which the same wine is believed by the participant to be more or less expensive [66]. This study suggests that the price of a product can influence associated BOLD activations in regions thought to mediate the experience of reward as well as the reported pleasure from consumption.

In the context of imaging analyses, parts of the brain can also become ROIs in different ways. The selection can be based on functional considerations as in the

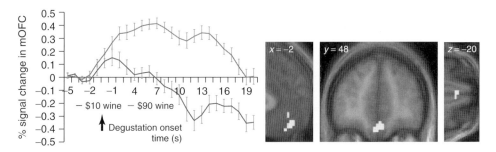

Figure 15.12 Development of activity during the tasting of wine. In the two conditions (blue and green plots in (a)), participants taste the same wine, believing that it cost either $10 or $90. The activity signal is extracted from an area of the medial prefrontal cortex (b), which is associated with the experience of rewards. (From Plassmann *et al.*, [66], their Fig. 2D and E).

wine tasting study [66] or on anatomical considerations. Studies may have a priori hypotheses about certain regions or structures because of prior research. This can have implications for the statistical thresholding, and acquisition of images. For example, imaging smaller structures can allow for higher spatial and temporal resolutions.

15.4.2.3 Limitations to Subtraction Paradigm

Using the subtraction paradigm as a basis of fMRI experimental design and analysis has been a very useful approach, as it led to numerous insights in cognitive neuroscience. However, the approach unquestionably has its limitations. On the one hand, it relies on an additive model of cognitive processing, which may not always apply. On the other hand, designing experiments with one condition containing exactly one process more than another can be very difficult, and increasingly so, the more complex the processes of interest get. This is not as much a feature of fMRI research as an assumption typically made in cognitive neuroscience. Experiments in perception are thus more suited for the subtraction paradigm than the study of social interaction phenomena. To overcome some of those limitations, a number of alternative approaches were developed. Those include matching the BOLD signal to activation patterns, rather than activation peaks, and combining data from fMRI experiments with other measures of neural activity.

15.4.2.4 Alternative Experimental Designs

15.4.2.4.1 Multivoxel Pattern Analysis

Using the subtraction paradigm to analyze fMRI data focuses on activation "peaks." That means that the approach is sensitive for finding areas that are widely activated by a certain cognitive process. At the same time, it may overlook areas that are activated by the same process in a specific spatial pattern. The multivoxel pattern analysis (MVPA) approach accounts for this possibility and analyzes spatial "shapes" of activity, rather than overall means, thus improving the spatial resolution of fMRI. The approach has been successfully used to address a range of questions, including those regarding visual processing and attention [67–69]. It is also probably the closest that neuroscience has come to mind-reading. The authors of one such study were able to conclude from the fMRI data (with accuracy slightly greater than chance), which of three object categories a participant was thinking about [70].

15.4.2.5 Analysis Based on Mathematical Models of Behavior

The subtraction paradigm points to an area that is more active in one condition than in another, but it does not necessarily tell us what process that difference in activity reflects, that is, what the area is busy doing while activated. Model-based fMRI is an analysis method, which applies the predictions of computational models of behavior to the BOLD signal. Computational models attempt to account for behaviors by hypothesizing mathematical operations that operate on environmental inputs and mental representations to give rise to behaviors. One then correlates activation levels with the values such a function would produce in a given trial and a given task. This approach improves the validity of conclusions based on fMRI data, as it allows finely distributed parametric predictions of fMRI signal and of behavior associated with a neural process [71].

15.4.2.6 Combination with EEG and TMS

In general, some limitations of fMRI can be overcome by combining fMRI with other neuroscientific methods. Electroencephalography (EEG) signal, which can be acquired simultaneously with the BOLD signal in an MRI scanner, displays excellent time resolution, while sacrificing spatial precision. This makes it a good candidate to compliment fMRI, which is precise spatially but has poor temporal resolution [72]. Similarly, the correlative nature of fMRI can be overcome by combining it with transcranial magnetic stimulation (TMS). In a typical fMRI study, the experimenter aims to manipulate some cognitive process and observes brain activity that goes along, or correlates, with that process. On the other hand, the relationship is not necessarily causal. One cannot be sure if the observed brain activity is essential to the cognitive process of interest or simply coincides with it. TMS uses the rapid application of a magnetic field to temporarily disrupt the functioning of small areas of the cortex. If used to disrupt an area previously identified with fMRI, it can demonstrate whether the function in question is compromised, providing evidence for a causal relationship between the neural activity and the cognitive process [73].

15.4.2.7 Recent Applications

The advancement and improved accessibility of fMRI technology, as well as user-friendly analysis tools, have contributed to an increased impact of the technique. In the last decade, the questions investigated with fMRI have increasingly pertained to areas outside classic cognitive neuroscience. Those areas include affective science, tackling questions about neural underpinnings of emotion, motivation, and their regulation [74–76] (Figure 15.11). Within social science, fMRI is used to investigate otherwise methodologically challenging questions such as prejudice [77]. Social interaction can be investigated with two or more participants being scanned simultaneously, something referred to as *hyperscanning* [78]. Furthermore, questions that economists have struggled to answer with their conventional tools can be aided by brain imaging [79, 81]. fMRI has also been used to investigate issues pertaining to law, justice, and politics [82–84] (Figure 15.13).

In psychiatry and clinical science, fMRI has been widely used to investigate the neural basis of behavioral deficits and abnormalities in patients. For a review, see Linden and Fallgatter [80]. Some advances have also been made toward clinical use of fMRI. DeCharms and colleagues [85] showed patients with chronic pain their real-time brain activity related to pain during a scanning session and enabled them to significantly reduce pain levels through self-control. (In analogy to biofeedback, this technique has been termed *neurofeedback*.) Technical development also allowed the creation of MRI scanners with particularly strong magnetic fields

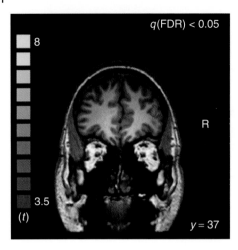

Figure 15.13 Activity in the right dorsolateral prefrontal cortex, corresponding to participants assessing responsibility for a crime. (From Buckholtz et al. 2008, their Figure 2A).

(e.g., 7 T, compared to more standard 3 T), improving their resolution and signal levels. Those high-field scanners for humans are, for example, able to show the precise location of single-digit activations in the somatosensory cortex [86] (Figure 15.14).

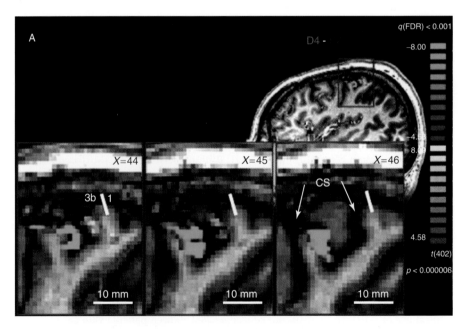

Figure 15.14 This high-resolution image shows the separation of activity related to digit 2 (blue and green) and digit 4 (orange and yellow) sensation in area 3b of the somatosensory cortex. (From Stringer et al. [86], their Fig. 2A).

15.4.2.8 **Limitations**

Brain imaging, and especially the use of fMRI, has made an important contribution to our understanding of brain function. Nevertheless, its usefulness and promise are restricted by a number of limitations. Some of them are linked to technological progress and will be overcome, while others are inherent to the technique. At the center of the limitations is the BOLD signal, which reflects blood oxygenation and is thus an indirect, and rather slow, index of brain activity. BOLD is also a relative, rather than an absolute measure, so comparisons must always be made within one experiment, rather than between experimental sessions or studies. Finally, brain imaging studies provide information on neural correlates of cognitive processing rather than their causes. Regarding more practical issues, MRI scanners are bulky and costly to purchase and maintain. Given that they rely on a electrical magnet that needs to create an incredibly strong field, this is likely to remain so in the future.

References

1. Lauterbur, P.C. (1973) Image formation by induced local interactions: examples employing nuclear magnetic resonance. *Nature*, **242**, 190–191.
2. Mansfield, P.G. and Grannell, P.K. (1973) NMR 'Diffraction' in solids? *J. Phys. C*, **6** (L422).
3. Belliveau, J.W. *et al.* (1991) Functional mapping of the human visual cortex by magnetic resonance imaging. *Science*, **254** (5032), 716–719.
4. Edelstein, W.A. *et al.* (1986) The intrinsic signal-to-noise ratio in NMR imaging. *Magn. Reson. Med.*, **3** (4), 604–618.
5. Norris, D.G. (2006) Principles of magnetic resonance assessment of brain function. *J. Magn. Reson. Imaging*, **23** (6), 794–807.
6. Slichter, C.P. (1990) *Principle of Magnetic Resonance*, Springer-Verlag, Berlin, Heidelberg.
7. Abragam, A. (1983) *Principles of Nuclear Magnetism (International Series of Monographs on Physics)*, Oxford University Press, p. 614.
8. Bitar, R. *et al.* (2006) MR pulse sequences: What every radiologist wants to know but is afraid to ask. *Radiographics*, **26** (2), 513–U15.
9. Viswanathan, S. *et al.* (2010) Alternatives to gadolinium-based metal chelates for magnetic resonance imaging. *Chem. Rev.*, **110** (5), 2960–3018.
10. Kiselev, V.G. (2001) On the theoretical basis of perfusion measurements by dynamic susceptibility contrast MRI. *Magn. Reson. Med.*, **46** (6), 1113–1122.
11. Brunecker, P. *et al.* (2008) Evaluation of an AIF correction algorithm for dynamic susceptibility contrast-enhanced perfusion MR1. *Magn. Reson. Med.*, **60** (1), 102–110.
12. Jun, Y.W., Seo, J.W., and Cheon, A. (2008) Nanoscaling laws of magnetic nanoparticles and their applicabilities in biomedical sciences. *Acc. Chem. Res.*, **41** (2), 179–189.
13. Banerjee, R. *et al.* (2010) Nanomedicine: magnetic nanoparticles and their biomedical applications. *Curr. Med. Chem.*, **17** (27), 3120–3141.
14. Golman, K. and Petersson, J.S. (2006) Metabolic imaging and other applications of hyperpolarized 13C1. *Acad. Radiol.*, **13** (8), 932–942.
15. McDermott, R. *et al.* (2004) Microtesla MRI with a superconducting quantum interference device. *Proc. Natl. Acad. Sci. U.S.A.*, **101** (21), 7857–7861.
16. Golman, K. *et al.* (2003) Molecular imaging with endogenous substances. *Proc. Natl. Acad. Sci. U.S.A.*, **100** (18), 10435–10439.

17. Mansson, S. *et al.* (2006) 13C imaging-a new diagnostic platform. *Eur. Radiol.*, **16** (1), 57–67.

18. Ernst, R.R. and Anderson, W.A. (1966) Application of fourier transform spectroscopy to magnetic resonance. *Rev. Sci. Instrum.*, **37** (1), 93–99.

19. Parker, D.L., Yuan, C., and Blatter, D.D. (1991) Mr angiography by multiple thin slab 3D acquisition. *Magn. Reson. Med.*, **17** (2), 434–451.

20. Wilson, G.J. *et al.* (2004) Parallel imaging in MR angiography. *Top. Magn. Reson. Imaging*, **15** (3), 169–185.

21. Dixon, W.T. *et al.* (1986) Projection angiograms of blood labeled by adiabatic fast passage. *Magn. Reson. Med.*, **3** (3), 454–462.

22. Detre, J.A. *et al.* (1992) Perfusion imaging. *Magn. Reson. Med.*, **23** (1), 37–45.

23. Williams, D.S. *et al.* (1992) Magnetic resonance imaging of perfusion using spin inversion of arterial water. *Proc. Natl. Acad. Sci. U.S.A.*, **89** (1), 212–216.

24. Ye, F.Q. *et al.* (1996) Perfusion imaging of the human brain at 1.5 T using a single-shot EPI spin tagging approach. *Magn. Reson. Med.*, **36** (2), 217–224.

25. Kerskens, C.M. *et al.* (1996) Ultrafast perfusion-weighted MRI of functional brain activation in rats during forepaw stimulation: comparison with T2 -weighted MRI. *NMR Biomed.*, **9** (1), 20–23.

26. Zhang, W. *et al.* (1995) NMR measurement of perfusion using arterial spin labeling without saturation of macromolecular spins. *Magn. Reson. Med.*, **33** (3), 370–376.

27. Bernstein, M.A. (2004) *Handbook of MRI Pulse Sequences*, Academic Press, Oxford.

28. Kerskens, C. (1998) *Entwicklung Theoretischer und Experimenteller Methoden zur Messung der Gehirndurchblutung mit Hilfe der Kernspintomographie*, 1st edn, Logos-Verlag Berlin, Berlin.

29. Zhernovoy, A.I. (1976) On fast adiabatic passage in nuclear magnetic resonance. *Physi. Status Solidi B*, **74** (1), K79–K80.

30. Zhang, W., Williams, D.S., and Koretsky, A.P. (1993) Measurement of rat brain perfusion by NMR using spin labeling of arterial water: in vivo determination of the degree of spin labeling. *Magn. Reson. Med.*, **29** (3), 416–421.

31. Trampel, R. *et al.* (2004) Efficiency of flow-driven adiabatic spin inversion under realistic experimental conditions: a computer simulation. *Magn. Reson. Med.*, **51** (6), 1187–1193.

32. Maccotta, L., Detre, J.A., and Alsop, D.C. (1997) The efficiency of adiabatic inversion for perfusion imaging by arterial spin labeling. *NMR Biomed.*, **10** (4–5), 216–221.

33. Utting, J.F. *et al.* (2003) Velocity-driven adiabatic fast passage for arterial spin labeling: results from a computer model. *Magn. Reson. Med.*, **49** (2), 398–401.

34. Pekar, J. *et al.* (1996) Perfusion imaging with compensation for asymmetric magnetization transfer effects. *Magn. Reson. Med.*, **35** (1), 70–79.

35. Alsop, D.C. and Detre, J.A. (1998) Multi-section cerebral blood flow MR imaging with continuous arterial spin labeling. *Radiology*, **208** (2), 410–416.

36. Edelman, R.R. *et al.* (1994) Qualitative mapping of cerebral blood flow and functional localization with echo-planar MR imaging and signal targeting with alternating radio frequency. *Radiology*, **192** (2), 513–520.

37. Golay, X. *et al.* (1999) Transfer insensitive labeling technique (TILT): application to multislice functional perfusion imaging. *J. Magn. Reson. Imaging*, **9** (3), 454–461.

38. Kwong, K.K. *et al.* (1995) MR perfusion studies with T1-weighted echo planar imaging. *Magn. Reson. Med.*, **34** (6), 878–887.

39. Kety, S.S. and Schmidt, C.F. (1948) The nitrous oxide method for the quantitative determination of cerebral blood flow in man: theory, procedure and normal values. *J. Clin. Invest.*, **27** (4), 476–483.

40. Calamante, F. *et al.* (1996) A model for quantification of perfusion in pulsed labelling techniques. *NMR Biomed.*, **9** (2), 79–83.

41. Buxton, R.B. *et al.* (1998) A general kinetic model for quantitative perfusion imaging with arterial spin

labeling. *Magn. Reson. Med.*, **40** (3), 383–396.

42. Meier, P. and Zierler, K.L. (1954) On the theory of the indicator-dilution method for measurement of blood flow and volume. *J. Appl. Physiol.*, **6** (12), 731–744.

43. Parkes, L.M. (2005) Quantification of cerebral perfusion using arterial spin labeling: two-compartment models. *J. Magn. Reson. Imaging*, **22** (6), 732–736.

44. Zhou, J. *et al.* (2001) Two-compartment exchange model for perfusion quantification using arterial spin tagging. *J. Cereb. Blood Flow Metabol.*, **21** (4), 440–455.

45. Parkes, L.M. and Tofts, P.S. (2002) Improved accuracy of human cerebral blood perfusion measurements using arterial spin labeling: accounting for capillary water permeability. *Magn. Reson. Med.*, **48** (1), 27–41.

46. Zappe, A.C. *et al.* (2007) Quantification of cerebral blood flow in nonhuman primates using arterial spin labeling and a two-compartment model. *Magn. Reson. Imaging*, **25** (6), 775–783.

47. Kelly, M.E., Blau, C.W., and Kerskens, C.M. (2009) Bolus-tracking arterial spin labelling: theoretical and experimental results. *Phys. Med. Biol.*, **54** (5), 1235–1251.

48. Calamante, F., Gadian, D.G., and Connelly, A. (2000) Delay and dispersion effects in dynamic susceptibility contrast MRI: simulations using singular value decomposition. *Magn. Reson. Med.*, **44** (3), 466–473.

49. Weisskoff*, R.M., Chesler, D., Boxerman, J.L., and Rosen, B.R., (1993) Pitfalls in MR measurement of tissue blood flow with intravascular tracers: Which mean transit time? *Magnetic Resonance in Medicine* **29** (4), 553–558.

50. Le Bihan, D. *et al.* (1988) Separation of diffusion and perfusion in intravoxel incoherent motion MR imaging. *Radiology*, **168** (2), 497–505.

51. Brunecker, P. *et al.* (2008) Evaluation of an AIF correction algorithm for dynamic susceptibility contrast-enhanced perfusion MRI. *Magn. Reson. Med.*, **60** (1), 102–110.

52. Zierler, K.L. (1965) Tracer-dilution techniques in the study of microvascular behavior. *Fed. Proc.*, **24** (5), 1085–1091.

53. Zierler, K.L. (1965) Equations for measuring blood flow by external monitoring of radioisotopes. *Circ. Res.*, **16**, 309–321.

54. Kelly, M.E. *et al.* (2010) Quantitative functional magnetic resonance imaging of brain activity using bolus-tracking arterial spin labeling. *J. Cereb. Blood Flow Meta.*, **30** (5), 913–922.

55. Brown, G.G., Clark, C., and Liu, T.T. (2007) Measurement of cerebral perfusion with arterial spin labeling: Part 2. Applications. *J. Int. Neuropsychol. Soc.*, **13** (3), 526–538.

56. Ogawa, S. *et al.* (1990) Oxygenation-sensitive contrast in magnetic resonance image of rodent brain at high magnetic fields. *Magn. Reson. Med.*, **14** (1), 68–78.

57. Ogawa, S. *et al.* (1990) Brain magnetic resonance imaging with contrast dependent on blood oxygenation. *Proc. Natl. Acad. Sci. U.S.A.*, **87** (24), 9868–9872.

58. Ogawa, S., Lee, T.M., and Barrere, B. (1993) The sensitivity of magnetic resonance image signals of a rat brain to changes in the cerebral venous blood oxygenation. *Magn. Reson. Med.*, **29** (2), 205–210.

59. Ogawa, S. *et al.* (1992) Intrinsic signal changes accompanying sensory stimulation: functional brain mapping with magnetic resonance imaging. *Proc. Natl. Acad. Sci. U.S.A.*, **89** (13), 5951–5955.

60. Kwong, K.K. *et al.* (1992) Dynamic magnetic resonance imaging of human brain activity during primary sensory stimulation. *Proc. Natl. Acad. Sci. U.S.A.*, **89** (12), 5675–5679.

61. Bandettini, P.A. *et al.* (1992) Time course EPI of human brain function during task activation. *Magn. Reson. Med.*, **25** (2), 390–397.

62. Fox, P.T. and Raichle, M.E. (1986) Focal physiological uncoupling of cerebral blood flow and oxidative metabolism

during somatosensory stimulation in human subjects. *Proc. Natl. Acad. Sci. U.S.A.*, **83** (4), 1140–1144.

63. Hoogenraad, F.G. and Pouwels, P.J., Hofman, M.B., Reichenbach, J.R., Sprenger, M., and Haacke, E.M. (2001) Quantitative differentiation between BOLD models in fMRI. *Magn Reson Med.*, **45** (2), 233–246.

64. Ogawa, S. *et al.* (1993) Functional brain mapping by blood oxygenation level-dependent contrast magnetic-resonance-imaging - a comparison of signal characteristics with a biophysical model. *Biophys. J.*, **64** (3), 803–812.

65. Downing, P.E. *et al.* (2001) A cortical area selective for visual processing of the human body. *Science*, **293** (5539), 2470–2473.

66. Plassmann, H. *et al.* (2008) Marketing actions can modulate neural representations of experienced pleasantness. *Proc. Natl. Acad. Sci.*, **105** (3), 1050.

67. Kamitani, Y. and Tong, F. (2005) Decoding the visual and subjective contents of the human brain. *Nat. Neurosci.*, **8** (5), 679–685.

68. Peelen, M.V. and Downing, P.E. (2007) Using multi-voxel pattern analysis of fMRI data to interpret overlapping functional activations. *Trends Cogn. Sci. (Regul. Ed.)*, **11** (1), 4–5.

69. Norman, K. *et al.* (2006) Beyond mind-reading: multi-voxel pattern analysis of fMRI data. *Trends Cogn. Sci.*, **10** (9), 424–430.

70. Polyn, S. *et al.* (2005) Category-specific cortical activity precedes retrieval during memory search. *Science*, **310** (5756), 1963.

71. O'Doherty, J., Hampton, A., and Kim, H. (2007) Model-based fMRI and its application to reward learning and decision making. *Ann. N.Y. Acad. Sci.*, **1104**, 35–53.

72. Bledowski, C. *et al.* (2004) Localizing P300 generators in visual target and distractor processing: a combined event-related potential and functional magnetic resonance imaging study. *J. Neurosci.*, **24** (42), 9353–9360.

73. van Koningsbruggen, M., Downing, P., and Rafal, R., (2009) The effect of theta

TMS over the FEF on fMRI activations. *J. Vision.* **9** (8), 378.

74. Piech, R.M. *et al.* (2009) Neural correlates of appetite and hunger-related evaluative judgments. *PLoS ONE*, **4** (8), e6581.

75. Morrison, I. *et al.* (2004) Vicarious responses to pain in anterior cingulate cortex: is empathy a multisensory issue? *Cogn. Affect. Behav. Neurosci.*, **4** (2), 270–278.

76. Ochsner, K. *et al.* (2002) Rethinking feelings: An fMRI study of the cognitive regulation of emotion. *J. Cogn. Neurosci.*, **14** (8), 1215–1229.

77. Freeman, J.B. *et al.* (2010) The neural origins of superficial and individuated judgments about ingroup and outgroup members. *Hum. Brain Mapp.*, **31** (1), 150–159.

78. King-Casas, B. *et al.* (2005) Getting to know you: reputation and trust in a two-person economic exchange. *Science*, **308** (5718), 78–83.

79. Plassmann, H., O'Doherty, J.P., and Rangel, A. (2007) Orbitofrontal cortex encodes willingness to pay in everyday economic transactions. *J. Neurosci.*, **27**(37), 9984–9988.

80. Linden, D.E.J. and Fallgatter, A.J. (2009) Neuroimaging in psychiatry: from bench to bedside. *Front. Hum. Neurosci.*, **3**, 49.

81. Sanfey, A.G. *et al.* (2006) Neuroeconomics: cross-currents in research on decision-making. *Trends. Cogn. Sci.*, **10**(3), 108–116.

82. Buckholtz, J.W., *et al.* (2008) The neural correlates of third-party punishment. *Neuron*, **60**(5), 930–940.

83. Lieberman, M.D., Schreiber, D., and Ochsner, K.N. (2003) Is political cognition like riding a bicycle? How cognitive neuroscience can inform research on political thinking. *Polit. Psychol.*, **24**(4), 681–704.

84. Meyer-Lindenberg, A. *et al.* (2006) Neural mechanisms of genetic risk for impulsivity and violence in humans. *Proc. Natl. Acad. Sci. U.S.A.*, **103**(16), 6269–6274.

85. DeCharms, R. *et al.* (2005) Control over brain activation and pain learned by using real-time functional MRI. *Proc. Natl. Acad. Sci. U.S.A.*, **102** (51), 18626.

86. Stringer, E. *et al.* (2010) Differentiation of somatosensory cortices by high resolution fMRI at 7 T. *NeuroImage.* **54** (2), 1012–1020.

87. Bellin, M.F. and Van Der Molen, A.J. (2008) Extracellular gadolinium-based contrast media: An overview. *Eur. J. Radiol.*, **66** (2), 160–167.

Index

Microcirculation Imaging, First Edition. Edited by Martin J. Leahy.
© 2012 Wiley-VCH Verlag GmbH & Co. KGaA. Published 2012 by Wiley-VCH Verlag GmbH & Co. KGaA.